YOGA, FASCIA, ANATOMY AND MOVEMENT

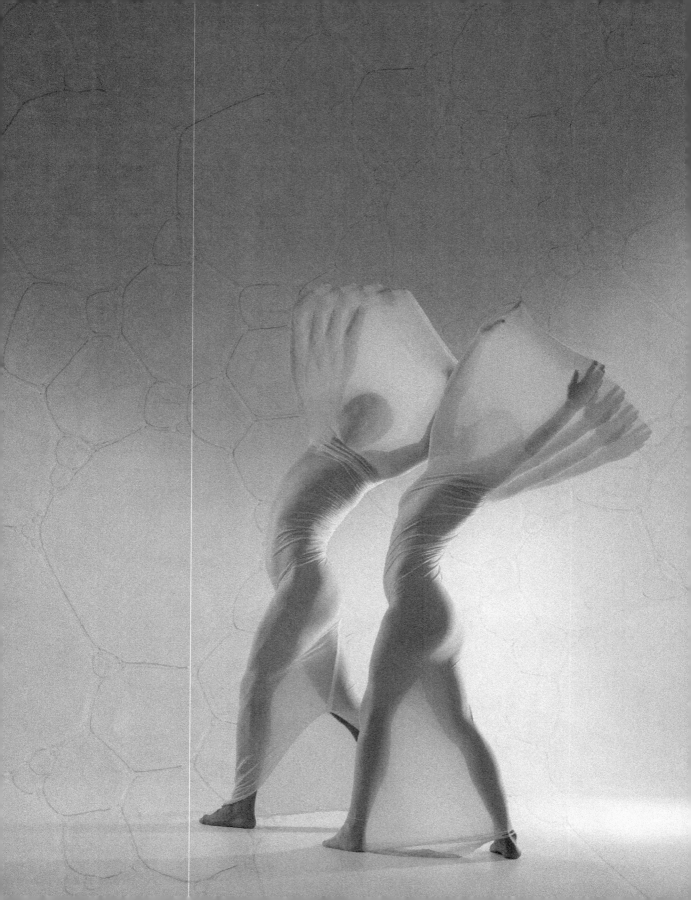

YOGA, FASCIA, ANATOMY AND MOVEMENT

Joanne Avison MSS

Yoga: E-RYT500, Structural Integration: KMI, CTK, CMED

Director: Art of Contemporary Yoga Ltd

Forewords
Thomas W Myers
Jill Miller
Jules Mitchell

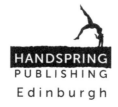

HANDSPRING
PUBLISHING
Edinburgh

SECOND EDITION

HANDSPRING PUBLISHING LIMITED
The Old Manse, Fountainhall,
Pencaitland, East Lothian
EH34 5EY, Scotland
Tel: +44 1875 341 859
Website: www.handspringpublishing.com

First published 2015 in the United Kingdom by Handspring Publishing
Second edition published 2021

ISBN 978-1-913426-04-0
ISBN Kindle eBook 978-1-913426-05-7

British Library Cataloguing in Publication Data
A catalogue record for this book is available from the British Library
Library of Congress Cataloguing in Publication Data
A catalog record for this book is available from the Library of Congress

Notice
Neither the Publisher nor the Author assumes any responsibility for any loss or injury and/or damage to
persons or property arising out of or relating to any use of the material contained in this book. It is the
responsibility of the treating practitioner, relying on independent expertise and knowledge of the patient, to
determine the best treatment and method of application for the patient.

Commissioning Editor Sarena Wolfaard
Cover design Bex Hawkins, Bex Hawks Creates
Artwork Joanne Avison (unless otherwise indicated)
Indexer: Avril Erlich
Typesetter: Amnet, India
Printer: Ashford Colour Press Ltd

The
Publisher's
policy is to use
paper manufactured
from sustainable forests

CONTENTS

DEDICATION

To Daddy-Billy-Willyum,

Your last words to me, on this side of the veil, carried me through this second edition. Thank you for teaching me, so very fundamentally, to love learning and to learn lovingly and with laughter, every day. You could not bear segregation of any sort and to that end, my guiding light has been a dedication to wholeness of body, mind and being; which in living, breathing life-on-earth are not segregated either. They only appear so in our inherited anatomy books. The mystical principle that *the one and the all is the same* is emerging in these "twenty-twenties" and with it, the new ways of understanding our living bodies.

I dedicate this effort to explaining that, scientifically and in practice, with love, light and the sound of laughter.

I love you for teaching me, at the age of six, this poem:

> *Scintillate, scintillate global vivific*
> *Fain would I fathom thy nature specific*
> *Loftily poised in the ether capacious*
> *Strongly resembling a gem carbonaceous*

and for reminding me it is this nursery rhyme: *it depends how you say it, right Pops*?

> *Twinkle, twinkle little star*
> *How I wonder what you are?*
> *Up above the world so high*
> *Like a diamond in the sky*

I dedicate this second edition to you and your grandson, who is my "little star". You both share a wicked sense of humour and a nobility of mind to stand for truth and grace and it is my privilege to be daughter and mother; the sandwich generation between two noblemen.

SYMBOL OF THE HU

Hu – the Sanskrit word for Divine.

Since we are **all** made of the same star dust; since you always said I began as a twinkle in your eye; since I hold you in my heart like a shining star ANYWAY – may this work shine light on the wholeness of humans being. I love you for eternity.

Baruch Bashan (the Blessings already are), MeX

ABOUT THE AUTHOR

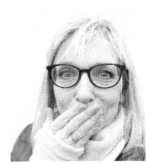

Joanne Avison MSS, C-IAYT, E-RYT500, KMI, CTK, CMED

Joanne is an international teacher of applied structural anatomy for movement and manual practitioners in a variety of fields. She is a professional Structural Integration practitioner, member of IASI (International Association of Structural Integrators) and certified teacher (KMI, Anatomy Trains 1998–2005: Tom Myers' school) and Director of the Art of Contemporary Yoga Teacher Training, London, UK. The school registration (2006 onwards) qualified as an RYS-500, with Yoga Alliance (US), European Yoga Alliance and Indian Federation of Yoga. As an advanced Yoga Practitioner and Certified Yoga Therapist, C-IAYT (Certified by International Association of Yoga Therapists), Joanne appreciates the art, craft and science of yoga and body architecture. Her Master's degree in Spiritual Sciences has deepened her understanding of yoga and the philosophy behind it, that relates closely to how the physical body integrates and animates form. For Joanne the study of philosophy and anatomy are not necessarily separate, which is a unique approach to integrated practice.

Joanne is also trained in Craniosacral Therapy, continuously working in ART (Autoimmune Response Testing) and FSM (Frequency Specific Microcurrent) to further her studies in complementary health and complementary medicine. She is also a graduate of the CMED Institute, USA. After over 20 years of manual and movement practice, she appreciates deeply the resonance field(s) the body animates *as a living form*.

As a member of the Biotensegrity Interest Group (BIG), Joanne is fascinated by the application of biotensegrity principles to the understanding of the human blueprint and natural structural organisation in motion. Her writing and workshops are devoted to making this emerging context for human movement applicable and clearly understood. "*It makes sense of how we make sense of our world, literally and symbolically.*"

"BioTensegrity is an emerging context for what I refer to as 'biomotional integrity'. That is – how we move the way we do. Understanding the fascia and the fabric of our form is relatively meaningless, without the architectural organisation of that fabric, explaining how it permits movement and indeed manages the movement forces we move (that move us). We are formed under tension; pre-stressed or pre-stiffened – but what does that mean to us as movement teachers or manual therapists? What are the implications of tensional forces through the matrix of our living, animated form? The fascia is a force transmission system. Biotensegrity offers a very compelling paradigm that makes sense of its many structures and functions and multifaceted assets. It also transforms our understanding of connection and resonance; with ourselves and others."

FOREWORD TO FIRST EDITION
Thomas W Myers

Yoga, along with martial arts and dance – all of which stretch back into the mists of pre-history – is certainly among the earliest organized attempts to change a person by means of body movement. Even though modern psychotherapy has largely abandoned a body-centred approach in favour of talk therapy and increasing amounts of pharmaceuticals, the positive effects of exercise on the psyche – Juvenal's *mens sana in corpore sano* – have been acknowledged for centuries. Yoga, at least in the developed texts and adepts, goes well beyond these general benefits that come from engaging the mind in a coordinated pumping of the muscles. It claims (and in my experience, often delivers) to advance our psychophysiology into positive territory, away from self-centred, fear-based chemistry to a more serene, objective and fully present state of bodymind.

The modern flowering of yoga owes a great deal to the late B.K.S. Iyengar, a lion of a man who wrestled both the postures and the breathing practices of yoga into an understandable and graduated discipline. Even current forms of yoga that have rejected the particulars of his practice owe him a deep debt – without him there would be no "art of contemporary yoga". With him, and with the interest that has followed and branched out from his work, yoga has taken many forms, and over the course of my working life has gone from a few hippies contorting themselves in an ashram to the current ubiquity of yoga classes in nearly every gym, village hall, street corner, and even school athletic programmes, corporate retreats, and senior centres. Yoga itself has diversified into hundreds of branches, ranging from the athletic Ashtanga to the flowing Vinyasa to Iyengar's precise positioning to more meditative approaches. These days, we are spoilt for choice in which yoga to choose for ourselves.

Inevitably, then, yoga comes up against science – "Prove it!" say the researchers. Joanne Avison – not a researcher in the laboratory sense, but rather a re-searcher – is uniquely positioned to help us understand the research we have already, as well as provide a framework to understand the studies to come. Joanne's background includes many years of teaching yoga in a variety of contexts, and with her quick mind and her ability to write clearly, this book provides the contemporary teacher and practitioner of yoga with a frankly astounding tour of current thinking that blends the spiritual with the scientific, and the sacred with the intensely practical.

Fascia – that long-ignored biological fabric that shapes us – has now become a buzzword, often used with more enthusiasm than understanding. This book takes on the developmental significance of what Dr Robert Schleip calls the "neuromyofascial web" in all its glory, without bogging the reader down in the details of anatomy or biochemistry, which are relevant to "afascianado" or biomechanist, but not necessary to daily practice.

The tradition of yoga has a great deal to teach us, but in another way these ancient texts and forms are entirely irrelevant. Industrialized, electronified humanity faces a challenge – a whole series of challenges – never before encountered by any previous era. One of these challenges is the loss of self-sense, a sense of alienation from the body and its whispered but essential messages, dulled in the roar of the planes, trains and automobiles, the blare of radio, TV and Internet, and the sheer weight of the number of people on this intricate planet. We must face the challenge of how we educate our children to move and feel in the natural world, and create a programme of what I have called "Kinesthetic Literacy" for this hyper, data-rich, information-poor era.

Read this book no matter what form of yoga you practice or teach – in fact, read this book if you happen to have a body. You will be pulled along a merrily flowing stream of ancient and contemporary thought, and you will emerge with a fresh explanation of why the many new interpretations of yoga can be so important in the revivification of our body and mind.

Thomas W Myers
Walpole, Maine, USA
tom@anatomytrains.com

November 2014

FOREWORD TO SECOND EDITION
Jill Miller

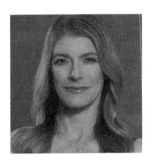

Decades ago, as a twenty-something yogini, I was initiated into practices of Yantra. Yantra are sacred geometric symbols with complex angles, dimension, color and architecture. I was to trace these Yantras, posters that my teacher taped to the wall, first with my eyes open. Then with closed eyes, recreating the pattern with the mind. Each line, vertex, curve and hollow space foiled me with its precision and exactness. I was not a visually oriented person. I am a touchy feely type. Memorizing the sketch of a complex symbol was definitely my edge.

These yantra images challenged me; I could not inflate the 2D graphic into 3D scope. Something blocked my translation of the illustration into an object with depth and dimension. I was literally stuck in my head about it and knew that either I was a deficient practitioner or perhaps I misunderstood how to anchor this esoteric practice into the matter of my body.

Practicing other limbs of yoga, I always enjoyed a deep sense of connection throughout my body and being. However, the Yantra practice felt external to me, like a computation of memory that my disconnected body could not engage with. It didn't feel like Yoga; frankly the leap from 2D to imagining 3D discombobulated me. I persevered, taking the practice home with me – but after months of frustration, I gave up. I surrendered to the uneasy notion that Yantra was not going to fulfil my Yogic punch card of practices. I had plenty others and I could settle with deepening my understanding of asana (poses), anatomy, technique, pranayama (breath practice), mantra (chanting), and meditation.

I had known about fascia during this time, but I didn't know the contextual shape of it. I knew that when I received or gave massage, I was swimming in fields of fascia and fluids and not just the muscles we all learn in classical anatomy. But I hadn't yet made the connection between the micro level of biological shapes and the essential geometry.

Enter Joanne Avison's book and an instant shift, via the science, into the esoteric universe, weaves that whole story together so you can wrap yourself in it. This woman's colossal understanding of dissection, movement arts and the scope of yoga practices illustrates the felt path of science and soma; whatever colors you choose for your own particular tapestry.

Joanne Avison has a way with words, she deftly weaves them to fold you into the pages of her book and into the very contours of her embodied mind. Her knowledge of the living body's self-development comforts the reader as you trace your way through the history of anatomy. She warms a stiff topic by delighting you into thought processes that have aged and transmuted across the millennia and matured into ideas that resonate with your experience of doing.

Her writing will regress you initially, as journeying through the embryo is the path of discovering how you unfold, recombine and expand into the shape you occupy now. The writing will touch you, in all of your senses, and help you peer out once again with a whole sense of be-ing.

As for Yantra practice, I've now transcribed it for myself. Rather than trapping myself in the visual loop that's difficult for my brain to "see" I locate cells, threads and molecules in my body, watch them vibrate and swim where they live. I dance a dervish dedicated to their shape.

Joanne's book confers the reader with permission to feel their way through their yoga no matter what style they practice. She encourages your own sensibility to inflect your experience so you can crawl into embodiment no matter what shape you take, and no matter what shape takes place.

To that point, the brilliance of Yantra practice was separate. It hadn't shown up as a way to journey into the body's impressive living representation of those paper posters and the exquisite story behind their ancient wisdom and deeper purpose.

The recognition of geometry "Gaia Metria" (meaning the Measure of Mother Earth) gave me permission to see those Yantras again, as if they resonate through me, for me. This fundamental basis of how fascia forms, takes the science of yoga full circle, through the practice, to the philosophy behind it. We dare to feel it and know it, for ourselves.

Jill Miller C-IAYT, ERYT
Author of *The Roll Model*
www.tuneupfitness.com

February 2021

FOREWORD TO SECOND EDITION
Jules Mitchell

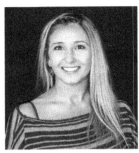

Photograph by Sabrina Pozzi
SabrinaPozzi.com

Throw out your stack of anatomy books! Joanne Avison is rewriting the way in which anatomy is taught to yoga teachers.

This book is an intellectual journey through yoga and anatomy, and also how we *talk* about yoga and anatomy. You can't help but be transformed as you turn the pages, pondering what it means to *live* in your body while reflecting on how great thinkers of past and present *explain* what it means to live in a body.

In my own studies of anatomy and biomechanics, I found the best teachers to be the philosophers. In fact, my interest in mathematics, physics, and engineering during my academic years was driven by the philosophical aspects. Calculating something with no limit to its value requires you to accept that infinity exists. Thinking in such a capacity easily carries over into the study of self, life, and existence. Hence the anatomy teachers who truly appreciate the complexity of the human form must, at some point, philosophize. This is the nature in which Joanne tells her story.

As with any great narrative, the history provides the context. Joanne explains to us how we evolved from *declaring* anatomy to *discovering* anatomy, and continually reminds us that our textbook anatomy and classical biomechanics instruction is based in declaration. From there, she deconstructs mainstream teachings, presents alternative explanations, and weaves them together in the same manner that fascia makes us whole.

Of course, the study of anatomy is incomplete without considering embryology. Joanne calls on this field at appropriate times and in appropriate doses, to remind us of our own wholeness. Gone are the days of memorizing attachment points, assigning "jobs" to individual muscles, and applying two-dimensional models. Joanne's anatomy lessons emerge from growth, movement, sensing, awareness, and becoming.

Finally, the study of anatomy is also incomplete without biotensegrity, a central theme in the text. Joanne's geometry lessons, fluid dynamics explanations, and movement-centered dialogue complete the reading experience. Your explanation of *how* and *why* yoga poses *are*, will never be the same. Joanne is creating a community of philosophers through her work.

Jules Mitchell MS, LMT, RYT
Yoga Educator, Research & Adjunct Faculty at Arizona State University
Author of *Yoga Biomechanics: Stretching Redefined*
www.JulesMitchell.com

February 2021

ACKNOWLEDGEMENTS

The list of acknowledgements since writing the first edition of this book has grown exponentially. It is with love that I acknowledge those who played key roles in the creation of this work – and with love that I acknowledge those who are not mentioned here. Forgive me and you know who you are. I love you anyway.

First and foremost, my son, Ben, my mother, Stephani, my sister Caroline and my brother-in-law Jim, I cherish all that you are for me, every day. A special loving word to Poupette, to all my family (you know who you are): To Malcolm, for all we created and for the artisan skills of the chocolatier; where I learned the liquid crystal nature of soft matter.

My dear friends and broader family; without your loving listening and encouragement this wouldn't have happened. In no particular order Philippa King, Zara Morrison, Jo Ellis, Jane Priddis, Jessica Brass, Annie Waite-Gilmer, Linda d'Antal, Gilly (Bean) Smith, Diane Ward, Shane McDermott, Martin Gordon, Susie Llewelyn, Karel Aerssons, Julie Margiotta, Petra Gommers, Clare Maddalena, Helen Moss, Michelle Martin, my beloved BLE buddies, Paul Kaye, Lesley Freeman and my Reverend Mama and wider family around the world. William Winram and Michèle Monico, Richard Tittensor, Sarah Sinclair, Helen Eadie and Bex Hawkins, Amy Very and Jake Clerk-Derby I thank you all for your loving support beyond the work we do together.

Professionally I thank all my teachers; those from whom I have learned by design (and those from whom I have learned, by default, what not to do). My profound thanks to each of the graduates at Art of Contemporary Yoga for teaching me more than you learned. It was a privilege to work with each of you. To the many people I have met through the work of ABC School and all my beloved facilitators around the world. Since the first edition I have travelled far and wide and made many friends whom I hold dear. John Sharkey and his family, Verena Tremel, Athina Vittori, Jaap van der Wal, Darrell Evans, Carol Davis, Karen Kirkness, Wilbour Kelsick and Christine Wushke. Everyone at NTC and everyone in the Biotensegrity Interest Group including Dr Stephen Levin, Chris Clancy, Susan Lowell, Leonid Blyum, Graham Scarr and Danielle-Claude Martin, to name a few. Neil Theise, Deane Juhan, Jill Miller, Sue Hitzmann, Bruce Schonfeld, Fran Phillips, Jo Phee and Ana Outsubo have all contributed and supported me materially or morally and I am deeply grateful. Thank you each.

The passing away of B.K.S. Iyengar, and the issues that have surrounded yoga in recent years since the first edition, brings me to an observation about the matriarchy behind Restorative Yoga. Iyengar taught Vanda Scaravelli one-to-one and their combination of masculine and feminine perspectives brought forth the work we animate today. My thanks and gratitude for their legacy. I have had the privilege of working with Elizabeth Pauncz and Diane Long, John Stirk and Peter Blackaby, all of whom have inspired me and encouraged my deep fascination with anatomy and biomechanics *and how they apply to real living bodies and humans being*. Actually, it was also frustration – which ignited the questions contained herein. My deepest appreciation to Caroline Myss for personally and professionally giving me the confidence to take those questions about the physical body and raise them to the level of the archetypal, the sacred and the mystical in down-to-earth, valuable ways that I treasure. To that end, my deepest appreciation to John-Roger for the teachings and the Grace that goes with them for us all.

To Phil and Patricia to say thank you for Bill Corsa my "special agent", without all of you I would have struggled more and giggled less. To Stephanie Pickering and Glenys Norquay for their meticulous editing care and attention to detail. Bex for exquisite design, presence and endless patience behind the scenes; and Helen for endless encouragement with every word. Thanks and love to you both and Wibbs Coulson and Amy for the cover shoot; the grace with which you all created it with me. Freddy for just being there, always. Sarena Wolfaard, Andrew Stevenson and everyone at Handspring Publishing, my huge appreciation for your guidance, patience and warmth.

With gratitude and grace
Joanne Sarah Avison
Brighton, England

February 2021

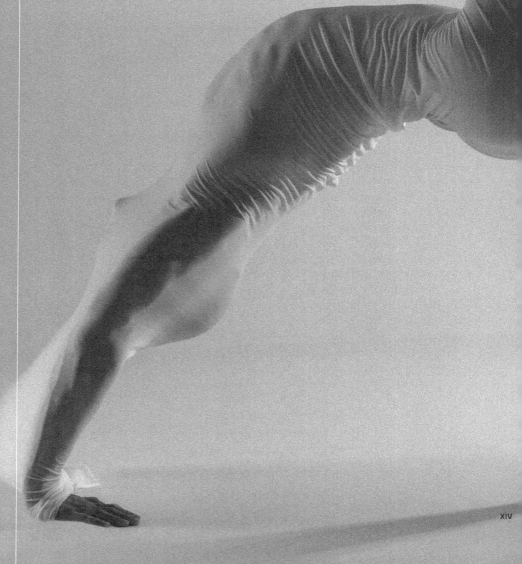

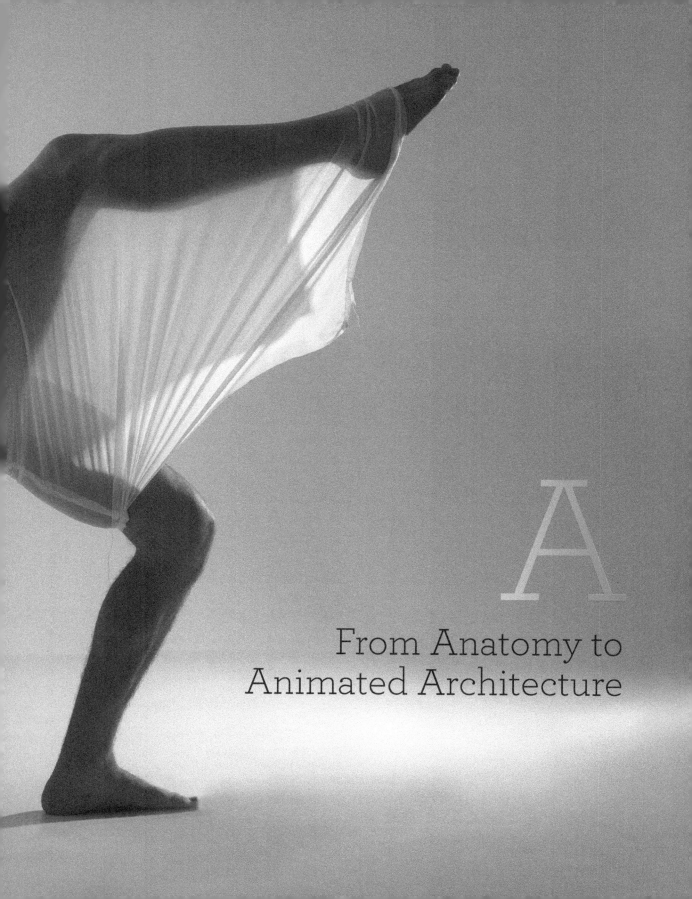

A

From Anatomy to
Animated Architecture

1

The Art of Contemporary Yoga

"Out beyond ideas of wrongdoing and rightdoing, there is a field. I will meet you there"[1]

Rumi (1207–1273)

Yoga means different things to different people. It can be as variously complex and straightforward as the individuals who practise it. It relies as much on its inherited wisdom as it retains exceptional relevance and value in a modern culture. Fascia is the *unifying* fabric of the body form and since yoga means "unifying", in one sense we could say it is the yoga of our forming, since we are a work in progress throughout our lives.

There are as many different styles of yoga and perspectives on yoga as there are people to interpret them. There are fast and slow practices, dynamic and static aspects, different cultures and applications. Some yogic forms embrace only physical postures, while others emphasise a more meditative approach. Any yoga teacher training includes philosophy and technique, ethics and practice, anatomy and physiology, as well as work on meditative approaches and the broader quest for expanding awareness and conscious understanding of what it is to be alive in a body. In truth, yoga can become as far reaching, profound and multi-faceted as we can. It seeks to account for body, mind and being as a context for health and vitality on many levels. Whatever your interest, there is far more to the art of yoga than a series of exercises or shapes-in-space on a mat; the medium in which you do it is that of your fascial body matrix.

Yoga has evolved from ancient principles that have never separated body, mind and being from each other, as we have in the West. We do not leave our minds at the desk, our hearts outside the door, and take only our functioning anatomical parts to the yoga class. Rather, we engage our many different aspects and faculties to arrive (and leave) whole and complete. We activate ourselves as one animated form, unique and essentially self-motivated.

Yoga is about movement and quality of motion as well as the power to be still and present. Much of its value resides in the ability to expand awareness and attention *beyond the mind* and its intellectual processing, to a state of presence in the body. We can begin to learn stillness through poise and balance, practising the art of *experiencing equanimity* in quiet reflection; a pathway perhaps, beyond the forms. This practice fosters the ability to quieten mind chatter (*chitta vritti*), taking our yoga beyond thinking and individual postures. It can invite fun in the physical realm, balance to the emotional and curiosity in the mental pursuit of the philosophy; animated by the form, but not reduced to its components. Once these aspects are woven together, we can become inspired by the breathing practices and beyond to the more esoteric aspects. Yoga can be a kind of portal to vitality and awareness. It takes more than theory, however, to makes sense of the experience, way beyond the exercise technique. It is in action, through the *medium* of our whole physical form, that we *animate* what is essentially our *own* yoga.

Movement is not an intellectual process, and nor is breathing, or meditation, or seeking awareness. They are heart-felt practices of a conscious being, animating a body. Our intellect, or thinking mind, is just one of our many gifts; yoga can bring awareness of all these myriad expressions of our living architecture. These include the thinking body, the moving body, the instinctive body and the emotional body, with all its sensory and intuitive abilities to experience *embodiment* essentially as a self-motivated being. Fascia, as the original fabric of our form, incorporates and organises all these aspects of us.

Anatomy of the Body

When we begin to study how the body is formed, scientifically, we (particularly in the West) tend to veer away from whole embodiment, preferring to examine the detail, separated or broken down into its component parts. We turn to various works based on long-held theories in the fields of anatomy, physiology and biomechanics. This approach requires the naming of our parts, understanding our physical systems and explaining how we move, *deduced from those parts*. We learn the locations, which parts are where (topography); we explain the systems in which those parts function (biology and chemistry) and describe the movement (locomotive) apparatus and how it works under various aspects of biomechanical and neurological theory. Muscle–bone–joint anatomy is the foundation on which we base our understanding of any movement modality. Awareness of the being inside the moving body is largely assigned to the study of psychology or more esoteric practices, *as if they are separate*.

To understand how we do the postures, we focus on the musculoskeletal system to name which muscles move which bones via their specific attachments. By learning how the nervous system works and assigning specific nerves to each muscle, we seek to explain which actions do which movements. This explains the postures accordingly. Or does it?

Musculoskeletal System

Once we have identified the muscles and bones, we name the ligaments attaching the bones of the skeleton to each other, the tendons attaching the muscles to those bones, and how, between them, they activate (via various types of leverage) the different types of joint. This is to study the form and function of the "*musculoskeletal system*".

I was in my early thirties, three years into learning yoga on a more formal basis, trying to make sense of anatomy. Having been trained by osteopaths, I considered anatomy and biomechanics to be a high priority but could not understand why there was such a rift between the books and the moving people actually doing yoga in my classroom. Into this confusion walked Tom Myers, presenting to a large group of yoga teachers. He announced to us all that "there ain't no muscle connected to no bone, nowhere, in no body". To give you a context, this was the late 1990s, in Brighton, England. Not only was this man apparently committing anatomical heresy, he was doing it with a big grin and an American accent. It shifted a few notions and ignited a curiosity in me that has only grown since.

In this "musculoskeletal" system, each muscle has a name and position, an origin, an insertion (or distal and proximal attachment) and an action assigned to it, via a nerve, responsible for that specific action or type of motion. The whole suite of muscle–bone–joint anatomy combines to motivate a system of levers and pendulums that provides explanations of how our bodies move around. We follow up on the biomechanics of those levers first, or the nervous system that apparently innervates their separate, respective functions. In either case, it becomes progressively more complex and difficult to divide up, or work out, which functions belong to which system. We require ever more complicated rules, for more detailed fragments. The ability to *make sense* of the wholeness that arrives in the classroom becomes increasingly elusive and confusing. Who looks forward to "learning their anatomy" and finds it easy to make sense of how the body moves from the icons in the books?

In yoga books on anatomy, these classical principles are usually presented via poses (asanas), with a related image showing which muscles are contracted, which stretched, and the point at which they are individually attached in their so-called "antagonistic pairs". Similarly, in the anatomy of the breath, we study the principles of the organs and muscles of breathing: how they attach to (and move) the rib cage and diaphragm. We learn by rote which muscles are for accessory breathing, shallow breathing and deep breathing, etc. A great deal has been studied and described from this particular perspective. However, although this perspective has been taught for centuries, it largely excludes an essential feature of body architecture. That essential feature is the significance and ubiquity of the fascia, historically assigned to the role of connecting tissue, as if that is merely a kind of "scaffolding" or inert packaging material.

The importance of fascia has become clearer and more differentiated only comparatively recently. "Fascia" is the name given to a specific (and variable) kind of connective tissue that is the subject of a rapidly increasing amount of research with regard to its range, capabilities and characteristics.[2] From 200 papers per year in the 1970s and 1980s, to almost 1,000 in 2010 on the subject; the following article in 2019 indicates the exponential rise in research and interest:

"While anatomy textbooks are slim on fascia a search on the Internet using the term "Fascia" on PubMed alone resulted in excess of 20,000 articles. Anatomical texts provide detailed images and descriptions of muscles, nerves, lymphatic's, organs and blood vessels while the very tissue connecting, supporting, nurturing, wrapping and investing them is most often not included. Recent research indicates the role of Fascia in the pathogenesis of a variety of conditions including Lumbago, inguinal hernia and the regulation of posture, muscular biomechanics, peripheral motor coordination and proprioception."

John Sharkey[3]

The fascia is what we might call the "stuff in between" all of the parts, that in traditional dissection has mostly been removed. It is scraped away in order to properly present the more important items, considered to be the muscles, joints, bones, vessels and materials of the musculoskeletal system. A similar focus in studying visceral anatomy includes removing fascia to study the "more important organs" that it wraps. What is perhaps ignored, is that everything in the human body is *made of fascia*. We will see in the following chapters how this has hidden, for so long, in the obvious. What is so vitally important, and growing in recognition, about this exceptional fabric of the human body?

What is Fascia?   The difficulty in answering that question is twofold. The first concern is that fascia is so many things. The second is that if fascia *really is* so many things, with such a tremendous influence on so much of our body, movements and systems, then how has it been overlooked, in terms of its significance, for so many centuries? These are good questions to consider, and this first part of the book will attempt to answer them.

We will discover that the increasing knowledge about the fascia is creating a sea change, transforming our understanding of anything to do with the body and motion. The scale of this effect is big enough to be described as a paradigm shift. It revolutionises our view of anatomy since modern technology reveals that fascia is not only ubiquitous (everywhere), but sensory in nature (see Ch. 5) and crucial to any part of any muscle connecting to any part of any bone in its locality (not to mention its neighbouring muscles). We begin to learn how essential the fascia is to truly understanding anatomy and movement since it is the universal tissue of relationship between all our parts, on every scale. What is more inspiring, however, is that we will find it begins to make perfect sense of the very wholeness that the *ancient* principles of yoga endorse and espouse (see Ch. 13). That includes the more subtle, energetic practices.

Fascia could be described as the fabric of our form (see Ch. 7). It literally joins every single part of us together, from the finest, microscopic level of detail within us, between the cells, to the outermost skin in which we are wrapped. In some places it is so fine it cannot be seen by the naked eye, while in others it forms thick, dense sheets making up a named entity such as the thoracolumbar fascia, which integrates the tissues of the lower and mid back. In some anatomical representations of the body it is presented in white against red muscles. What is usually less obvious is that it is invested throughout those muscles and forms the membranes between them and within them; as muscle fibre. It is continuous with, rather than separate from, the tendinous attachments, and much more besides as we will explore.

The fascia is essentially made up of various types of collagen and elastin fibres bound together, with bound water, to form a variety of living tissue expressions. (It also includes reticulin, which is immature collagen.) Together, all these tissues combine to form one tensional matrix that contains every part of us, on every scale.

Fascia includes, for example, tendinous sheets (aponeuroses) and chords (tendons), connecting webs (some strong and some gossamer-like) and the boundaries that distinguish one part from another. The various types of tissues have different densities and contribute to the formation and continuity of joints, attachments, relating membranes; even the fibres and fibrils of the

All fascia is connective tissue. However, not all that is described as connective tissue in the body is necessarily fascia; there are some distinguishing points. For example: blood is considered to be a connective tissue, but it is not fascia. (There is a distinction made between biology and biomechanics.) There are detailed discussions of the naming of different fascial tissues and academic considerations for what can and cannot be called fascia (see Chs 3 and 7). However, many of the pioneers of fascia research seek a global term for these connective tissues to restore a perspective of wholeness to the living body that correlates with the experience of manual therapy and movement.[9] *In vivo* examination (see Chs 2 and 3) reveals that fascia is continuously connected and related throughout our systems, from micro to macro levels of scale. This will be explored and referenced throughout Part A.

muscle units we name are essentially formed in the fascia's connected continuity throughout our bodies.

It has been suggested that the entire body is made up of variations on this tissue theme: from bone (as a calcified form of fascia at its thickest, hardest and most compressed[4]), to cartilage, with high hyaline content, with a nylon-like[5] behaviour. Ligament and tendon behave as sheets and cords of various "condensation" and myofascia (muscle) contains numerous muscle fibres[6] wrapping the red protein, of the muscle. These issues of exactly what is and what is not fascia are now being thoughtfully debated (see Ch. 7, where we also investigate its fluid properties). Certainly, it can be considered the main building material in our bodies, varying in thickness and density, including even the softest and most delicate of membranes, such as the eardrum. Whether or not there is universal agreement about exactly what is or is not fascia, the recognition of this tissue as *significant* represents a huge shift in perspective. We are "crossing the Rubicon"[7] from studying the individual components, as if they can exist separately, to appreciating the wholeness of the architecture holding *all* of them *all* together.

Whatever the different parts of it are named (there is much conjecture around this – see Chs 3 and 7), the fascia certainly forms what can only be described as a matrix that surrounds everything, connects everything, yet paradoxically *disconnects* everything, by distinguishing it from everything else! In other words, it *distinguishes* one part of our body from another, containing all parts by wrapping them. It also holds together the extracellular matrix, that is, the more fluid domain in which the cells that make up our organs and parts reside (see Ch. 7). The fascia contains them and our bodily "colloids and emulsions"[8] in its variety of expressions as the basic tissue of our whole structure, or human architecture.

The fascia envelops every organ; it is part of what forms our vessels (it is the dura of the nerve vessels, the tunicae of the blood vessels) and keeps them in place. It covers the microscopic muscle fibrils at its finest, the fibres in their bundles and the whole muscle forms, as well as groups of muscles. It forms the back of the skin, the soft gliding between the skin and underlying structures. It forms the architecture of the heart, it wraps the lungs, the viscera, the brain and sensory organs. It begins *as one original piece* embryologically and continuously develops throughout our lives (see Ch. 4) and our entire body form, *as a continuity*. If the rest of us were to be removed, we would remain recognisably us, with just our fascia forming a ghost[10] of our entire body in its finest detail and fullness (see Fig. 7.3). All of these fascial structures have individual names, and some are studied from different perspectives, for their distinct roles in the body. Although they are studied under the designation of separate systems and subjects, however, *they are not experienced that way* in the living body.

Among several things, perhaps, that have been sometimes overlooked when fascia is removed post-mortem is this *universal continuity*. Study of fascia does not replace musculoskeletal anatomy but includes, enhances and evolves it. From a yoga perspective, studying what we could call "fascial anatomy"

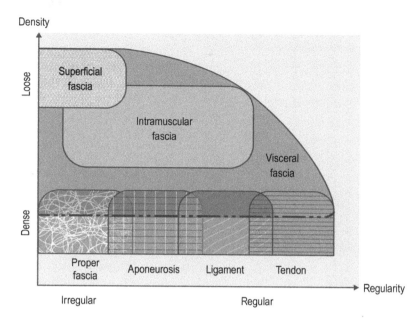

Figure 1.1

This image shows the different types of connective tissues considered to be included in the term "fascia".

Image reproduced with kind permission from Robert Schleip, fascialnet.com.

(variously, if unofficially, termed osteo-myofascial and neuro-myofascial anatomy) makes complete sense of yoga and brings the art of yoga into a powerful contemporary focus and holistic relevance.

Figure 1.1 shows the different types of connective tissues considered by Schleip and colleagues to be included in the term fascia. (Terminology referred to here is discussed in Chapter 7):

"a more encompassing definition of the term fascia was recently proposed as a basis for the first Fascia Research Congress (Findley & Schleip 2007) and was further developed (Huijing & Langevin 2009) for the following congresses. The term fascia here describes the 'soft tissue component of the connective tissue system that permeates the human body'. One could also describe these as fibrous collagenous tissues which are part of a body-wide tensional force transmission system."[11]

Collagen fibres can have different densities and directional alignments depending upon which kind of fascial tissues they express. This is influenced by what we do, how we do it, and how frequently we do it (i.e. the usage patterns or local loading history) as

Traditionally, the "white stuff" (fascia and connective tissue) and the "yellow stuff" (adipose tissue, or fat) are removed in the anatomy laboratory in order to provide "clean" dissection and reveal the important parts for the study of anatomy of the locomotor system. Biomechanics, anatomy and the related physiological basis of structure and function have all been, at least in part, deduced in the absence of this "in-between" fabric or wrapping. Historically, it has been assigned to the cadaveric bins.

Far from Inert

The fascia is now considered to be far from simply an inert packaging material or just a discrete unit, such as the thoracolumbar fascia or other specific parts of dense fascial fibres to be found in the body. Fascia is also considered to occupy well as locality in the body and the amount of body weight and forces put through a particular tissue. Ligaments and tendons in the ankle, for example, will always be stronger and therefore denser than visceral fascia, wrapping organs. (This will be explored further in Chapter 3.)

This does not mean that the subject of fascia is not taught in anatomy classes. It refers to the much larger context considering that fascia is routinely removed in order to reveal the underlying or embedded structures, and thus there is a possibility that its full significance has been vastly underestimated and overlooked. Once the tissue has been thrown away, it cannot be reinstated as a part of the whole structural integrity. It is into this gap that the contemporary research has revealed a new recognition of the roles, importance and variation in fascial tissues in terms of our functions and the profoundly significant relationships to structure (and vice versa). How we negotiate forces moving through our form, from moment to moment, is profoundly related to the fascial matrix.

the incredibly complex world of the "in-between"[12] and forms a single, body-wide, tensional network in all dimensions (see Ch. 7). The organs, vessels, muscles and bones are contained within it. Indeed, we will discover in Chapter 4, they arise from it. The fascia could be described as "the common architectural and morphological denominator of our unified form". (In other words, everything is made from it, wrapped in it, organised by it structurally and shaped by its structure.) Until recent decades, the idea that its removal was effectively distorting the theories of structure, function and locomotion upon which the study of human movement has been (and still is) built in the West would have been too challenging. Now the fascia can no longer be ignored, as we continue to experience the ever-increasing body of research that is gradually changing the basis of medical practice and of movement and manual therapies.[13] Studies of fascia are igniting new questions and transforming the foundations upon which classic theories of anatomy, physiology and biomechanics are based. Indeed, the study of proprioception is igniting the relevance of the structural tissue, to aspects of study more commonly assigned to psychology (which we will explore in Chapter 5).

Fascial anatomy, as a body-wide architecture, makes complete sense of the study of yoga in all its contemporary forms. It is a system that unifies the body, upgrades our appreciation of movement and confers exactly the kind of wisdom and congruency we seek in the philosophy of yoga. From the postures (yogasana) to the ability to manage various physiological systems (such as respiration) and more refined practices of meditation and self-awareness. We will discover that the fascia plays an intimate role in our living human sentient experience.

The significance of the fascia to studies of the human body has been quite astonishingly underestimated given that (1) it is alive and anything but passive, (2) it is a sensory organ (see Ch. 5), (3) it is literally everywhere, (4) it is continuous throughout our form, on every scale, joining and relating everything to everything else and (5) its architectural status affords the recognition of geometry; deep to the patterns of nature, within this, our universal matrix. As such, it invites the pursuit of unity – reflecting the patterns of the Yantras in the organisations of the physical form. Therein lie the resonance fields of the mantras, all of which play a part in the practice of yoga, previously considered separate from the study of anatomy. It is an invitation beyond unity, to the universal nature of forms, which we will explore in Chapter 13.

This combination of characteristics amounts to the recognition of the fascia as the master of our sense of where we are in space. This sense is additional to the commonly held belief that we are five-sensory creatures. It is developing as the basis of our sixth, very important sense: the one that tells us where we are relative to our environment and ourselves at any point in time. This self-sensing awareness is known as *proprioception* and it provides an essential key in the role of self-regulation (see Ch. 5).

Proprioception

Proprioception is the sense that tells us where we are in space at any given moment, feeling the cup we lift to drink from and the amount of energy it takes to place it accurately and sip, making tiny subtle renegotiations as the volume goes down and we put it back on a surface. (As we will see in Chapter 7, it also plays a part in our inner sense of how much we have drunk, its temperature and materials.) Proprioception is at work when we move our fingers over the keyboard we tap to write an email, or the strings we pluck to play a musical instrument or simply send a text message on a smart phone. Fascia is referred to as our organ of organisation and its proprioceptive qualities are subtle and extensive. In yoga it is essentially the sensing of every part of us, in any given pose, relative to every other part and the mat – and the air we breathe while we are doing it. It speaks the instinctive language of movement because the body literally senses where it is and what it does all the time, regardless of our ability to analyse it intellectually. The matrix self-balances faster than we can think about it; self-regulation instinctively happens much more rapidly in life than we can describe it on paper.

Interoception includes the internal awareness or "gut knowing" we often refer to as our "instinctive" sense. Putting it very simply, the sensory nature of the fascial matrix and the particular structure of our formation actively keep us in touch with that feeling of "knowing"; be it a "gut reaction" or an even more subtle inner awareness. New research about the sensory receptors (mechanoreceptors) of the fascial tissues (including those in the gut) are influencing the terms under which this quality of self-awareness is understood.[14]

Current fascia research challenges our traditional general notions of anatomy, physiology and biomechanics and shakes the foundations of many classical principles. At the same time, it offers a new context that unifies not only the different parts of the body but also the physical and metaphysical aspects of the being that resides within it. This is an exciting time to be a yoga teacher, since union is such a founding, ancient basis of yogic wisdom and so fundamental to the contemporary art of yoga in all its variety. We are – and remain – one; connected to all the other ones.

The Art of Contemporary Yoga

The brand of yoga, the way a pose is performed, the anatomy, physiology and philosophical origins of the posture or meditation, is not always the key. You are. Each one of us is seeking our own expression of balance and congruency, a refinement of our proprioceptive awareness and experience. That is uniquely and never in the same place and time twice. Yoga does not bring you to a particular state so much as it accumulates an inner knowledge of the states you are capable of being in. It can expand the facility to explore your range of potentials and the possibilities you consider yourself to embody. How we connect these many aspects is fascinating and the discovery that we do so through this sensitive connecting fabric of our form, as a medium or interface, enhances the founding principles of yoga and expands our appreciation of this inner-sensing[15] ability of self-organisation, on every scale.

Yoga does not respond well to being fragmented, and neither do we. Nor is a static state of fragmentation like life. Essentially, even if our journey is one of distinguishing the parts, it only makes sense in the context of a process of becoming whole. Can we unite, or reunite our sense of who and how we are, at any point in time, once we identify the "cogs" we seek to literally and symbolically re-*cog*-nise ourselves?

"Proprio" comes from the Latin propius, meaning "one's own", and "ception" comes from perception. So, the translation of *proprioception* is "one's own, or self, perception". Innate to the term is its meaning as a sensory feedback signaling system (Ch. 5). The word "*appropriate*" comes from the same origins. So, a self-appropriate practice is one in which our proprioceptive sense guides us to congruency; at any given time. This is the invitation for us to find our own kind of yoga, one that speaks the language of our own essential body dialect, written in its fascial form. That form is inclusive of the muscles and wraps the bones, profoundly invested with fascia and embedded in the wholeness of our multi-dimensional matrix. We will explore this principle throughout the book.

Our yoga practice changes as we do, ebbing and flowing with our lives, as an intimate part of us that simply keeps us awake and aware. It offers us the opportunity to know and develop ourselves, once we find the right type of yoga for our own particular form and fascia type (see Ch. 17), at any point or period in time. It remains entirely personal: a unique practice that we can foster and develop to deepen our sense of being, through postures and sequences, movements and meditations. It can be a beautiful opportunity to realise our potentials at any age and at any stage in life. It changes with us. We can explore and grow together, in every sense.

There are many ways of doing this, and yoga is but one of them. Upon exploration, we discover yoga can be a very rewarding pathway along which to seek that congruency and unity of body, mind and being – particularly when we understand the fascial matrix; profound knowledge about a tissue that has been there since the beginning and knows us, precisely, as we know ourselves. The treasure of comfortable motion, at whatever level we can embody, is well worth the expedition to find this congruency. This is the journey from the vitality of movement itself to its fullest expression into stillness and presence. We can even carve a path of self-esteem once we explore becoming *conscious of being,* beyond *"adept at doing"* yoga. It is a beautiful means to an endless possibility that the fascia, as the "page" upon which we write our journey in the body's story, is written large in its multi-dimensional architecture.

Learning Anatomy and Physiology and Biomechanics

Yoga was never divided up in the way that anatomy, physiology and biomechanics have been, in the Western study of these academic subjects. Not only was the yogic body treated as a breathing, moving whole, but the mind, body and spirit did not undergo the intellectual, political and religious segregation practised in Western medical and biomechanical academies. In Chapter 2 we will discuss how this fragmentation came about, in a historical context. However, we can note here that this legacy sits awkwardly with a practice as naturally integrated and intuitively tuned as yoga was originally designed to be. The growing understanding of the fascial matrix as the foundation of our entire movement apparatus (in all its detail) makes much more sense of the foundations of yoga and what actually happens in a yoga class, whatever style you practise.

We will explore the shift from anatomy to understanding the soft tissue architecture, in Part A. We begin whole, we end whole, and at all stages between we remain whole. The question is how do we animate well? How do we anticipate, navigate and negotiate suitable change, *as a whole*? How do we do that in an appropriate way at the time?

As the fascia is revealed as the basic tissue of relationship in the body, joining everything to everything else in one continuous tensional network, it is redefining our understanding of how any part moves and experiences sensation, relative to another. It is offering new explanations of how forces are transmitted throughout our structure, modified and balanced by our innate kinaesthetic intelligence. This forms the new foundation of Biomechanics (Part B) that takes us to the natural geometry of motion – as living Tensegrity-based architectures. Biotensegrity provides an understanding of how we form and how living things move in the round. Essentially, we live, breathe and move as soft tissue volumes, subject to the rules of fluid-dynamic organisations, like every other living thing in the cosmos.

The evolving understanding of fascia invites us to see and assess movement in whole gestures and consider the relationships of the parts to each other as paramount. How we put this into practice and move better (gradually becoming aware at different levels of subtlety and sensitivity) are explored in Part C, as we mark a pathway from "classical to connected" in the classroom. How can we honour this remarkable tissue, through our teaching?

In contemporary yoga, knowledge of the fascia expands and changes how we apply anatomical understanding in a relevant way to our actual human experience of the postures. Soft tissue plays a profound role in our ability to adapt and sustain useful adaptations. At the same time, we can release compensations that are less than optimal, if we can learn to recognise them as such. While human beings share many aspects in common, the fascia of each one of us behaves uniquely, depending upon how we use it, as we will see in later chapters.

Into Three Dimensions

We occupy space in three dimensions, although our culture often resides in a domain of duality, preferring a more two-dimensional thinking. In anatomy and physiology we talk about specific oppositions and about "equal and opposite forces" (see Newton, Ch. 2 and Chs 6 and 7) that are activated in nature. Muscles are classically described in terms of antagonistic pairs. We think of muscles and bones as the protagonists of the locomotor system and the breath is often described in terms of the inhale and the exhale, as if we do one or the other (see Ch. 11).

In a paradox, two opposing ideas can coexist at the same time; however, beyond paradox, we enter the *field*. This field is inclusive of both polarities, both opposite forces; providing a kind of "platform" yielding a combination that is simultaneously "both" and "neither". We are calling this the "neutral field" or the "witness state". Essentially it takes us beyond duality, into the 3- or multi-dimensional form in which we live. This becomes very important because, unless we upgrade the conversation to *include this language of paradox*, we will not fully understand the impact of fascia on form or function. It will elude us if we stay within the old language of two-dimensional thinking because this is a whole new paradigm. It is the third dimension (and beyond) of the locomotor system; which is only ever a volume in all aspects of our form.

Medical textbooks are often illustrated with two-dimensional iconographic images in order to express things in understandable ways (see Ch. 3). This may not be wrong necessarily; however, in the light of fascial research it is insufficient. We might also expand our understanding to include and recognise the wholeness we experience. Visually, this is very complex; intellectually, it is easier to draw only one conclusion at a time. However, the body works instinctively and intuitively in wholeness, so fascia provides some very compelling invitations to consider it anatomically as the tissue that weaves us together *as a whole,* from the beginning.

Neutral is not a default condition, resulting from the failure to make a decision between two alternatives. Rather it is an actively generated state which expands the point of view to include all possibilities (see Ch. 12). These are challenging notions because they go beyond the mind to include the being. The intellectual mind may prefer the pendulum-swinging metronome, oscillating between right and wrong, up and down, forward and back; antagonistic pairs. This is where we find our rhythm. However, the pairs are included as an underlying pattern in the larger paradigm, where that rhythm finds *expression* and by incorporating both aspects, contains them *in a larger field* (see opening chapter quote).

Beyond Polarity

Consider a circle. A series of overlapping circles can make a beautiful pattern (Fig. 1.2). (We will see the significance of this in Chapter 12.) The moment you see that series of circles represented in three dimensions as a series of spheres, it absorbs the pattern the circles made (Fig. 1.3). There are fewer lines in the literal sense, but, symbolically, there is more volume represented.

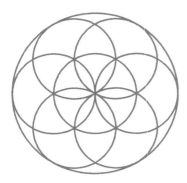

Figure 1.2

This is a three-dimensional diagram of the same eight spheres seen in Figure 1.3.

The Renaissance

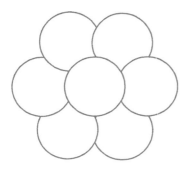

Figure 1.3

This series of overlapping circles is a two-dimensional diagram of eight spheres; one sits behind the centre circle.

Image by Martin Gordon, www.mothmedia.co.uk

Yet the circular pattern remains within the spheres, albeit innately hidden within them. What has changed is your point of view and the expansion of awareness to portray depth of field. There is more dimension implied, with fewer lines to see it. Your kinaesthetic ability to interact with the object is transformed. The kinaesthetic sense of animation, or movement, occupies a domain that not only lives in three (or more) dimensions but also operates at a rate many thousands[16] of times faster than intellectual thinking. (See Margin note.)

The three-dimensional perspective, the neutral field, includes the circles within the spheres. This perspective becomes essential to understanding fascia and how it integrates our fully functional movement, *in the round*. It represents our embodiment of those rhythmical sums of our parts. We make the shapes in yoga in order to enquire how we move and shape space (and shape ourselves within it) in all our aspects and wholeness. We are the sum of the up and the down, the lateral and medial, the inner and outer. We are the in-between interface, the membrane responding through forms, the domain in which both can occur as polarities and find themselves united, expressing as us. We are the unpredictable sum; greater than the individual parts.

The representation of human beings in three dimensions, rather than two, was part of a huge shift in culture, affecting every area of the Western world during the Renaissance. It was shown in art and in our understanding of Earth as we sailed to new lands. This period marked a turning point in the history of European thought, when science and medicine became studies in their own right. The whole period between 1400 and 1800 was a time of immense change in every field of endeavour in the Western hemisphere. It produced many of the philosophers and scientists upon whose genius our current beliefs rest, for much of our knowledge in the arts and sciences. We will consider them in Chapter 2, to provide a context for the changes we are seeing in our current age. Indeed, some suggest we are in a new period of Renaissance or rebirth, entering the next dimension of seeing.

Part A of this book examines some of the impacts of past and present changes in thinking on anatomy, physiology and biomechanics, considering how essential it is to understand the triune nature of our wholeness on every level. Nowhere does this become clearer than in understanding the structural principles of nature's geometry and how we animate the rules of living tensegrity (see Ch. 6). Triangulation is presented as a basis of our architectural wholeness and its forming. The chapter on embryology (Ch. 4) presents the essence of it all, evolving beyond two-dimensional thinking, to embrace and recognise ourselves as volumes.

What we cannot forget in all this is that the practice of yoga originated in the Eastern hemisphere. As such, bringing it to the West is an invitation to expand our thinking to include the far-reaching nature of its potential. If we do not, we risk reducing and diminishing it. The range of studies and the

If you try to instruct someone new to yoga, or they use a book, with only verbal or written cues and no recourse to demonstration, you will bump into the divide between intellect and instinct and their respective speeds. Participation and practice bring the moves into the instinctive realm so that eventually, we do not have to think about them. Fascia brings our understanding of the living structure and function into *being*. It could also be described as a kind of interface between things, including our inspiration to animate, from intention to gesture to performance.

pioneers developing the field of fascia research[17] have made that reductionism unnecessary.

The tensional network of the human form unites anatomy and physiology. It makes sense of the biomechanics and clearly forms the sensory basis of our instincts to move. It transforms our understanding of yoga, while yoga itself can actively transform the fascial matrix. This includes the muscles and bones, but is by no means limited to them. Like the spheres absorbing the circles, the fascia includes the organs of movement, unifying them with the whole of the body; from vessels to viscera, heart to hamstrings, ground to crown.

Yoga is not restricted to postures or authentically limited to making shapes using the bony framework of the axial and appendicular skeleton. Our being moves us in every sense and on every level, in our own ways. It becomes clear that yoga and fascia sit congruently together, making sense of each other and of our personal, unique organisation within the space–time continuum.

Yoga is really about sentient beings, but unless we can step into (and beyond) neutral and see how we are being, detached from the illusion of what we make that mean, we cannot easily realise our own potency to co-create our lives and recognise our full grace and potential. That possibility resides in the difficulty and sweetness, the complexity and simplicity of movement and stillness, as they are. We can observe both at the same time. Uniting the multiple aspects of ourselves and witnessing that journey is the invitation to the field of grace that Rumi refers to in the quotation at the head of this chapter. It is the field "out beyond ideas of right doings and wrong doings". As a fellow yoga practitioner, I would love to meet you there.

Notes

1. Jelaluddin Rumi, *The Essential Rumi*, translated by Coleman Barks with John Moyne, A.J. Arberry and Reynold Nicholson, HarperCollins, San Francisco, 1995.
2. The number of papers on fascia indexed in Ovid, the MEDLINE and Scopus databases has grown from 200 per year in the 1970s and 1980s to almost 1000 in 2010 (Robert Schleip, Thomas W. Findley, Leon Chaitow and Peter A. Huijing, *Fascia: The Tensional Network of the Human Body*, Churchill Livingstone/Elsevier, Edinburgh, 2012) and upward of 20,000 since 2010 (see Note 3).
3. John Sharkey. Can Medical Education be Enhanced by the World's First 3d Printed Fascia Models and Plastinated Specimens of Fascia Superficialis and Profundus. *Biomed J Sci & Tech Res* 15(4)-2019. BJSTR. MS.ID.002749.
4. John Sharkey (2019). Letter to the Editor. *Journal of Bodywork & Movement Therapies* 23: 6e8.
    Article by Stephen M. Levin - 2018/08/21, SP , Bone is Fascia - published on ResearchGate and as a special contribution within the Introduction of Susan C. Lowell de Solórzano's *Everything Moves: How Biotensegrity Informs Human Movement*. Handspring Publishing Ltd, Pencaitland, 2020.
5. Deane Juhan, *Job's Body: A Handbook for Bodywork*, Station Hill Press, Barrytown, NY, 1987, "Connective Tissue", Ch. 3.
6. For an excellent overview see Thomas W. Myers, *Anatomy Trains: Myofascial Meridians for Manual and Movement Therapists*, 4th edition, Churchill Livingstone, Edinburgh, 2021.
7. "Crossing the Rubicon" is a phrase that Dr Caroline Myss uses as a symbolic reference to the "crossing over" from "unconscious" notions to more conscious awareness. It originates from Roman Times, 49 BC, when Julius Caesar made a significant crossing, from one side of the River Rubicon to the other (named in Italian, for the red earth of the region), beginning his reign, a significant step in the formation of the Roman Empire.
8. Stephen Levin, www.biotensegrity.com
9. Introduction to Robert Schleip, Thomas W. Findley, Leon Chaitow and Peter A. Huijing, *Fascia: The Tensional Network of the Human Body*, Churchill Livingstone/Elsevier, Edinburgh, 2012.
10. The image of the Ghost Heart and a link to the work of Dr Doris Taylor can be found here, showing how the heart (once dipped into an acid bath that removes all tissues except the fascia) allows us to see the detailed connective tissue architecture. This work is having a profound influence on the role of human architecture and tissue morphology upon stem cell therapy. https://www.tmc.edu/news/2019/06/in-the-lab-with-scientist-doris-taylor-and-ghost-hearts/

11. Ibid.

12. P.C. Benias, R.G. Wells, B. Sackey-Aboagye, et al (2018) Structure and distribution of an unrecognized interstitium in human tissues. *Sci Rep* 8: 4947.

13. In August 2019, Clinical Anatomist John Sharkey led a team of Fascia experts presenting a Fascia Symposium to the 19th Congress of the International Federation of Associations of Anatomists (IFAA) which is held every 5 years. In 2019 the Congress was held, for only the second time, in London, England. The IFAA Congress is a unique opportunity for medical professionals to share research and new developments in anatomy and anatomy research. Applications are peer-reviewed; presentations undergo rigorous scientific scrutiny, before being accepted for presentation. In the event, a presentation by John Sharkey and Drs Carla Stecco, Vladimir Cheremnsky, Rafael De Caro, Veronica Macchi and Andrea Porzionato was enthusiastically received by the large number of delegates at this prestigious event. In the same year the professional journal of anatomists, *Clinical Anatomy*, produced a Special Issue journal, [reference Volume 32, Issue 7. October 2019, pp. 896–902] devoted entirely to the topic and science of Fascia. This is scientific progress with a capital "P" and is referred to in more detail in later chapters in Part A.

14. Robert Schleip and Heike Jäger, "Interoception: A New Correlate for Intricate Connections Between Fascial Receptors, Emotion and Self Recognition", Ch. 2.3 in Robert Schleip, Thomas W. Findley, Leon Chaitow and Peter A. Huijing, *Fascia: The Tensional Network of the Human Body*. Churchill Livingstone/Elsevier, Edinburgh, 2012.

15. Ibid

16. Alexander Filmer-Lorch, *Inside Meditation: In Search of the Unchanging Nature Within*. Matador, Kibworth Beauchamp, 2012.

17. International Fascia Research Congresses 2007, 2009, 2012: www.fasciacongress.org and Fascia Research Society: www.fasciaresearchsociety.org.

2

Ancient Wisdom and New Knowledge

"Seeing how geometry shapes nature, you can understand why ancient artists, architects and craftspeople of many cultures were impressed by its power and its ability to ennoble human creations. The ancients were aware of nature's geometric language and purposefully employed it in their arts, crafts, architecture, philosophy, myth, natural science, religion and structures of society from prehistoric times through the Renaissance. The world today needs scholars and researchers who give the ancients credit for their intelligence and understanding, to view their art and entire cultures in the light of its mathematical symbolism."[1]

Michael S. Schneider

There is a rich story behind the evolution of anatomy. Early anatomists worked in a way that tended to reduce our soft architectural individuality to the lowest common denominators. The discovery of how important the fascial matrix is in reuniting those same parts and recognising the significance of their natural architecture has come at a time in our culture when we understand networks – and invisible ones, at that. While the Internet enables communication and education around the world, the "internal-net" is being recognised as global in terms of the body's world.[2] It lifts the game of anatomy from the page and places it on the mat, where yoga plays it and each being animates it, as a self-motivated form, in their own way.

How the fabric of the fascial web is structured as the basis of our physical three-dimensional architecture will be considered in the next chapter and throughout Parts A and B, anatomically and biomechanically. What follows in this chapter is some of the cultural background, showing how the wholeness of human anatomy came to be fragmented into parts in the first place. This chapter begins to answer the question we asked in Chapter 1 as to how the fascia was generally overlooked for so many centuries. It also provides some clues as to how the questions that were asked at the time were closely related to the culture in which they were raised.

Early Western Medicine

To some extent the system of "humours" shared similarities with the Ayurvedic principles that are still practised in Eastern medicine. However, such "body typing" (somatotypes) was eventually almost entirely abandoned in the West in the late nineteenth century with the discovery of the cell as the "primary unit of life" (see Virchow below) as a founding contextual shift in the field of medicine.

Hippocrates (approx. 460–377 BC) is often credited with being the founding father of Western medicine and with making medical and anatomical studies a distinct profession. Human dissection was strictly forbidden under Greek law, so medical practice was developed by carefully taking notes concerning the patient's living experience. This built up a body of knowledge gained from due consideration of ailments and a logical study of the stages an illness or condition and a patient went through.

The Hippocratic School united both the Asclepian principles of intervention (the doctor) and the Hygeian (the healer; meaning "to make whole") notion of facilitation whereby the patient made some contribution to their own healing process. The system of the so-called "humours" was developed based on classifying each individual into types according to the way their body held its fluids. Balance was the key to managing the person's health (according to their type) and various other conditions such as temperament and a suitable environment in which to heal.

In ancient times, the study of the human body was not restricted or confined to a particular science. Like the study of art and architecture, it also required an extensive knowledge of nature, form, movement and structure in all living and crafted things. The ideas of philosophers (as the founding fathers were known) and the extent of their knowledge was wide by contemporary standards but perhaps less restricted to any single area of specialisation. In earlier times the nature of a philosopher's religious faith was closely tied into the fabric of his life. Notably, the reproduction of text or image was made by hand, a process which was very expensive. Artists and craftsmen were patronised by the wealthy or apprenticed to a master, so they often had to follow the faith and social or cultural rules of their patron to thrive. Thus the sanction of the church, the emperor or the sovereign had great influence over how knowledge progressed. Let us consider some examples, in chronological order.

Vitruvius

One philosopher who enjoyed the favour of the first Roman emperor, Augustus, was Vitruvius (born approx. 80 BC). The date of his death is unknown. An architect and engineer, who served in the Roman army, Vitruvius was the first to provide written volumes on architecture. His work included a broad scope, such as the architecture of instruments for making music, the study of human form in its proportions as well as more classical aspects associated with the architecture of constructing buildings. His detailed *study of nature* as the *source* of understanding form, included how proportion mattered in balancing physical forces and aesthetic structural integrity, with sensory perception. In perceiving and presenting beauty in form and function, the architect studied and portrayed nature and its forces, which were considered essential to any architectural undertaking. Every design in nature, according to Vitruvius, included the three principles an architect must follow in anything he created:

"Firmitas, utilitas, venustas"

Firmitas, utilitas, venustas (Vitruvian design principles that suggest a design should be: solid (structurally sound), useful (useable, suitable for its specific purpose) and beautiful (aesthetically pleasing))

Divine Proportion gave rise to the harmony of nature and therefore dictated the ideal proportions of a building, based upon appropriate geometric ratios. This was particularly important as the blueprint for a temple or church, designed to honour the divine. The rules of form were applied to far more than buildings, however. Whether for aesthetic harmony to the eye or ear, or the experience of a shape or form, these laws were considered necessary to assure "*firmitas, utilitas, venustas*" in everything (see Margin Note), from designing an instrument, bridge or tool, to a piece of furniture. Vitruvius took from Plato and Pythagoras the principles of "Sacred Geometry", which described the proportions and ratios of the Platonic Solids. These form the foundation, or essence, of the regular shapes of matter in living dimension. These are the regular polyhedrons inherent to all crystals making up forms in nature, and we will consider their importance to fascial formation in later chapters (see Ch. 12 for Archetypal Geometries).

The Golden Ratio was found everywhere in nature, so to use it in the broad spectrum of design in ancient architecture was actually to recognise the essence of natural (and therefore sacred) form. The architect did not seek to dominate or authorise this sacred form but rather to capture or recreate its essence and beauty, by mimicking nature. Man was considered to be the ultimate expression of Divine Proportion, the embodiment of nature's purest geometries. Vitruvius set an extraordinary challenge, whose solution remains a powerful symbol today:

"To any artist or architect to draw the human body with its arms outstretched such that both feet and hands could simultaneously touch the perimeter of the circle and the square" (of the same area)."[3]

This conundrum of Divine Proportion in relation to the human body was not solved until the fifteenth century, when Leonardo da Vinci completed a drawing which answered the challenge visually (see later in this chapter).

The Renaissance

Between classical antiquity and the Renaissance, human bodies came to be considered in very different ways in Western culture, at a time long before yoga (an aspect of Ayurvedic Wisdom) was known there. From the aesthetic sensibilities and sensitivities of the arts to the anaesthetic objectivity of medicine and anatomy, all such studies of the human form in the West were authorised by the church, since religion was considered the supreme guardian of the human spirit and its highest interests.

The period of the Renaissance in Europe was an exceptional era of expansion and development in many fields throughout the continent. During the Middle Ages, the church's dominance was reflected in social class structures and in the systems that governed organisations and cultures. Education was not accessible to the masses, but remained a relatively restricted privilege of the nobility and the clergy and those wealthy enough to afford it (or lucky enough to find a patron).

Communication other than by word of mouth relied to a great extent on skilled use of pen and ink on expensive parchment. Rare, handmade books were the domain of an educated elite, wealthy enough to travel, read and write or patronise such undertakings. As one of the primary patrons of the arts, the church's development of religious symbolism was one of its main means of disseminating religious ideals. The church also sanctioned the fields of education that developed, for without ecclesiastical approval, any theory or practice could be judged heretical and the theorist would not only no longer

Academic fields in former times were unlike those of today. Many philosophers (a term formerly used for both scientists and artists) had what we would now consider to be multidisciplinary skills. Human dissection, for example, was strictly forbidden under religious law, so early scientific development of anatomy and biomechanics was restricted to the study of animals, and theories were derived from such diverse fields as mathematics and the study of clock mechanisms (horology).

Polarity

The large-scale persecution, prosecution and execution of witches in these centuries was an extraordinary phenomenon. It is also an episode of European history that has spawned many myths and much inaccuracy. [Nevertheless]…between 1482 and 1782, around 100,000 people across Europe were accused of witchcraft, and some 40–50,000 were executed.[6]

be patronised, but might even be punished. Artistic endeavours had to be approved.

Gutenberg's[5] invention of the printing press in 1440 began an era of mass communication that changed society. His 1455 Bible is revered for its beauty of design and illustration and its iconic status as the first major printed book. The popularity of relatively economically produced printed books over subsequent decades (albeit very slowly) would eventually extend education beyond the elite; information and ideas began to be circulated. This gradually gave rise to new waves of scholarly investigation and popular culture was changed by what was to diversify into the arts and the sciences. The ability to print and publish their theories allowed the founding philosophers, writers, artists, musicians and scholars in a wide variety of different fields to *communicate their concepts and interpretations*. Their ability to explore and develop their ideas, however, was intimately related to whether they were able to gain sanction or patronage from the church or from local noblemen. For centuries to come, the church's influence over all aspects of academic and social development was profound.

The sixteenth century was a very significant time for all aspects of European culture. Bear in mind this was also, historically, an era in which Western society as a whole was emerging from the darkness of the medieval ages of superstition.

This era of emergence was particularly true for the birth of what we now call science. From this period onwards, change was rapid and many of the great philosophers were to become the so-called fathers of various fields of modern science and medicine.

The volume and depth of information being discovered with new instrumentation, when telescopes and then microscopes brought the worlds of both heavenly and living bodies into new perspectives, generated exponential growth in opposite directions. One field grew on the scale of the cosmos and the other on the scale of the microcosmos; the universe inside a cell. Such polarities naturally stretched the space between them and gave rise to fast and vast growth in every area of Western culture.

A great divide began to arise between man and nature; his own nature. Due in part, ironically, to the way in which the study of human anatomy eventually came to be sanctioned by the church, Descartes (see later in this chapter) created what is referred to today as "Cartesian Reductionism". Soft tissue was removed from the physical body when human dissection was eventually permitted. Since it was not recognised as playing any kind of significant role in physical, mental or emotional realms, it was relegated to a kind of unclassified hinterland, where it remained for centuries to come. In short, it was overlooked and discarded.

While artists such as Leonardo da Vinci and Michelangelo changed the aesthetic aspect of how human form was presented, Descartes and Borelli theorised over the anaesthetic domain of "mechanical function" and formalised anatomical study. The kinaesthetic aspects of experience were somewhat lost in translation.

We will next consider some of the key pioneers (in chronological order) from earlier centuries in order to show the significance of what is happening in this, the third millennium. A groundswell of change is shaping our very different worlds. The huge impact of printing in the fifteenth century is echoed by that of personal computing in the twenty-first. Both inventions have transformed the rate and reach of information. In the fifteenth century it was disseminated at walking pace and now, at the speed of light. Can we somehow distinguish the ancient wisdom that enhances contemporary knowledge?

The Cutting Edge

Galen (AD 129 – approx. 217) was a prominent physician and philosopher at the court of the Roman emperors; a society or civilization initiated by Julius Caesar's "crossing the Rubicon". Galen's reputation was gained from his extensive anatomical studies, although since human dissection was strictly forbidden under the laws of Rome the subjects of his dissections were often Barbary apes on the grounds that they were "similar to humans". Galen's theories followed those of Hippocrates and remained unchallenged for centuries until the work of Vesalius in the seventeenth century (see later in this chapter).

It was during the period of the Renaissance that the long-established principles of antiquity began to evolve more rapidly into new areas of advanced study. Creative and scientific development was opened up and ideas could, by this time be disseminated more easily.

"The Renaissance was the rebirth of man out of the dark years of medieval superstitions and belief and a return to the light of human reason. Italy and particularly Florence were at the heart of this reawakening of the human spirit. What more promising time or place could have existed as Leonardo's milieu?"[7]

Leonardo da Vinci (1452–1519) (born around the time of the printing press first being invented) is considered to be one of the finest examples of the archetypal Renaissance Man. It was Leonardo who eventually solved the circle and the square riddle posed by Vitruvius, 1500 years earlier, by placing their centres at different points on the human form (Fig. 2.1). Every other draughtsman who had attempted to solve this riddle had assumed the centre point of the circle and the square were the same. Leonardo's Vitruvian Man sets the centre of the square on the pubic bone and the centre of the circle at the navel. This drawing has profound significance in terms of Sacred Geometry (see Margin Note). Perhaps it also represents a symbolic "crossing of the Rubicon" in its invitation to explore seeing mankind as a spiritual creature, rather than necessarily a religious one. There is deep symbolic reference behind this image, as was the case for many Renaissance artists, who used their work to thinly veil their ideals and personal commentary, while avoiding political, social and ecclesiastical criticism. Vitruvian Man includes detailed measures of the ratio of the moon to the earth, nature's geometries and other cosmological details that were not necessarily sanctioned by the church at the time.

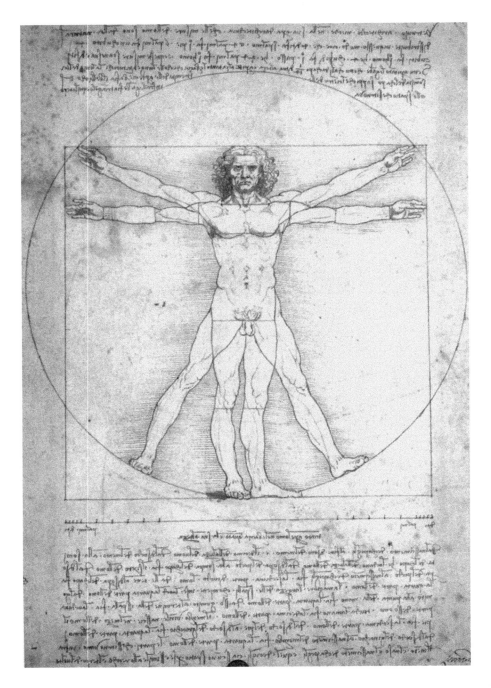

Figure 2.1

Leonardo da Vinci's Vitruvian Man. Leonardo's knowledge went beyond the ordinary and his ability to both literally and symbolically think outside the box demonstrated his unique mind and the breadth of his insight.

The hallmark of Renaissance humanism was its complete departure from the medieval culture of iconic symbolism that preceded it. The Renaissance artists sought to achieve a vivid sense of animation in portraying their living subjects. Leonardo was a leading figure in the transformation of the artist as a craftsman to the study of art as a science and the elevation of aesthetic principles.

"artists wanted to learn all they could about the inner structure of the human body in order to come up to the level of expertise of the ancient Greco-Roman artists in representing the human form. The Church had forbidden any such dissections, since it considered the human body a divine mystery. In addition, it was still leery of perfect representations of human and mythological figures, which it thought might lead to a sort of spiritual recidivism, a return to pagan idolatry. This is the reason that medieval portrayals of the human figure seem so flat and unnatural compared to those found in Classical and Renaissance artwork."[8]

We find out how essential the study of geometry is, to truly understanding human motion, in the following chapters. It is something innate to (and consciously concealed in) da Vinci's work. Not least the careful study of perspective in all his paintings, but deeper than this is evidence of Divine Proportion and Ratio, that goes beyond secular and even symbolic mathematics, to the mysteries behind Sacred Geometry (see Ch. 12).

According to his own notes, Leonardo did not want to draw muscles as "bulging shapes"[9] without understanding how the "tendinous function" caused them to actually behave in physical movement. He dissected human cadavers, illegally, to deepen his study of form as well as making extensive studies of living bodies in motion. This was to explore how the whole body in "action" expressed movement naturally (structurally) before it was transferred onto canvas or fresco, to be represented artistically. Structure and function were intimately related, and a profound understanding of fundamental principles of geometry and mathematics was translated into his engineering and architectural designs, as well as his drawings, paintings and sculptures.

Leonardo's studies also included Sacred Geometry and through his deep understanding of nature (and number) he was able to capture the essence of his subjects as well as their form. His sense of the three-dimensional space and light around and within those he portrayed is exceptional. For Leonardo, the body had a vital architecture. It was not just a shape, nor did it function mechanically. He understood that structure and function were profoundly related to geometry and motion. His paintings also evoke an emotional response and the sense that the Mona Lisa is following you around the room is palpable. It went beyond the aesthetic to include the kinaesthetic, evoking the felt sense from the observer. This was an essential aspect of Renaissance art: to capture the charisma ("charism" meaning soul-essence) of the subject(s) permanently.

The foundation of Leonardo's skills included mathematical deduction and geometry. The complex and mathematically accurate studies by Leonardo of the five Platonic Solids (Figs 2.2 and 2.3) are also exceptional; even by modern standards, with the use of computerised animation. They relate directly to the study of biotensegrity (see Ch. 6) and the most contemporary research into human motion and the fascial matrix.

The subject of Leonardo's mastery, whether a body or a building, was considered from the point of view of its aesthetic, its function and its form. Its

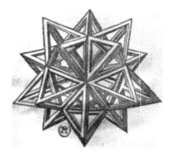

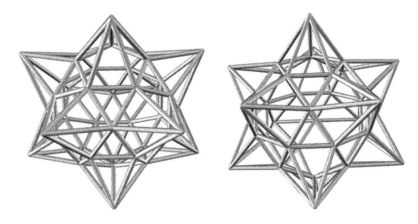

Figure 2.2

The small marginal image is a visual reference to one of Leonardo da Vinci's geometrical drawings in the book *De divina proportione*. Only two copies of this book exist: one in Biblioteca Ambrosiana in Milan, the other in Bibliothèque de Genève in Geneva. (Various Leonardo da Vinci geometrical images are available online from the Bridgeman Art Library.) In an attempt to draw this complex geometry with computer graphics the other images were produced – however, they are not entirely accurate. Leonardo "saw" beyond the page to create this with only a pencil and the instruments available to him. They present something far more sophisticated than technical draughtsman's skills.

Images by Martin Gordon (www.mothmedia.co.uk).

It is notable that, over the ensuing centuries, the realism the Renaissance artists were striving for was gradually replaced in the study of anatomy by ever more iconic renditions of schematic diagrams. This is partly why the connecting tissue continued to be overlooked. Clean dissection and clean, diagrammatic or graphic representation of what is dissected have underlined the focus on content over context. This is an important factor in understanding fascia. We have been mesmerised by iconic images of clean red muscles attaching to defined bones, much as our predecessors were seduced

whole architecture and purpose were integrated and the fundamental origins and ultimate "utilitas" of the structural shapes were recognised and presented with artistic conscience; always including "formitas" and "venustas" to respect Vitruvian wisdom.

Leonardo developed art as a science, even though he did not observe for a medical purpose. He portrayed the vitality of the subject, how movement was captured in a moment of stillness, implying a sense of life force and concealing social commentary. He designed machines, instruments, vehicles and buildings as well as being a prolific painter and craftsman. At this period the absolute division between art and science had not yet become part of accepted dogma. It could be said that da Vinci sought to understand how the soft tissue architecture made sense of motion and the ability to capture it in a "still frame" to use in his paintings. His anatomy studies are often considered exceptionally accurate, given the limitations within which he worked.

Andreas Vesalius (1514–1564) was the first to challenge 1500 years of tradition, upheld by Galen, in the field of anatomy. Vesalius acquired rare and special dispensation from a local judge to work with human cadavers. He also directly compared human bodies with those of certain non-human primate specimens, challenging the *differences* rather than upholding the similarities. In the Theatrum Anatomicum in Italy, at the University of Padua (the first anatomical theatre), Vesalius' anatomy demonstrations drew an audience from around Europe, including artists, scholars and members of the medical profession. Despite the fact that he was able to show the significant difference between the relatively straight lumbar spine of the ape and the curved human lumbar spine (lordosis), he was highly criticised for his views by many at the time. This observation significantly impacts explanations of motion and implicitly challenges the use of the word "column" in reference to the human vertebral organisation (columns don't tend to be curved). In a culture dominated by doctrine, "proof by demonstration" did not necessarily counter "tradition by declaration".

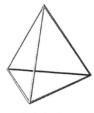
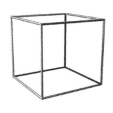
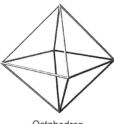
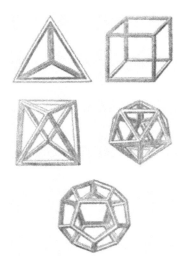

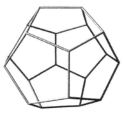
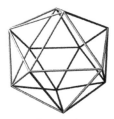
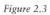

Tetrahedron
4 vertices; 6 edges; 4 faces

Cube
8 vertices; 12 edges; 6 faces

Octahedron
6 vertices; 12 edges; 8 faces

Dodecahedron
20 vertices; 30 edges; 12 faces

Icosahedron
12 vertices; 30 edges; 20 faces

Figure 2.3

The marginal image is a reference for Leonardo's exceptional drawings of the five Platonic Solids, cleverly portrayed in three-dimensional perspective. The main image conveys the same solids using computerised graphics – pointing to the exceptional vision at the heart of Leonardo's profound understanding of all nature's forms, something he sought to translate into fresco, painting, instrument design, machine design and elaborate architectural ventures.

Images by Martin Gordon (www.mothmedia.co.uk).

by Christian iconographic symbols. On every level, we are now invited to reconsider our perspective to one that is more inclusive of the context. It is a profound shift across the divide from topography to topology (see Ch. 3).

Anatomical drawings relied heavily on excellent artists to produce them. After a century of development, refined printing techniques meant that the work done by Vesalius could be more easily reproduced and publicised. Though acceptance of his work was not universal, it represented an exceptional breakthrough at the time in several ways. First, he challenged the 1500 years of acceptance of Galen's work on apes as the basis of human anatomy. Second, he considered the study of anatomy an essential basis for surgery, which was a revolutionary notion at the time. Third, he publicly presented his findings by demonstration and observation. (This was also exceptional at the time.)

These events have to be seen in the context of their era. They were extraordinary challenges to the fifteen *centuries* of belief they sought to evolve. Vesalius redirected the course of anatomical study of the human body from its established tradition and asserted its relevance to medicine. In 1543 he published his groundbreaking work *De Humani Corporis Fabrica*, literally meaning "the material/workings of the human form" or "made from the human body". ("Fabric" is a word derived from this Latin-based origin.) This implies the "making of" (and inadvertently refers to) *the fabric of that form*, which will be explored later. The book was based largely on human dissection which was done in a particular way. The scalpel was focused upon what it *cut to* rather than what it *cut through*. Nevertheless, anatomy was transformed into a subject that relied upon detailed and careful observation and meticulous dissection, making it as much an art and a skill, as a science. This legacy, linking the relevance of anatomy to surgery, was available in print and thus contributed to the expansion of the whole field of medicine, surgery and anatomy across Europe. Many universities opened anatomical theatres as a result, to further develop the study of anatomy both as a subject in its own right and as the basis of medical practice. Padua remains, to this day, at the forefront of anatomical authority, maintaining the official archives on human anatomy. Whatever his contemporaries thought about his views, through his style of dissection Vesalius radically changed the point of view regarding human form and the significance of anatomical organisation. His use of the scalpel in cutting up parts, regardless of the context or continuities in which they reside, became the assumed basis of the study of anatomy.[10]

Galileo Galilei (1564–1642) first studied medicine at the University of Pisa but changed to philosophy and mathematics, becoming Professor of Mathematics at the University of Padua in 1592, more than 30 years after Vesalius lived. He is most famous for supporting the Copernican theory that the sun was at the centre of the universe, not the earth, as the prevailing orthodoxy had upheld it. The church forbade such heretical ideas, which Galileo nevertheless put into print. His work is thought to have influenced Descartes and Newton (see later). The key point here is that his focus was via the telescope (in one direction), seeking to view the earth in the context of a universal scale. Importantly, the developing science of astronomy explained the movement of the planets through complex epicycles, to justify their earth-centred (geocentric) motion. Through Galileo's recognition of a sun-centred (heliocentric) universe, the epicycle theories were made redundant. They were transcended. This could act as a metaphor for the impact of current theories of the significance of fascia, which is evolving to transcend many classical anatomical notions and biomechanical concepts (as we will see in Chs 3 & 6).[11]

Descartes (1596–1650) was primarily a philosopher. At the time, instrumentation enabled the seeing of the heavenly bodies and that of greater detail within the human body. Great store was set upon breaking things down into their component parts in order to understand how they were assembled and then, according to Dr Candace Pert,[12] "extrapolat[ing] over-arching theories about the whole". This included human beings. According to Descartes the mind was demonstrably separate from the body and thinking and being were upheld as synonymous. He is most famous for his phrase "*Cogito, ergo sum*" (commonly held to mean: *I think therefore I am* (see Margin Note).

Although he is known as the father of modern medicine and science, Descartes' subjects of study included clocks (horology) and he was a mathematician in geometry and laws of motion. He applied the same intellectual reasoning to human behaviour and movement, considering the body to function completely separately from the mind. Descartes sought sanction directly from the Pope to use human bodies for his dissections, to study anatomy and properly demonstrate his point of view and analysis of function. *He argued that human behaviour itself was evidence of the fact that the mind and the*

This philosophy is significant in terms of the Age of Reason that ensued in Western culture. In the Eastern world of the yogic sages, the intellectual mind and its powers of reasoning are distinct, although not separate, from the mysteries of the being and the spirit therein; animating the body in the physical realm. Regardless of the religious, theoretical or political preferences, Descartes' meditations influenced the emerging cultural notion that wisdom resided in the reasoning mind and scholarly, academic pursuit of science. In other words; body and mind were (and could be treated as) separate.

In fact, according to Jaap van der Wal, *Cogito ergo sum*, means "I **doubt**, therefore I am" which suggests a much more subtle awareness or consciousness than Descartes is generally given credit for. He also wrote "*Doubt is the origin of wisdom*" and "*if you would be a real seeker after truth, it is necessary that at least once in your life you doubt, as far as possible, all things*"

The human ability to be self-conscious seems to have become lost in translation, over the centuries. Furthermore, Descartes' use of the word "automaton" actually translates to a "self-motivated" entity. In those days, clocks were an example of a self-motivated machinery. Unlike us, they need some sort of winding up, or mechanical/electrical intervention, however it makes more sense of the subtlety Descartes was exploring, to be in a state of wonder, rather than conviction. Nevertheless, wonder was destined to become a segregated issue from the being that was wondering; curiosity, awe and doubt are invisible! Such invisible forces were formerly placed under ecclesiastical authority.

body were entirely separate. The Pope sanctioned dissection on the grounds that the church retained jurisdiction over the invisible forces of the thinking and feeling realms of human experience. It was a confirmation of Descartes' larger philosophy (and possibly an act of guardianship for the soul) to sanctify the science. Body and being became legitimately considered as separate domains.

Descartes argued that bodily human motion is based on similar workings to those found in a clock mechanism and declared the body to move like any other "automaton" (from Greek automatos, meaning "self-moving" or "self-acting"). Thus, his reasoning effectively reduced the movement of the human body to that of a purely automated system of mechanical function, albeit self-motivated. Although the spirit of that "self" belonged to the church, human form reduced down to the biomechanical sum of its anatomical parts.

This philosophy proposed that the mind was distinct and could be elevated through study, the soul belonged to God, so was clearly under the domain of the church, and the body could be authentically broken down into its component parts for scientific analysis. Science could therefore justify furthering intellectual knowledge of anything under examination through the lens of "objective realism". The anatomical parts of the automated system could then be legitimately labelled and assigned their function and all (invisible) aspects of a human being would thus be understood and correctly assigned to the appropriate authority. Whatever the subtleties, naming parts became crucial in the pursuit of mending function: the early iterations of what developed into mechanistic views.

"I desire you to consider, I say, that these functions imitate those of a real man as perfectly as possible and that they follow naturally in this machine entirely from the disposition of the organs no more nor less than do the movements of a clock or other automaton, from the arrangement of its counter-weights and wheels."[13]

It is important to note again at this point that yoga did not develop under the influence of reductionist segregation of the human experience. The study of Ancient Psychology (as it was called) in the mystery schools or Wisdom School teachings abroad were not practised under these particular influences.[14]

The Italian physiologist Giovanni Alfonso Borelli (1608–1679) was a philosopher, mathematician and astronomer with a special interest in animal biomechanics. The two parts of his major work *De Motu Animalium* ("On the Movement of Animals") were published posthumously but his investigations into the field of movement led to his being called the father of biomechanics. In accordance with ideas of the time, Borelli's analysis of animal movement was based upon linear mechanics and two-dimensional deduction, while his theories were validated mathematically, based upon mechanical working parts (of machines). He stated that "*muscles do not exercise vital movement otherwise than by contracting*", extrapolating that the body moved forward by shifting its centre of balance via the joint angles acting as various kinds of *levers*. This principle is still alive in current research. It is still harboured as part of the classical model of biomechanical movement of the human gait and structure, despite its iteration of a two-dimensional, two-bar open-chain model. By reducing the nature of human motion to a single flat plane (as if human joints were pin-joints), Borelli described the mechanism of a wooden puppet, rather than a living being. It was accepted nonetheless.

Sir Isaac Newton (1642–1727) was, among many other things, a scientist and an alchemist. He devoted much time to discovering the philosopher's stone, as well as studies in the fields of theology, mathematics, astronomy, optics and numerous other scientific investigations. He is most famous for his formulation (or recognition) of the laws of gravity, and his work on the light spectrum and laws of motion and speed that were to become the basis of modern physics. Newton understood the principles of force and counter-force. Now considered as one of the most influential scholars in the history of science, in his day, Newton was revered in some academic circles but ridiculed in others as the "great geometer". He proposed the powerful distinction that "to every known action in the universe there is an equal and opposite reaction". (We will consider the influence of his particular genius (regarding the invention of calculus) in Chapter 6.)

Newton sought to understand man and motion in the context of nature as a whole, formulating the common physical laws of energy that govern individual and celestial bodies. He did not invent gravity so much as distinguish it. The Renaissance period saw the invention of both telescope and microscope, opening the cultural perspective to include a kind of "zoom lens". It distinguished scale from the telescope ("zoomed out") to the microscope ("zoomed in") as an asset or common denominator to all nature and forms. This context of scale is very important in understanding the body from a point of view of the soft tissues in current research. At this period in history, however, its novelty did not prevail.

Bernard Siegfried Albinus (1697–1770) was a lecturer on anatomy and surgery and one of the most famous teachers of anatomy in Europe, as was his father. He was appointed professor in 1745 and worked with draughtsman and illustrator Jan Wandelaar to produce exquisite anatomical drawings (Fig. 2.4).[15] The printing press was now 300 years old and considerably more sophisticated, so the speed of change and availability of information was expanding more rapidly. Nevertheless, the reproduction of information retained an aesthetic value. In order to be true to the human form, Albinus and Wandelaar would hang webbing with a grid marked upon it behind the suspended cadavers to give an accurate representation of scale and perspective. Their presentations included a sense of wholeness and continuity; as well as uprightness of posture, that made sense of the living aspect of human structure, within its environment. The principles of Renaissance humanism were retained. The images kept a sense of their original wholeness, representing continuity within the whole living body, separated out for medical purposes but nonetheless displaying a context for their original form. Albinus' famous work *Tabulae Sceleti et Musculorum Corporis Humani* (*Plates [illustrations] of the Skeleton and Muscles of the Human Body*) was published in 1747 but garnered much criticism of the "frivolous" backgrounds to the drawings. It seems

What was also developing, rather than a universal understanding, were the different fields of specialisation that we encounter today. Disciplines such as physics, chemistry, biology, botany, mathematics, biomechanics, physiology, medicine and anatomy were dividing according to religious and social orders, political and philosophical differences. The power of communication of knowledge was increasing and with it the value placed on theoretical reasoning. Standards of learning were developing too, as education became more available to a broader range of people, although it still relied heavily on social status, patronage, gender and politics. Fragmentation was occurring at many levels.

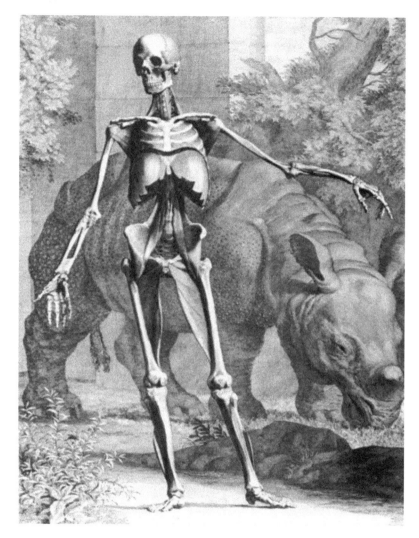

Figure 2.4

Albinus on Anatomy includes beautiful drawings of the bones and musculature. The original work shows whole-body presentations of the musculoskeletal anatomy at various depths and includes many exquisite drawings of the compartments and their relationships, such as this one of the diaphragm and its connectivity. Upwards (cranially) its continuity embraces the intercostals, subscapularis and scalenes, through to the deep cranium. Downwards (caudally) it continues through the deep psoas and adductors and deep crural compartment to the ground.

that by the later eighteenth century aesthetics were considered to be out of place in the serious academic study of anatomy and medicine. Other branches of science were also detaching body content from the context of wholeness; the gap between human experience (human being) and the separate facts about function (human doing) was widening.

With the increase in information availability and the cultural changes accompanying the Industrial Revolution there was a rapid expansion of education. Increasing specialisation brought about a further separation of the arts and the sciences. The study of anatomy began to be respected for its own sake and the hallmark of excellence in the field was to create "clean dissection", with images of the detail completely separated from their place in the context of the whole body or their original nature. Everything other than the key elements (bone, muscle, vessel, organ, gland or tendon and ligament), such as the layers of adipose tissue (fat) or scruffy bits of fascia and connective tissue between things, were considered to be "inert packaging material" largely irrelevant to the study of structure, function and motion. Apart from certain specific, discrete elements (separately named, such as the thoraco-lumbar fascia, for example), the looser fascia around and between things was removed and discarded as irrelevant. **In the anatomical laboratories fascia was largely consigned to the cadaveric bins. It was, and still is, literally thrown away; disregarded as insignificant.**

This was the general trend of anatomical study, in the growing fields of medical and surgical practice. However, there were notable exceptions.

John D. Godman (1794–1830) was an anatomist and naturalist who died young and was known, if at all, for his outstanding anatomical drawings and studies of the natural world. He came from a less than traditional medical background but his passion and enthusiasm for true anatomy were themes in his drawings, paintings and writings at the time. In his book *Anatomical Investigations comprising descriptions of various Fasciae of the Human Body* (1824),[16] he espoused a principle of honest observation of all that was in front of the student. Thus they could fully appreciate the connected nature of nature, including all the anatomical parts they were asked to study and understand. He insisted they ignored preconceived notions of named systems and looked at the parts, within the whole, in their context of this continuous tissue, the fascia. He went on to detail the class observations of this tissue as a connected whole throughout the entire body.

"The following investigations were begun without reference to any system, and without the slightest wish to support any preconceived opinions. The conclusions drawn were unavoidable, even at first inspection, and their correctness was more firmly established by every subsequent examination."[17]

It was almost 200 years ago that John Godman wrote, presciently, at the end of his introduction:

"The novelty of these descriptions will, perhaps, be the greatest impediments to their general acceptation, for it has been very correctly remarked by an illustrious anatomist, Geoffroy Saint Hilaire, that there are many persons who become furious at the mere annunciation of new ideas – like him, however we shall wait patiently, convinced that time fixes everything in its place."[18]

The cell came to be the centre of many branches of scientific enquiry and generally considered as the unit of life. The parts being examined were getting ever smaller and the quantity of information was expanding exponentially. This, in itself, raised difficulties of scale and focus. There were ever more powerful telescopes to see the farthest reaches of the cosmos and ever more powerful microscopes to see our smallest universe, inside an individual cell. What happened to the context in which, or from which, both are observed; the pattern of the matter in which they (all) reside?

Rudolf Virchow (1821–1902), considered to be the father of modern pathology, developed microscopy further and stated that the cell was the basic unit of life: the single unit of the body that had to be studied to understand disease (Fig. 2.5). This was a significant turning point as the focus in medicine narrowed even more, concentrating on the smaller components (see Appendix B), distinct from their natural structural context.

Science, medicine and anatomy were about discovering what is "true" and objectively, measurably accurate. However, they diverted attention from a perspective that was inclusive of wholeness, or whole-body function and structure as a united and complete being-in-action.

Andrew Taylor Still (1828–1917) was a physician and surgeon who became the founding father of osteopathy. Interestingly, Still referred to the body as a machine but offered the idea that it was designed to heal itself, by a force greater than itself. He wrote of the inclusive aspect of the soul, rather than segregating it.

"This life is surely too short to solve the uses of the fascia in animal forms. It penetrates even its own finest fibers to supply and assist its gliding elasticity. Just a thought of the completeness and universality in all parts, even though you turn the visions of your mind to follow the infinitely fine nerves. There you see the fascia, and in your wonder and surprise, you exclaim, 'Omnipresent in man and all other living beings of the land and sea …Other great questions come to haunt the mind with joy and admiration, and we can see all the beauties of life on exhibition by that great power with which the fascia is endowed. The soul of man with all the streams of pure living water seems to dwell in the fascia of his body."[19]

Writing from a view that harks back to Hippocrates in its values of working with the human experience as well as the condition being presented at the time, Still suggested the innate human capacity for self-healing.

"The Fascia: I know of no part of the body that equals the fascia as a hunting ground. I believe that more rich golden thought will appear to the mind's eye as the study of the fascia is pursued than any division of the body. Still one part is just as great and useful as any other in its place. No part can be dispensed with. But the fascia is the ground in which all causes of death do the destruction of life. Every view we take, a wonder appears … I dislike to write, and only do so, when I think my productions will go into the hands of kind-hearted geniuses who read, not to find a book of quotations, but to go with the soul of the subject that is being explored for its merits, – weigh all truths and help bring its uses front for the good of man."[20]

We have outlined some of the highlights of the rich story behind the evolution of anatomy in the West. Now, after a long divorce between the pieces of the person and the persona, fascia research is materially changing the view

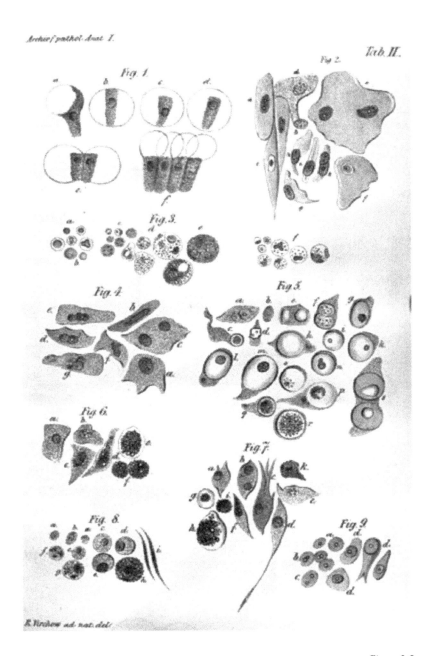

Figure 2.5

Image of Virchow's cell biology. It suggests cells are separate from each other and does not reference the context of the surrounding milieu upon which they rely for structure, function and survival.

It could be said that Still conceived the genesis of the science of body architecture. His work had the authority to give birth to a new school of medical thought. His writings on the fascia, now over 100 years old, showed a deep sense of awareness of this fabric of the human form and its profound relationship to the being as a sacred, living, fluid matrix. The most recent research can be seen to validate much of what he, and John Godman before him, asserted. They researched the fascia anatomically and practically, finding considerable evidence for its continuity and significance through their work and experiences, one and two hundred years ago, respectively.

and the language of the body, written in its own kinaesthetic dialect. The soft architecture of our unique, animated movement signature is an exciting field to explore, restoring the wholeness that yoga and all movement practices invite us to perceive and express, as self-motivated beings. Yoga, in particular, given its emphasis upon finding stillness as well as mobility as a foundation to embodiment, fosters such wisdom.

There are many scientists and genius minds that have not been included in this selection of the "ancient wisdom" upon which current "new knowledge" is growing; especially in reference to understanding fascia. From a structural point of view, of the geometry of form, we should include D'arcy Wentworth Thompson (1860–1948), and his works *On Growth and Form* and the mathematics behind biology. He sought to explore "synergy" (which refers to the *unpredictable* behaviour of a system that is more than the sum of its parts – but rather governed or explained by the emergent properties of their interactions – see Ch. 7). His appreciation of shape (morphology) as an essential aspect of differentiation and function is fundamentally significant in understanding why fascia is so key to yoga, oriented as it is on shape. This was also a subject deep to Buckminster Fuller's heart as we will explore in Chapter 6 on Biotensegrity.

Another key prediction, over 100 years ago, is that of Sir William Bates Hardy. Quoting from Eric Rideal's[21] commemorative piece: "…Hardy once observed a cell divide and wondered why. This led him into enquiries in the physico-chemical properties of the proteins and the behaviour of matter in what Hardy called the 'the boundary state'. More specifically, his first enquiries arising out of the properties of protoplasm were on sols and gels." According to Gerald Pollack (see Ch. 7), Hardy was the first to suggest that there may be a fourth phase of water, which (if we are to appreciate the subtle ubiquity of the fascial matrix) calls for a new vision of how fascia holds our watery inner world together. (Note the quotation above from Andrew Taylor Still.[19, 20])

If fascia does anything, it offers us the opportunity to evolve *our perspective* to include and transcend all that precedes it. We cannot just throw out the muscles and bones or beautiful dissections of many an anatomical book. We can, however, regard them in their unifying context. Although they have often been painstakingly depicted **in the absence** of that fabric that enfolds them (that they enfold), we are invited to consider it was **hidden in the obvious**. The parts depicted **only** exist in the presence of their intimate weave, the living, fluidic, collagen matrix without which they have neither structure nor function. The science of body architecture emerges as a triumvirate in many ways, calling upon a new perspective from which to re-present all that we thought we knew. From the microscopic to the telescopic level, we are seeking a scale-free model that makes sense of the wholeness which includes all of our parts; animated as they are, by us. The wholeness of this interconnected, fluid, sensory and structural fabric unifies. Its daily triumph is to form what we present *as us – as a living volume!* At the same time, paradoxically, fascia distinguishes those parts from each other. The next chapter examines the paradigm shift fascia research is inviting and its echoes of new "Renaissance principles" bringing an entirely new perspective. It is one of inclusivity, connectivity and unity. What makes us all the same is that we are all unique, all connected and all part of the wholeness from which we emerge (and to which we return).

Notes

1. Michael S. Schneider, *A Beginner's Guide to Constructing the Universe: The Mathematical Archetypes of Nature, Art, and Science*, HarperCollins, New York, 1994.
2. N.D. Theise, et al (2018) Structure and distribution of an unrecognized interstitium in human tissue. *Science Reports* March 27.
3. There is speculation that Leonardo had help from a dear friend, a young architect well versed in Vitruvian principles named Giacoma Andrea (Toby Lester, "The Other Vitruvian Man", Smithsonianmag.com February 2012).
4. Benjamin Blech and Roy Doliner, *The Sistine Secrets*, HarperCollins, New York, 2008.
5. Johannes Gensfleisch zur Laden zum Gutenberg (c. 1400–1468) is credited with inventing and introducing the printing press to Europe in the 15th century. He was a goldsmith, blacksmith and an inventor whose name is associated with the first bible to be formerly printed.
6. Professor Suzannah Lipscomb, MA, MSt, DPhil (Oxon), F.R.Hist.S., FHEA, Professor of History at the University of Roehampton. https://www.historyextra.com/period/history-witches-facts-burned-hanged/ Article for BBC History Magazine, A very brief history of witches, October 2nd 2019, accessed 15th June 2020.
7. Silvio A. Bedini, *The Unknown Leonardo*. 1974, McGraw-Hill Book Co. UK Ltd, Maidenhead, England. ISBN 0-07-037196-2,
8. Benjamin Blech and Roy Doliner, *The Sistine Secrets*, HarperCollins, New York, 2008.
9. Translated from Leonardo's notes. In: *The Unknown Leonardo*. Silvio A. Bedini, *The Unknown Leonardo*. 1974, McGraw-Hill Book Co. Uk Ltd, Maidenhead, England. ISBN 0-07-037196-2.
10. Ch. 1 in Thomas W. Myers, *Anatomy Trains: Myofascial Meridians for Manual and Movement Therapists*, 2nd edition, Churchill Livingstone, Edinburgh, 2009.
11. In *Cells, Gels and the Engines of Life*, Gerald Pollack uses a similar metaphor for the changes currently being demonstrated in cellular biology and the structure of water (Gerald H. Pollack, *Cells, Gels and the Engines of Life*, Ebner and Sons, Seattle, 2001).
12. Candace Pert, *Molecules of Emotion: The Science Behind Mind-Body Medicine*, foreword by Deepak Chopra, Scribner, New York, 1997.
13. René Descartes [published in French in 1664], *Treatise of Man*, Harvard University Press, Cambridge, MA, 1972.
14. Alexander Filmer-Lorch, *Inside Meditation: In Search of the Unchanging Nature Within*. Matador, Kibworth Beauchamp, 2012.
15. Robert Beverly Hale and Terence Coyle, *Albinus on Anatomy*, Dover Books, New York, 1988.
16. *Anatomical Investigations, comprising descriptions of various Fasciae of the Human Body* (http://www.biodiversitylibrary.org/item/89909#page/7/mode/1up), originally published in 1824 in Philadelphia by Carey and Lea. Digitized by the Internet Archive in 2010 with funding from Boston Library Consortium Member Library.
17. Ibid
18. Ibid
19. "The Fascia", in Andrew T. Still, *Philosophy of Osteopathy*, A.T. Still, Kirksville, 1899.
20. Andrew T. Still, *Philosophy of Osteopathy*, A.T. Still, Kirksville, 1899. Ch. 10.
21. In memorium: Sir William Bate Hardy, F.R.S.k 1864–1964 by Eric K Rideal, Commemorative Meeting, Cambridge, 16–17th June 1964, p. 55.

3

From Anatomy to Architecture

"We shape our dwellings and afterwards our dwellings shape us."[1]

Winston Churchill

Fascia Research

The story of fascia is taking some time to filter through some layers of our culture, although many areas of medicine, movement and manual therapy are in the process of recognising the work of fascia research pioneers and changing their approach as its significance is being re-evaluated. As it was for Vesalius and Newton, new ideas are not always greeted with enthusiasm, often due to a lack of understanding. Evidence by demonstration disturbs "truth by declaration", especially if institutions have built themselves upon the "truth" of what they thought they knew. We have our very own twenty-first-century Vesalius, or at least a suitable candidate to challenge the preceding history and change the way the scalpel is used to define the tissues. Jaap van der Wal's pioneering work has become a powerful resource for the other explorers in this rapidly growing field. What he found is also palpable and demonstrable now that we have the refined technology with which to "see", and even measure, the finer aspects of the fabric of the fascia.

A Modern Vesalius?

In the late 1980s, for his doctoral research, Jaap van der Wal, MD PhD, Associate Professor of Anatomy and Embryology (now retired), carried out a tissue-sparing dissection of the human elbow. In other words, he did the opposite of the required "clean dissection". Instead of removing the scruffy, fibrous "stuff" in the way of the muscles and bones around the joint capsule of the elbow, he spared the tissue and meticulously removed the muscles, in order to see what the "fibrous scaffolding" looked like on its own. He *revealed* something extraordinary; namely, that the connective tissue material formed a complete and continuous whole architecture. There was nowhere that it stopped, changed angle abruptly or failed to enclose the whole elbow organisation in all its detail. There were different densifications of the tissues. However there was no part of the joint that was not under continuous tension, or omitted from the ensheathing, encapsulating integrity of the whole connective tissue architecture of the joint and the arm. He suggests that a different view might be that the arm is continuous and the elbow represents an architectural "disjoint" in that continuity, thus permitting motion.

Jaap van der Wal was Associate Anatomy Professor at the University of Maastricht in the Netherlands. The new method of dissection he used in his research project was developed by one of his colleagues, H. van Mameren, in the 1970s. Jaap van der Wal came to work in the laboratory of Professor Drukker (then Chairman), where van Mameren did his studies, and under his supervision van der Wal started to follow the same procedure and researched the importance of this connective tissue or fascial architecture *investigating the process of proprioception*. It came about that this "continuity thinking", in architectural terms, fitted the way our proprioception and body sensing is (self-)organised in natural motion. It made sense of our motion sense, so to speak. "*It was not the anatomy of bones and muscles that was instrumental for proprioception, but the architecture of continuity*."[2]

That is a huge statement! This discovery shone a totally different light upon anatomical study itself and it did (and still does) stimulate whole new issues of how we explain how we move. What van der Wal and his colleagues did was a complete reversal of standard procedure. In a sense, he dissected the "negative space" – in simple terms, he did not cut out the "stuff" to get to the "thing", rather, he removed the "thing" to see the "stuff". This constituted a shock to the traditional view not wholly dissimilar to what happened in the sixteenth century, when Vesalius acquired special dispensation to dissect a human cadaver. For the previous 1500 years, Galen's work based upon Barbary apes (on the basis that they had "similar" structure to humans) was unquestioned. Great consternation arose when Vesalius queried Galen's basis for describing human anatomy at that time (see Ch. 2). Once again, centuries of assumptions had been hugely challenged by a new context of curiosity. This was as threatening as any paradigm shift. (See Figs 3.21 and 3.22 showing the "negative space" of the traditional style of iconic muscle images.)

Van der Wal's findings, in the 1980s (440 years later), were not embraced immediately, any more than Vesalius' work was. (As a result van der Wal turned his attention towards embryology.) In truth, van der Wal's earlier work is only just beginning to filter into the anatomy publications in this new millennium. After three decades the message is gradually being acknowledged through manual and movement practitioners and researchers working in fascia, rather than as a universally accepted basis for medical anatomy. The implications of this work, sparing the fascia, were huge at the time and their impact is still authorising change in the hallowed halls of anatomy education.[3,4] Van der Wal described what he revealed as "*the transanatomical architecture [of the human elbow] and its proprioceptive substrate*".[5] Transanatomical in this sense means something beyond the (traditional) anatomical distinctions, inclusive of all of them. (Trans means "across", so this encompasses, evolves and includes all distinctions.)

Transanatomical Architecture

The implications of this continuity of tissue were that the separately named muscle-to-tendon, bony periosteum, ligament and joint capsule together formed one *continuous* architecture. It was thickened, vascularised, innervated and invested with different *qualities* at different points of connection *and disconnection*. Nevertheless, the tissue in, around and beyond the joint was uninterrupted, containing and continuing the different facilities for movement afforded by muscle–tendon–bone–ligament and joint space. It is all fascia, of one expression or another. On examination, it was also found to be sensory in nature with a density of sensors (mechanoreceptors) around the joint and between the fabric depths. This suggested that the perception of gliding motion within the tissue matrix is relevant to the self-sensing matrix and it raised a host of questions about the information system *that is the fascial organisation* (see Ch. 5, wherein we explore the sensory nature of the tissues specifically).

Van der Wal's work pointed to the idea that the naming of certain ligaments, and the particular way in which they are cut out from their neighbouring (whole) myotendinous joint architecture and bone, makes them more of an *artefact* than a distinct *fact*. He suggests that most (not all) ligaments are part of a larger architecture including elements that (despite the fact they are named separately) do not function or exist separately in the body. It implies that the anatomist is using his knife to *design* and name a part of the body (assigning it the role of a particular named ligament, for example) by the act of cutting it, *anatomically*, out of its *architecture* rather than using that knife to reveal the architecture exactly as it is *in life*. In life it is whole and combined as an integrated complex unit van der Wal refers to as a "dynament" (a "dynamic ligament"). This is a very interesting revelation in a field that threw out aesthetics several centuries ago in an earnest pursuit of the facts behind anatomy. It is not actually saying there are no ligamentous attachments. (Please note the cruciate and nuchal ligaments are considered "true" ligaments, by Van der Wal, as they are the main six that can really be said to *ONLY* attach bone to bone). Rather, the term is including the ligamentous attachments, or ligamentous type of fascial tissues, *as part of a particular continuity*: an entire architecture that does not separate the ligamentous attachment, since it essentially remains *inherent* to the integrity of the whole [joint] structure.

Jaap van der Wal coined the term "dynament" as an inclusive name that better represents the muscle–tendon–bone–ligament–synovial joint relationship from a functional, *architectural* point of view, given the tissue continuity he established at every joint in the body. He derived this concept from the place it originates; by studying the embryo, in which one could also state that muscle tissue is a dynamic specialisation (which we will explore in Ch. 4). He is suggesting that muscle, or any specific tissue, arises from within the fascial matrix, according to the blueprint and embryonic growth function. He suggests that to use or label "*a 'synovial joint'* [as such] *is a contradiction in terms. It is not a joint. It is a dis-joint. Here connective tissue (cartilage) enables space and therefore motion*" (Jaap van der Wal).[6]

Suggesting any anatomist (or several generations of them) might be wrong, or worse, *designing anatomy* (instead of revealing it), rocked a very big boat. If every animal on the planet is a self-sensing fascial matrix, not a mechanical construction, then Borelli's *De Motu Animalium* (see Ch. 2) would need to be rewritten in fascial webs and tensional matrices. The fact remains that Dr van

Calling ligaments "dynaments" is a *contextual* change which impacts how we view the *content*. That means it impacts which questions we ask, how we look for the answers and upon which parameters we do research. That is the basis of this paradigm shift. Fascia becomes the architectural context in which we view the anatomical content. Once again, this is not new (see John Godman, in Ch. 2), but it is not classically how we learn anatomy either, as the basis of any movement discipline or manual therapy.

Sharkey's dissection and subsequent image of the Superficial Fascia (including the digits: see Fig. 3.1) played a direct role in what was to shape the FNPP Project from its inception: In Dr Robert Schleip's own words about this image: "…the fantastic photo of the superficial fascia dissection (as one piece) shaped the FNPP from the very beginning." Schleip had included the image in the very first project descriptions, that were discussed in the early meetings with Rurik von Hagens and team before starting the project….

Schleip wrote "For many important reasons, including your continued significant influence on this project. It is such a joy, to see the project continuing its drive." Perhaps for any true pioneers, it takes decades of determination (even with ridicule) to make the incremental changes that eventually cause the sea-change this book seeks to

A Practical Demonstration

navigate. My personal gratitude to John Sharkey is based in no small part on his devotion to education and generosity of spirit in sharing his extensive knowledge of movement, manual and medical practices. He never makes anyone else feel small for "not knowing." As a student who was once embarrassed and humiliated by her anatomy teachers, both publicly and privately, the guidance and inspiration from someone as qualified as John has been a gift to me personally and professionally – as it is to the world of fascia and optimum health.

der Wal was revealing the body as it is, inclusive of all that is in the anatomy books but in full-bodied three-dimensional architecture with its substrate intact. He revealed how it is architecturally organised, before it is anatomically cut, with the "white stuff" left in place – rather than disposed of, into the cadaveric bins.

John Sharkey is a clinical anatomist and exercise physiologist, responsible for the curriculum of a Masters Degree in Neuromuscular Therapy (originated with his much esteemed colleague, the late Dr Leon Chaitow),[7] accredited by the University of Chester.[8] Somewhat aligned with van der Wal's research, Sharkey has been studying the human body (and teaching standard medical anatomy[9]), including his own unique model entitled *Anatomy for the 21st Century*, for several decades. Focused on fascia in his own research (enough to earn him the nickname "Fascia Man" amongst his colleagues in the University of Dundee, Scotland; Department of Anatomy and Human Identification), Sharkey has hosted dissection courses internationally and advanced fascia-focused surgical technique trainings, in which he specifically focuses on demonstrating the ubiquity and interconnected nature of the fascial matrix and its surgical significance. In 2010 John Sharkey attempted to produce and plastinate the world's first fascia specimens of the superficial and deep fascia (Fig. 3.1), supported by Professor Hong-Jin Sui and a team of anatomists from the Department of Anatomy, Zhongshan College of Dalian Medical University, Dalian, P. R. China, and Dalian Hoffen Bio-Technique Co. Ltd., Dalian. However, at the time this first project did not come to fruition due to lack of funding. It was not until 2018, when Dr Robert Schleip invited Sharkey to be a project leader in the Human Fascial Net Plastination Project (later shortened to the FNPP) in conjunction with the von Hagen's Plastinarium in Guben, Germany, that such specimens have become a reality (this project also included fascia experts Professor Carla Stecco and Emeritus Associate Professor Jaap van der Wal, to name but two).

When you drum your fingers on the table, or type at your keyboard, the shadows you see on the back of your hand as you make the movements are where the tethers and expressions of different aspects of the fascial architecture permit or inhibit glide. Turn your hand over and you will see much less apparent movement within the tissues. They have different characteristics and *texture*. The fascia tethers the palm more because you use it differently. When you see muscles defined, it is the borders where the different fascial depths meet and connect that you are seeing in the hollows and grooves of the skin. It is what gives us our shape and our form (see box).

You have just touched upon your inner architecture, experienced its sensory feedback mechanism, demonstrated to yourself the responsive subtleties of movement your body does all the time and seen that it restored itself immediately. You might now be more conscious of the hand that felt you, or the hand you felt, but they have gone back to their original shape as rapidly as you let go.

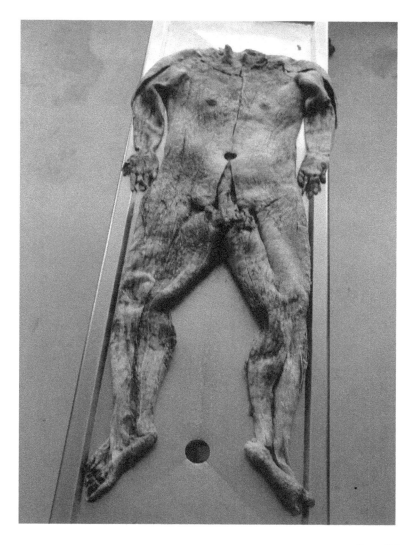

Figure 3.1

Dissected representation of the superficial fascia completed by clinical anatomist John Sharkey as part of a project in 2010 to produce the world's first fascia specimens for education purposes. Please note the exceptional presentation here of the digits (fingers and toes). While some consider this image to be of the skin, it is in fact on the next table; this is the entire fabric of the Superficial Fascia immediately beneath the skin, with the exception of the neck, face and cranium.

Reproduced with kind permission from John Sharkey.

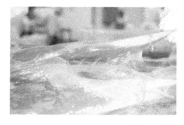

Figure 3.2

Palmaris longus. A small muscle of the hand, profoundly connected in all directions to its surrounding structures.

All that gliding is the superficial fascia, which is effectively the back of the skin, moving over the deep fascia, which is over the muscles enclosing the bones. Between them is a zone of what is called "loose connective tissue",

If you gently hold your hand, so that your left fingers are across the back of your right hand ... and wiggle your right fingers, you will feel the wave-like rippling of tendons, muscles and bones gliding under the skin (Fig. 3.3). Pretend you are drumming the table with your right hand but in mid-air. If you squeeze a little harder with your left hand you will find the tissues still glide, if slightly less easily, but you can feel other structures underneath which are deeper tissue arrangements. There are several things going on at once here:

- You can feel the tissues gliding in the back of the hand inside the fluid and gel-like matrix of (and between) the fascial structures.
- You can feel a different quality of gliding in the palm of the hand. Notice it is stiffer and thicker and slower.
- If you slow down or speed up the movements of your fingers (right hand) ever so slightly you can modify the speed readily and change the sense of the movements by timing them differently, at will, in an instant.
- The fingers of your left hand are sensing every one of these subtle differences.

Try the exercise to feel the glide. Notice that everywhere in your body, the skin glides over the structures underneath it and then restores itself to where it was before. Note that you can feel one quality of gliding at your ear lobes (it will be different for every individual) – how the back and front of each one glide over each other (or not) – and another quality entirely between your scalp and your skull bones or over the back of your elbow or the front of your knee.

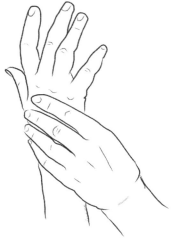

Figure 3.3

I have, since the first edition of this book, had the privilege to work with these two illustrious anatomists in Dundee University, working with soft-fix Theil cadaveric specimens. Having now done many such tissue-sparing

or "areolar tissue" sometimes referred to as the "shearing zone" (see Fig. 3.1 for the entire, body-wide presentation of the tissue that we are referring to). This depth of loose connective tissue arises between various structures of the body and plays a key role in mechanoreception (see Ch. 8). It forms part of the matrix that, notwithstanding its precise location in the body or particular characteristics, is everywhere (Fig. 3.4).

Sharkey has further demonstrated his commitment to fascia science by producing the world's first render of the living human thigh to be "3D printed". (Full details and further images of this render are explored in Ch. 7.) Sharkey shares similar anatomical reverence for van der Wal's view of the matrix as the original tissue of the human form and one that self-organises in complete continuity. Sharkey's focus is upon the tensional properties of the fascia (which forms the basis of our enquiry in Chapter 6), since he is also an exercise physiologist, devoted to how we actually animate this ubiquitous tissue in movement and manual practice – as well as how we treat it surgically.

Actually, these projects represent Progress with a capital "P". Of course it is essential for surgeons and anatomists to be able to name tiny sections of our anatomy with specificity and topographical accuracy, placing them on the map of the body in refined detail. However, it transforms our application of

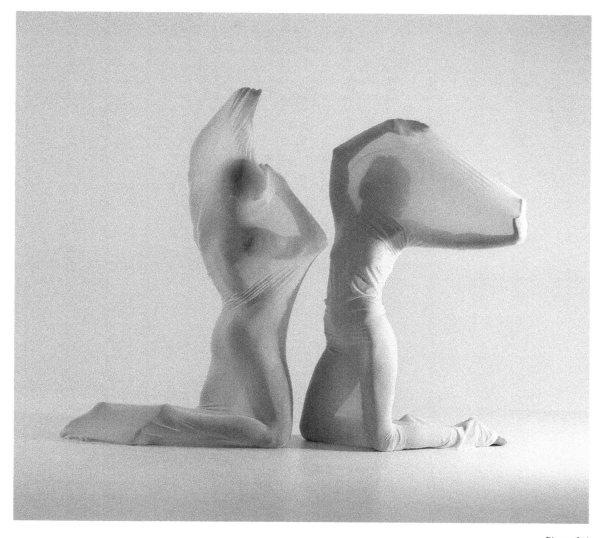

Figure 3.4

The internal net and tensional network is hard to see, or even to imagine in the context of its wholeness and ubiquity. This image was created to give the sense, albeit externally, of the moving depths responding as a whole soft, tensional architecture or internal fabric throughout the form, whatever shapes it is engaged in making.

Photographer: Amy Very. Models: Helen Eadie and Wibbs Coulson.

dissections, I am writing this second edition, with a different kind of confidence and understanding in what made sense to me before. Now it seems even more urgently required as a recognised basis of expanding the study of living beings, from anatomy (albeit a living anatomy and physiology *in motion* to know that the original territory is all (all ways and always) one piece, in all its dimensions and directions, under the skin (in ALL of us). That changes everything. Whatever names you give the anatomical and sub-anatomical details, the transanatomical architecture is structurally unified *at the same time*. **We are a unity walking around with named parts, not distinct parts longing for unity.**

useful foundation) to architecture – as the wholeness, that invariably presents itself on the yoga mat, includes all that the fascia shows up as. ALL of it! For ALL of us! No lines, not even continuous anatomical "trains" (see Ch. 18). Only volumes, contained in pockets of continuously connected weaves of the same, if variously tensioned, densified and compressed, fascia! It is the same for everyone; regardless of race, colour or culture. This is the tissue immediately under the skin, in complete continuity with everything to the core of the bone marrow and every cell nucleus. It is ubiquitous (everywhere).

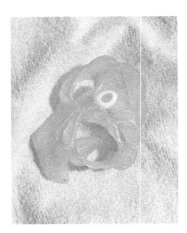

Figure 3.5

Render of human thigh sample.

Completed in 2019, this is a 3D print, rendered from an fMRI of the living human (female) thigh. It is a way of visualising, albeit in a model form, the tissue-sparing dissection principle that Dr van der Wal did in his laboratory in 1985. For more details of this model render, see Chapter 7.[10] Image reproduced with kind permission from John Sharkey.

Living Architecture

Topology is mathematically defined as the study of geometrical properties and spatial relations unaffected by the continuous change of shape or size of

Jaap van der Wal and John Sharkey echo the early nineteenth century work of John Godman, who invited his students to observe a subject of anatomical study without engaging preconceived ideas of systems (see Ch. 2) and, by imposing, *cut* them (out of the body). **This means that naming structural parts – and assigning functions to them – shifts and expands to appreciating structural integrity and realising that function emerges from it.** It is a major contextual shift.

Jaap van der Wal went on to discover that the nature of the tissue itself made it far more than a connector. It formed "a proprioceptive substrate", (more an "intelligent lining") around the joint that can feel, or sense, *itself*. It knows where it is in space via the tensional network (see Ch. 6), with a distribution of mechanoreceptors in the tissues, particularly prolific at myotendinous junctions and "dynaments". (Mechanoreceptors might be said to act something like multiple, movement-detecting antennae.) We will explore the sensory nature of the tissues in a chapter of their own (Ch. 5) with the relevant research. Suffice to say here that it shifts the classical perspective of a separate nervous system, to recognising the exquisite detail of the proprioceptive sense as *the sensory nature of the architecture itself*. That includes the neural net, because dura is made of fascia; however it extends the facility of self-sensory awareness to the fabric of the actual architecture. That means the body wall/cell walls/organ walls/vessel walls are alive!

This points to very particular sensitivity in monitoring movement and organisation, from deep within the architecture itself, "*the branch offices of the brain*",[11] which we will explore in Part B and consider in motion and application in Part C.

This makes sense of the yoga postures and our ability to do them and make tiny adjustments in order to organise or sustain a pose. The postures explore range, balance and coordination at multiple angles and directions, from detailed, subtle changes to gross ones. A demonstrable theory that sees this detail as part of one whole organisation makes obvious sense, particularly given that the word yoga means "unifying". A theory suggesting versatility, adaptability and flexibility with the integrity of the joints in tensional balance at all angles is akin to the practice of yoga itself (Fig. 3.6) or any movement, be it everyday motions or studied forms. This does not mean there is no need to learn your anatomy. It does ask us to make a new distinction – that of a (topographical) map within a continuous changing topological territory that senses itself in space and in response to gravity, *all the time*: "*read in your anatomy the neglected story between the lines; that is the continuity*".[12]

Van der Wal's work was not publicly presented until the Second International Fascia Research Congress in Amsterdam (in 2009), two and a half decades after he wrote his PhD thesis. It has been a key part of a momentous change in focus over recent decades. During this time, a hand surgeon in France, Dr Jean-Claude Guimberteau, has made further progress, in terms of visualisation, by

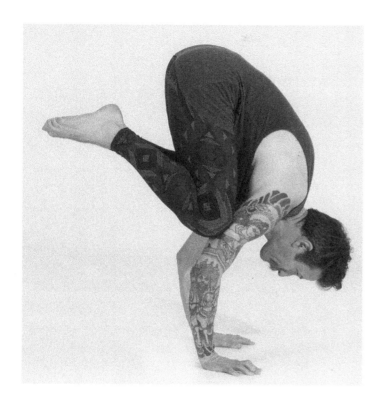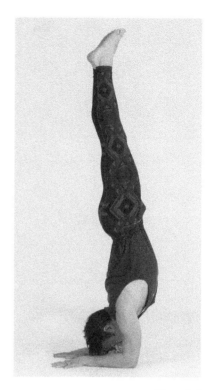

Figure 3.6

Crow pose (A) and elbow stand (B). These poses require tensional integrity of the system at all angles through the elbow throughout the posture, whether during preparation, execution, completion or release. Whichever yogic style, tissue integrity is required through the organisation of the muscles and the bones at the joints throughout the body.

Photographer Amy Very, Model: Wibbs Coulson.

figures; it refers to the way in which constituent parts are interrelated or arranged. Wikipedia offers the following definition. In mathematics, topology is concerned with the properties of a geometric object that are preserved under continuous deformations, such as stretching, twisting, crumpling and bending, but not tearing or gluing. Basically this refers to the original toroid of the embryo, twisting and folding into the architecture of the embryo, without adding on any additional parts, by gluing, sticking, tearing, cutting, pasting or editing. It is a topological, multi-dimensional performance, in the round. When we name those parts, separately,

confirming the continuity of the tissue, this time by making it possible to view it within the living body (Figs 3.7 and 3.8).

Using the endoscopic tools of the most advanced science to unravel the deeper questions of a tendon's ability to glide, Dr Guimberteau and his team of surgeons and researchers produced a revelatory movie called *Strolling under the Skin*, which was followed by *Muscle Attitudes* and then *Interior Architectures*, with more since.[13]

Guimberteau has transformed our view of the fascial matrix through his exceptional work in hand surgery and most particularly tendon transplants.[14] He discovered internal mobility and characteristics at the different levels of tissues under the skin that challenged many of the classical theoretical notions about movement of tendons and their ability to glide within their surrounding tissue matrix. With the use of the endoscopic camera during surgery, he was able to view living tissues. His films of what happens under the skin, throughout the muscle and in and around joints show the gel-like

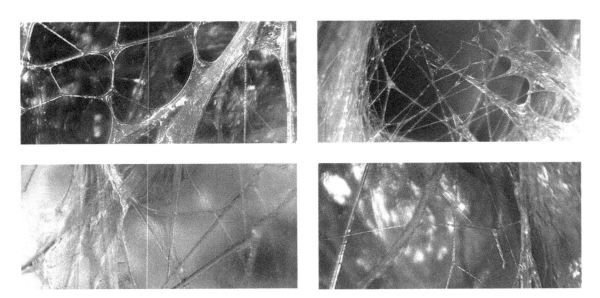

Figures 3.7 and 3.8

These images show the "transanatomical architecture", found under the skin throughout the body.

From: Strolling Under the Skin, a DVD by Dr Jean-Claude Guimberteau (www.endovivo.com/en/dvds.php). FIG INT.1 / 2.5 /2.6
AFT.4. Reproduced with kind permission from J-C Guimberteau and Endovivo Productions.

we are describing a *topographical* map – which is essentially 2D and won't get us to the wholeness without a quantum leap into morphological volumes: "Like what we are" at all times, ages and stages of our self-development.

I have had the privilege of working with Dr Guimberteau at Dundee University under the anatomical guidance of Clinical Anatomist, John Sharkey. Usually, as he works *in vivo*, Dr Guimberteau is restricted to the area of investigation relevant to/permitted by his patient – based upon his role as a hand surgeon. In Dundee, however, we were able to use the advantage of soft-fix Theil Dissection. The cadavers are not fixed as in the formalin examples upon which many classical anatomical studies are based. In these cases, fascia appears dried and fibrous – as in *The Fuzz* presented by Gil Hedley and often quoted as if fascia is only fibrous. In soft-fix methods, it is possible to see that it is gel-like and fluidic, sometimes dense and sometimes not; much more of a fluid, changing matrix organisation.

fibrillar network of the fascial matrix everywhere (Figs 3.7 and 3.8). This permits movement between structures, so that tendons in the hand can move independently of blood vessels, for example, just as you can feel them move in your own hand in the practical demonstration exercise (see box on p. 38). They always return to their original position via the fabric and the architectural design of the fascial matrix. Guimberteau's work has changed the view of gliding structures in the body and recognises a deep shift in understanding internal motion and motility throughout the living body, which we will consider more later.[15]

Guimberteau's[16] book and films reveal what appears as fractal chaos under the skin. The connections of the soft tissues directly beneath the surface (that you feel gliding under your hand if you do the demonstration exercise below) softly break and reform in a diaphanous, fractal dance of the fluid fibrillar matrix. This is what can be seen in the films made by Guimberteau and it was equally obvious in the soft-fix cadaveric dissection examples, everywhere in the body. The apparent chaos contains an order of its own, throughout the living system; as ever, it is a perfect paradox. In a way, we rediscover, repeatedly, the Vitruvian principles of architecture that we explored in Chapter 2: "*Firmitas, utilitas, venustas*", that is, formation and deformation to usefully perform and then reform to the

Thus, the term from Dr Guimberteau of "fibrillar network" rather than "fibrous" is preferred. In Dundee,

Why Is This So Important to Any Yoga Practice? Form, Deform, Reform

Dr Guimberteau was able to investigate other areas of the body and with the endoscopic camera under the skin near the ear, for example, we could see fluid responses from making distal movements at the leg. This was not done in a setting of formal research; however, the implications were that the containment principles of the fluid matrix, within the skin, are held together in total communion and communication. We will explore the evidence for this throughout Parts A and B, putting it into practical experience through application in Part C. (First we will think about it and then we will do it so that you can feel it!)

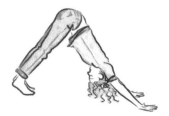

Figure 3.9

From Downward Dog (Urdhva Mukha Svanasana) to transition into a Low Lunge (Anjaneyasana) as part of a flow of movements, the whole body adapts to accomplish the sequence.

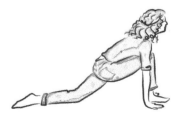

Figure 3.10

Forward Lunge (flexion) into a low lunge (Anjaneyasana) (extension).

original structural integrity, once the task or movement is complete. It is fit for purpose – your purpose at the time – and it is the form, which is very beautiful.

Form, Deform, Reform is the basis of natural elasticity, which we will explore in Part B. However, this subject (of reformation of shape and internal gliding) is of huge interest to a yoga practitioner or any movement teacher and the work referred to above changes how we understand its significance. At the simplest level of observation, if we move from a Downward Dog (Urdhva Mukha Svanasana) (flexion) through to a Low Lunge (Anjaneyasana) (extension), we rely upon the body's ability as a whole structure to glide internally, at all the joints, throughout the form, in order to carry out both poses with grace and poise (Figs 3.9–3.11) in a continuous sequence. There need not be anything disjointed or fragmented about the effort or the transition once we have practised and mastered any series. We take this wholly for granted; yet many meters of tubing, vessels and internal structures have to glide fluently with the movements and change with our intention to carry out any asana practice – *as a whole (referring to our bodies and the sequence!)*.

We expect the body to do this "deform–reform" or "disorganise and reorganise", always returning to a state of equilibrium, if it can, restoring the neutral field of homeostasis. Sharkey suggests a better word is "allostasis". This aspect of internal gliding is happily assumed as natural motion. It is when tissue does *not* glide that we notice it. "Sticky" tissue (a kinaesthetic term) can include (or cause) micro-tears, dehydration, inflammation or adhesion, and it is when we cannot do something easily that it becomes an issue. We do not generally expect our students standing in Eagle Pose (Garudasana) to get locked in that position to one side and not be able to do the other side because the body cannot translate *undoing* the movements. We naturally expect that to the extent we can do a pose, we can undo it (Fig. 3.12).

Even in the yoga forms that require a posture to be held for long minutes we know the extent to which we can do it *and are able to undo it*. There is a system taking care of that ability and it is not the muscles alone. They are just *part* of an orchestra of architecturally organised tissues. What holds them together and to each other, what holds them apart and relates them to everything else makes a huge difference to their ability to make such changes and reverse a pose, transition to another pose and "do (and undo) till we drop." Transition is fundamental and it is about the instinctive function of the whole structure; the entire organising architecture. The tissues are not separate; the need for them to glide over each other and remain contained overall is primary.

This approach changes the foundations of study of the so-called musculoskeletal system and the physiology of muscle, of sensory communication, of force transmission and of movement management. We will consider the sensory communication (Ch. 5) and the biomechanics (Part B) in more detail

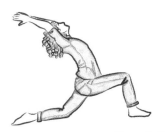

Figure 3.11

From a Forward Lunge posture, it is an effortless glide into extension (Anjaneyasana) once we have mastered the transition.

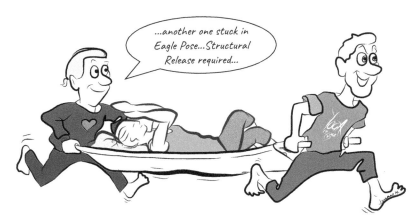

Figure 3.12

later, as they deserve chapters of their own. For now, let us explore the musculoskeletal aspect in a little more detail, to fully understand why this expanded view, shifting from anatomy to architecture, is so essential.

Classical Anatomy View

Perhaps a better word than "homeostasis" is "allostasis". It is one John Sharkey uses a lot, referring to the constant rebalancing of a moving body, rather than suggesting a 'static' state of homeostasis. (*Allostasis* is defined as the process of maintaining homeostasis through the adaptive change of the organism's internal environment to meet perceived and anticipated demands. From: *Stress: Concepts, Cognition, Emotion, and Behavior*, 2016.)

The classic skeleton used in schools is a traditional teaching tool in many yoga classrooms and certainly in the study of anatomy and physiology (Fig. 3.13). It is designed to demonstrate the approximately 206 bones of the adult human body, the bony landmarks on the living body, and how the spine is organised. It is also there for you to learn the attachment sites of muscles. In short, it provides the basics of the axial (excluding girdles and limbs) and appendicular (girdles and limbs) skeleton.

Looking at this particular configuration of the bones, we have no need to consider the connecting wires without which we would, in fact, be looking at a pile of rods and knuckles on the table. What is holding the whole thing up, or together, or suspended? (That is apart from wires and a pole where the spinal cord should be in most classroom models!)

We must not think about that too literally because of course we "know" that what is missing from this model is the muscles. We have stripped the skeleton so that we can learn where the muscles attach to the bones and work out how they move them. Some models even have blue and red markings to show us the points of attachment of each muscle.

However, if we were to stick the "muscles" on to these bones, at their blue and red attachment sites, on the classroom skeleton (without its wires and the pole up its spine) – they still couldn't hold it up!!! **That is an important statement.** We *assume* that movement would be available if the muscles were holding the bones together and each able to do their antagonistic "pair dance", which would then set those bones ready for motion at these various joints. That is, of course, according to the actions traditionally assigned to those muscle components of the locomotor system via the nervous system. We could then say it would all work when we have the neural wiring in place. However – *we still don't have a*

Connective tissue is present as missing in this classical model; because it was scraped away in dissection and its significance discarded. That significance means we have to *pretend* the skeleton is capable of representing the living body, with just a few wires and a pole. In living fact, it never exists without the ensheathing organisation of the bony wrapping (periosteum), which wraps every bone and does not stop at the muscles surrounding them, but forms an interface between the muscles and bones, in a continuous ensheathing.

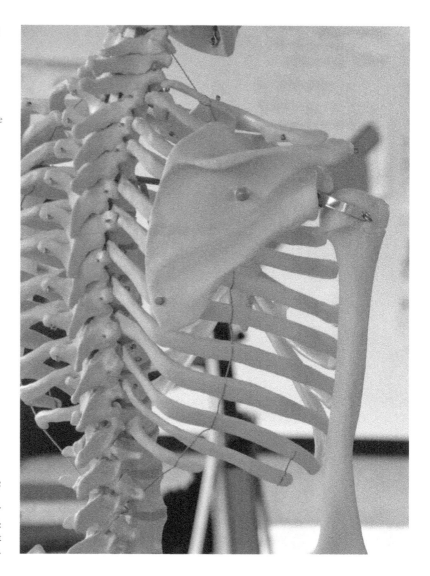

Figure 3.13

A classic classroom skeleton.

Photographer Bex Hawkins. Model: Max, Courtesy of Verena Tremel at Studio Rituel, Paris.

basic musculoskeletal form that binds itself together and can hold itself up in space. Remember, in this classroom model, the muscles are only attached at either end of their length; by the tendinous part, known as the proximal (closest to the spine) or distal (furthest from the spine) attachment. Musculoskeletal anatomical icons present muscles as if the muscle belly (gastric) is detached.

Traditionally then, once we learn the bones, we can go on to work out the origin and insertion points (proximal and distal attachments at either end) of

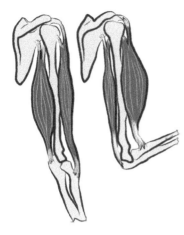

Figure 3.14

This is a common style of schematic, showing clean red muscles (the biceps and triceps brachii in this example) attached to clearly defined bones, touching each other at specific points. The whiter bits indicate the tendons. This is an iconic artefact of dissection.

the approximately 600 muscles attached to them. We then learn the individual actions, according to the charts, of each of these separate muscle units. Then we have to group them into suites, such as the "rotator cuff muscles" or the "quadriceps", as we seek to link the anatomy-of-the-parts into an organised system of functioning groups, where appropriate.

The problem is, the model has already failed. You will have a bigger pile of knuckles and rods, with lots of "muscle bags" attached at each end, "joining them" at end-points. They need something more, to effectively replace the wires or the rod that is making your classroom skeleton *appear* to be joined together and able to hold its structure in place. Muscles are not *only* attached at the origin and insertion! They arise *within* the matrix that enfolds them, is invested through them and wraps them entirely, everywhere *to the bones and to each other*. The whole muscle is attached, including the belly and every micromillimeter of protein it contains.

Figure 3.14 shows one such typical presentation of the muscles. Muscles are often shown as working in antagonistic pairs, as here in the upper arm, typically demonstrating the relationship between the triceps and biceps brachii muscles. They are presented as iconic, clean, red features, with clear separated tendons attaching to the bones. This is typical of the vast majority of anatomy teaching manuals. Muscles are thought to contract and relax; therefore, the image suggests that when the biceps contract they stretch the (relaxing) triceps, and vice versa. This explains a lever, which is a two-bar open chain mechanical device. (This actually means it explains how it might move if someone else was moving it and it was a hard-matter lever, which it cannot be in the human body, since there are no two-bar open chains [definition of a lever] and it isn't made of hard matter.) All this is classically displayed in tables, showing how each muscle functions according to its specific connections to the bony framework (at the attachments), via the actions assigned to it from the nervous system. So, in summary, from the schematics, we would learn something like the information shown in Figures 3.15 and 3.16.

In some resources, a cross-section of a real cadaver is included to endorse the positioning of these muscles within the arm. As soon as you see the image of a cross-section such as the one shown in Figure 3.17, it begs one *serious* question for the schematic representation, namely, *which bit in this cross-section is **not attached**?* The evidence, for the inaccuracy of the schematic, is right there in the photograph of the cross-section.

Continuous Anatomy

From skin to bone marrow in Figure 3.17 appears to be continuous and cross-section after cross-section is the same, however finely they are sliced. You might be forgiven for thinking (from the schematics) that once in the anatomy laboratory, you would be able to just "unhook" or "cut" a muscle at its origin and insertion points and lift it away from the skeleton. However, the first thing that would strike you in the anatomy laboratory is that these points and separations are not evident. Nor are the muscles separate from their surroundings in the body *anywhere*. There is no such thing! In a human dissection programme[17] it takes literally hours to dissect a single muscle *out of*

Figure 3.15

A table adapted from a typical example in Wikipedia.

Latin	*musculus triceps brachii*
Gray's	(Subject reference)
Origin	**Long head**: infraglenoid tubercle of scapula **Lateral head**: above the radial sulcus **Medial head**: below the radial sulcus
Insertion	Olecranon process of ulna
Artery	Deep brachial artery (Profunda brachii)
Nerve	Radial nerve and axillary nerve (long head)
Actions	Extends forearm. Long head extends shoulder
Antagonist	Biceps brachii muscle

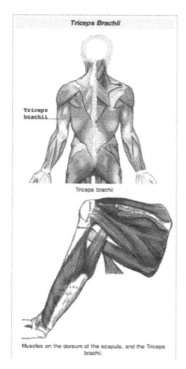

Muscles on the dorsum of the scapula, and the Triceps brachii.

Figure 3.16

Again, this is typical of what you would expect to find in traditional sources of information about the muscles. This image is from Gray's Anatomy via Wikipedia.

Nothing in the living body is like Figure 3.16, ever. Moreover, the "white stuff" actually runs through the entire muscle (we call it muscle fibre) on every scale (micro to macro) and wraps the bones in a continuum of enveloping tissue. We use our musculoskeletal system in life as it exists *before dissection*, not as shown in schematic diagrams. We "know" this, but how do we interpret the difference if all we are taught suggests the muscles are clear, separate units – yet they are not? Ever!

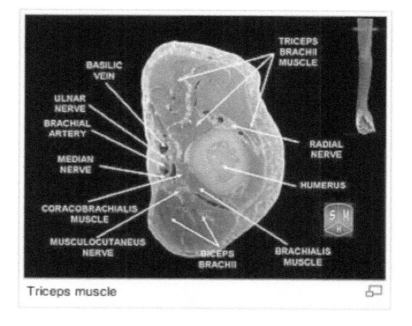

Figure 3.17

Cross-section of the upper arm showing triceps muscle. This is what you would expect to find in traditional sources of information; this image is from Wikipedia.

Recent research, as a whole, moves us very far from seeing the body as a series of stacked bony blocks with two hanging appendages (arms) and two supporting appendages (legs), balancing the axial stack (spine, torso and head) in a compression structure. That foundational shift then influences how we see muscles as the contractors, working in pairs or groups, to lift and change the angles of those stacked bones. This in turn changes how we

its surrounding tissue – anywhere and everywhere in the human body. Muscles have to be taken out of that original context, the one in which they invariably reside. Origins and insertions, if you leave the soft tissue respectfully where it belongs, look more like continuous attachments, with densifications, where the muscle fibres "condense" into tendinous continuities with their neighbouring structures. The densifications form more continuous attachments and so it goes on. Nothing is entirely separate *or separable* from the whole. That is just as it appears in any cross-section of the limb. As ever, it depends how you look and what you are looking for. The origins and insertions simply *don't exist as such* (any more than they are visible in a photograph on any cross-section). As Jaap van der Wal shows in tissue-sparing methodology (and Jean-Claude Guimberteau shows in endoscopy), there is nothing but ubiquitous continuity.

The Paradigm Shift: Dismantling the Classical Assumptions

"The simple questions discussed in musculoskeletal textbooks 'which muscles' are participating in a particular movement thus becomes almost obsolete. Muscles are not functional units, no matter how common this misconception may be. Rather, most muscular movements are generated by many individual motor units, which are distributed over some portions of one muscle, plus other portions of other muscles. The tensional forces of these motor units are then transmitted to a complex network of fascial sheets, bags and strings that convert them into the final body movement."[18]

interpret biomechanical movement and challenges the lever system and the pendulum explanation (upright inverted or otherwise) that is often used as a metaphor to explain the walking gait of the bipedal human. It renders it more than inadequate. (Jaap van der Wal taught his students about a "posturing and locomoting system" rather than talking about locomotion or the locomotor system as such. It is a distinction that makes sense in yoga, which we will explore throughout this work; as we are a living work in continuous performance.)

What is being revealed, at the most fundamental level, is that the connecting wires we *pretend are not there* in the classroom skeleton are the *only* reason that the bones stand up. It becomes a crucial omission in the light of this complete change of context, provided by the study of fascia as a significant tissue. Furthermore, the muscles are not actually directly connected to the bones other than via this fascial interface. It contains them, integrates and interconnects them all, as well as distinguishing them from each other, by texture. It may be more significant than we think to the nature of our fluid, sensory architecture – which will be explored in more detail in Ch. 7.

This challenges *our attachments* (pun intended) to many classical concepts of anatomy, physiology and biomechanics and urges us to evolve them. If those concepts rely upon the idea that individual muscles have assigned actions, the discovery that they do not work that way re-organises notions upon which many long-accepted movement theories are based, whatever the modality. It simply cannot be accurate.

The Challenge to Anatomy

To give you a simple way to see this anatomical continuity, Figure 3.18 shows how an orange looks in cross-section. Figure 3.19 is how it looks along the lengths of the segments. The hydration of the fruit has a lot to do with how its

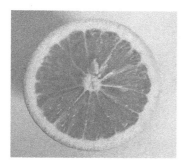

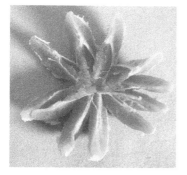

Figure 3.19

This is the three-dimensional view of an orange cross-section, bearing little or no resemblance to the two-dimensional version. Notably each segment has its own pockets, thus making the lines between the segments in the cross-section (see Fig. 3.18) very fine double laminae. Note each droplet of juice also has its own finer "pocket" of thin connective tissue material.

Figure 3.20

The form of the soft tissue in the orange provides a metaphor for the containment of fluids, in fascia of different densities and regularity, as a continuous architecture. Just as the segments are all attached along their lengths, so too are muscles. As the juice droplets are all closely packed in their particular organisation with the segments, so too are muscle fibres within the muscles.

"soft tissue" behaves, how plump it is and how tightly interwoven the segments are. If you can separate them carefully you will see each one is surrounded. It is contained in its own pocket-within-a-pocket from one end to the other (in the round!). Nowhere in any cross-section are they separate.

Within each segment are the juice droplets. They too reside in pockets of very much finer connecting tissues than that of the segment, which is finer than that of the pith, between the skin and the body of the whole fruit. Pockets, within pockets, within pockets is a forming principle in nature that we see recapitulated everywhere, including our own, human architecture (see Ch. 4).

Figure 3.20 can symbolise a model for soft tissue formation (see Ch. 7).

What is even more striking in a human dissection laboratory is that besides everything being connected everywhere, no two cadavers are quite the same. As noted in Chapter 4, biological systems honour the laws of biological self-assembly.[19] In the case of oranges, while the majority have the same overall format, you are unlikely to find an orange grove full of identical fruit. When you open them you may sometimes find there are extra little segments where their soft tissue divided them slightly differently to a sibling on the same tree. They may all be in the same family but (thank heaven) they are all slightly different.

We humans are not machines. We do not do straight lines, flat surfaces or exact symmetry anywhere in the body and no two of us are exactly the same. We might be very similar, but that is as near identical as we get. Take a long look in the mirror, then look at everyone else. It goes without saying that every Dog Pose, performed on your mat, or in the yoga classroom, is unique, as is the face of every person performing it. Same goes for their anatomy.

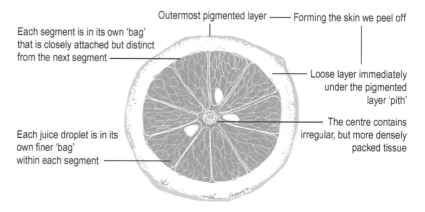

Outermost pigmented layer —— Forming the skin we peel off

Each segment is in its own 'bag' that is closely attached but distinct from the next segment ——

Loose layer immediately under the pigmented layer 'pith'

Each juice droplet is in its own finer 'bag' within each segment ——

The centre contains irregular, but more densely packed tissue

The 24/7 Tissue: An Overview of this Contextual Shift

We are being invited to consider the fascia as a ubiquitous, body-wide matrix, but not so much an additional "feature" of the musculoskeletal system, as if it was separate (or separable) in some way from muscle or bone. Let's consider that the fascia itself could be the *original* matrix, or *architecture* that in fact *contains* muscle proteins (and shows up as muscles), hyaline (and shows up as cartilage), calcium and mineral salts (and shows up as bone) and self-develops in variations on the theme, to form vessels, organ wrappings and tightly-knit ligaments (or dynaments, if you include the entire joint capsules) to hold the bones apart (because in healthy bodies they don't touch each other directly). What if this fascinating matrix can manifest itself *as* various thicknesses and materials that we selectively name "muscle" or "cartilage" or "bone" or "tendon", as a function of cutting them out? These ideas will be explored throughout this book.

There is now a new level of understanding of the tissues of the "internal net". It seems these tissues work 24 hours a day to determine where we are in space, even as we sleep. Indeed, they appear to be the tissues that organised our primal form and *forming process* (see Ch. 4). No muscle or bone anywhere in the body ever works without them (all); indeed, they arise from one net embryologically. In a manner of speaking, muscles, bones, ligaments and tendons *are* fascia, with different textures (see Appendices and Ch. 7). It is difficult to see the fascial matrix as merely connecting tissues, like a sort of fibrous scaffolding. Rather they are an active, inter-tensioned or inter-compressed, sensory fibrillar network (see Chs 5 & 6). They are in deep organisational relationship with the neural network, hydrated and vascularised by the circulatory matrices they are so intimately interwoven with in complex and profound arrangements of *fluid dynamics* (see Ch. 7). What is important to note here is that everything we thought was true shifts context in a new paradigm and it takes a while to re-orientate the knowledge. We therefore have to find some new coordinates and new language to describe them.

The Story Behind the Science

It is little wonder the fascia is being called the "Cinderella tissue" of the locomotor system and orthopaedic medicine: "*After several decades of severe neglect, this ubiquitous tissue has transformed from the 'Cinderella of Orthopaedic science' into an almost super star position within medical research.*"[20] Like Cinderella, she has been ignored, left to her own devices, but nonetheless relied upon. We are invited by the research to learn that in the body, the musculoskeletal system literally does not exist without the fascia. Anywhere. Ever.

Far from having only two attachment sites per item, muscles and bones do not have *any ability to connect to each other* without the tissues that hold them together (and apart), on *every scale of the network of networks they form together*. Not one single microscopic fibril of muscle escapes this ubiquitous fascial web that weaves us together. Cinderella, it seems, has a big heart and it includes everything and everyone in the entire body system. The scale of this shift is huge – and it may be part of the problem.

It appears that the fascia may be the primary tissue of the body (which we will explore in Chapter 4) and *muscle protein arises within it*. It may in fact be *how* we grow from the dot-sized being we are at conception and, without question, how we get to develop into someone who can "live happily ever after", thanks to the devotion of this neutral servant of our form in time and space – the "Cinderella tissue". Without it we do not move or function, and we certainly do not retain our shape; we wouldn't have any "material" to animate! Muscles and bones get to be in the limelight because "the Cinderella tissue" has the good grace and patience to watch out for them and keep them together, much as she does her "step-sisters" in the original fairy tale. The notion that motion is only down to muscles and bones is a fairy story, not science (see Fig. 3.2).

Like Cinderella to her family, your fascia is the neutral servant of all that you embody, containing every (micro- and macroscopic) detail of you. It responds with exquisite sensitivity to your ways, your woes and your wisdom, as they are at any given time; managing and responding to everything around and within you; seeking balance between them. How you express yourself physically, every moment and movement of the day, is recorded and recognised by the fascial network, and animated by it. (Or perhaps we could say it is the medium in which we express our animation.) At its best, it is how we restore ourselves to balance, and it seems it plays the sovereign role in defining what shape we are in. Morphology, the study of shape, is perhaps more significant than is usually thought.[21] It matters, it is why fascia matters and it takes us on a journey that makes sense of how we can move better, by shifting our focus from lists of parts with assigned functions to an integrated, sensitive structure from which they arise.

It has taken well over a century for Andrew Taylor Still's ideas on fascial structure and function to be researched enough to be treated with the significance he bestowed upon these tissues (see Ch. 2). One of the reasons is the ability to see and measure in detail, which we will consider later in Part B, in considering biomechanics.

On the micro scale, what is now apparent is that every single muscle fibril, or group of fibrils forming fibres, or group of fibres forming bundles, or group of fibre bundles and the proteins within and around them forming the muscle belly (and continuously extending beyond the muscle belly to form the tendinous part of the muscle) is fascia. Fascia is what holds the muscle proteins together, enfolds all groups of muscles together, attaches them through cross-links, as a group or individually, to another group, or to the wrapping around the bone (periosteum). Not at one little red or blue marker on a stick of bone; but as an intimately related system of biological origami, that folded and enfolded into form, originally; one piece in millions of pockets. It is fascia that wraps every bone and forms that periosteum and the joint capsule and plays its part in the so-called ligamentous bed between the bones. Even more emphatically, the embryo shows us that the *"primary space in the body is fascia"*.[22] It is the matrix in which all the other organs[23] are embedded (see Ch. 4). It is evident that everything arises from within the primary fascial matrix. (According to many protagonists, that includes bone *as fascia,* with mineral salts added.[24])

At the macro level, fascia forms the connective tissue wrapping around the organs (visceral fascia), between the depths of tissues that form us. We

The word "matrix" derives from "mother" and it is the "mothering sea" in which we form, in which the primary fascial architecture arises (see Ch. 7). The conceptus is a symbol of that unifying feminine egg, the "fruit" within which the masculine seed (see Ch. 4) animates the growing embryonic structures that emerge from the matrix and are uniquely nurtured and ripened there until birth. It is symbolic in nature and literally presented as such, *as us.*

Understanding fascia does not replace our understanding of muscle or bone but reconfigures our point of view of how they work together and apart; in other words, how they are related and organised. This is the tissue of relationships and relatedness and we have to be cautious when we study it. It is very tempting to get excited about fascia at the expense of the muscle–bone working team. The whole team works together in a triumvirate, rather than as a duo or in isolation. They are not separate parts of us; this is an upgrade, including all that precedes it – evolving us to new dimensions of understanding. It doesn't divide the anatomy into more detail, so much as it multiplies anatomical architecture towards unity.

New Views

"Peri" means outer, "os" means bone, "myo" is muscle, so periosteum is the tissue around the bone and perimysium is the tissue around the muscle. "Epi" means on or around, so epimysium is what you can see around the muscle fibres and bundles, within the perimysium. "Endo" means inner, and the endomysium, which is not visible to the human eye, is right inside the muscle fibrils as the gossamer webbing within the gossamer webbing. It forms an inner matrix, but not separate from any other depth in the rest of the matrix.

call the wrapping of the blood vessels "tunicae" and the tubing around the nerves, "dura". Both are part of the fascial matrix expressed in different weaves and densities, but nonetheless interconnecting forms (neurovascular tracts). Fascia attaches our skin to us, containing the subcutaneous tissue (superficial fascia) underneath it (see Figs 3.1 and 3.2), the skin ligaments that attach it to the underlying tissues and the adipose (fat) pockets in between, forming a body-wide web that has as many roles as it has characteristics to perform them. Fascia is the essence of our soft architectural variability and it takes various forms according to the requirement of a given territory in the body.

From heart to hamstrings, from cell chamber to body chamber, it is organising and forming our inside-out and outside-in architecture, including what is in between. Recent research into the "Interstitium[25]", as an organ of the organism (the "in-between"), is now significantly appreciated as fascial in its properties. It communicates, signals and organises us in a fluid medium, continuously, in continuity and in concert (see Ch. 7, exploring the fluid dynamics, and Appendix B).

The fascia blends the physical with the instinctive and emotional aspects of us *in motion, stillness and presence*. It provides the medium of, at the very least, our physical expression as a moving form.

The discovery that the fascia is among the largest sensory organs of the body[26] (see Ch. 5) makes it literally and symbolically our common sensory organ. We did not invent this important connective tissue; we overlooked it. We woke up to seeing it. The hard part is restructuring what we make it mean (given what we have made it mean historically) in terms of how each one of us moves as a whole being.

After the Renaissance had moved the visual perspective of an artist from two to three dimensions (including a more natural environment in perspective), the Cubists painted the spaces between and around things: that which gave them their three-dimensional definition or boundaries. Shapes were essentially revealed by *negative space*, or the surrounding environment, representing volume, shapes and movements by *what they were not*. This will become important in Part B because we actually rely on just that when we assess form in a classroom. In fact, it is a useful way to "realise" the fascial matrix invested through muscle; it is the negative space, so to speak.

If we look at Figures 3.21 and 3.22 we can see that if we take the structure of a muscle and switch how it is drawn, we get the "negative view". What you see defined in black in Figure 3.22 are the different depths and densities of the fascia: the perimysium, epimysium and endomysium, depending on which tubular depth you are referring to. The point is that they are all connected, all the time. It is a continuous web throughout the muscle (literally everywhere), as symbolised by the orange's segmental nature. It is a model that works throughout nature, making sense of movement, as we will go on to explore.

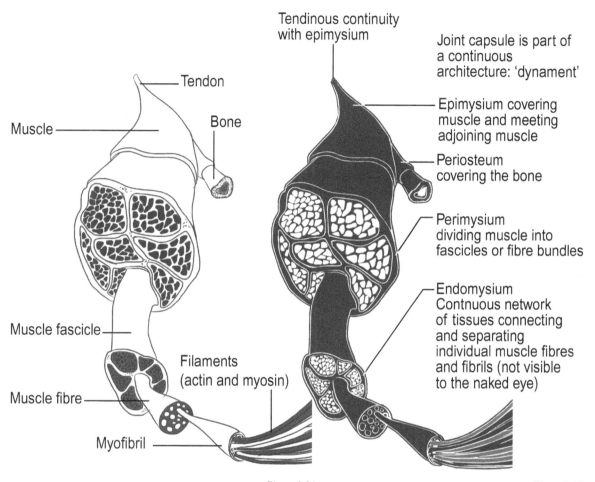

Figure 3.21

This is how a muscle is usually shown in an exploded diagram schematic on the physiology of muscles.

Figure 3.22

The same drawing as shown in Figure 3.21 has been used to highlight the fascia of the inner (endomysium), intermediate (epimysium) and outer (perimysium) fascial sheaths.

Endomysium (Fig. 3.23) looks like a loofah brush, although be careful if you use that particular metaphorical model, because a loofah is dry and stiff, whereas healthy living human connective tissue resides in (and forms) a vital fluid medium (see Ch. 7), held under tension and compression forces in very particular ways (see Ch. 6).

"as to the periosteum, the situation is even more clear; Bones are not 'passively' enveloped by a periosteum. The periosteum is the skeletal element itself that deposited the hard osseous tissue and serves the insertion of muscle and connective tissue. It mediates."[27-35]

Figure 3.23

This drawing is taken from a photograph of an electromyographic image of the endomysium once the myofibrils have been removed. The endomysium is the deepest aspect and cannot be seen with the naked eye. The image shows the long hollow spaces where the myofibrils were and reveals the continuity of the architecture in which they reside. It has a slightly randomly shaped honeycomb structure and clearly acts as a part of the communication and coordination faculty of what is commonly called the "musculoskeletal system". In the living body it is completely continuous with the epimysium, perimysium, loose connective tissue and skin. There are no separate layers *in vivo*; they are an artefact of fixed cadaveric preservation. They may also be a language of convenience; however, they do not explain motion of living beings in bodies.

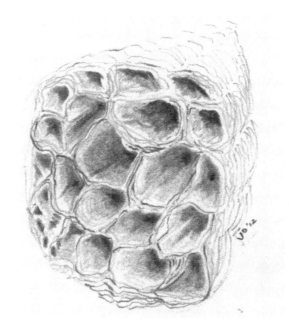

New View -- Same Architecture

The difficult thing to grasp is that, in a way, nothing has actually changed, only the point of view from which we are looking at and analysing the body and the context of how it is presented and learned. We can call this new way of seeing the "science of body architecture", to distinguish it from the old way of seeing. It is revealing what was always there, fascia is not new – as has been said – it is newly *recognised*. We are now "off the planar side elevation" on the drawing board, and showing the body full blown into multi-dimensional animated life. (Precisely how bodies show up in our classrooms!)

There is at the present time much discussion about what fascia is where and the different types of fasciae and their relative roles and collagen types. However, the question of detailed terminology remains a subject of debate around how exactly all these types are differentiated into named parts of the entire fascial matrix or tensional network.

"The Continuity: Functional anatomy now describes integrated systems, when in the past we only thought in terms of independent structures, and the various fascias of the body are now recognized as part of a "fascial system". As we move away from thinking of muscles as isolated structures, we must recognize that muscles are useless unless they pull against something. A functional support and motor system must include the compression elements such as bones. In a musculoskeletal system, where does a muscle end and the bone begin? Unless the muscle cell pulls on fascia, and fascia pulls on bone, nothing much can happen. As Guimberteau and Delage[36] (2012), Huijing and Baan[37] (2001), and van der Wal[38] (2009) have shown, boundaries in the body are artificial,

arbitrary, descriptive conveniences. Tissues in the body are not contiguous, just sharing borders, but continuous, transmuting into one another (Sharkey[39] (2016)). The body is an open-office plan, a union of organs united under one roof. The distinction between the muscle parenchyma and its various -mysiums is a subjective one that is inconsistent with its function. Where endo-/peri-/epimysium ends and tendon, ligament or periosteum begins is arbitrary. Like a doorway connecting rooms in an apartment, the periosteum is continuous with both the fascia of the muscle and the matrix of bone".

Stephen Levin, MD, *Bone is Fascia*[40]

"Bone is "continuous" with the bone matrix. The Sharpey's fibers do not merely penetrate into bone, they become the bone matrix. If fascia is a continuum, as described by the IFRC committee, then the ligaments and tendons (by their definition of "fascia") must continue on into the interstices of the bone and the bone matrix and out the other end."

The fascia itself presents a profound difficulty when it comes to naming its parts since it is essentially ubiquitous and continuous. That is the key to the codex! John Sharkey points out there is only one "fascia" [41]; a legitimate statement given its total continuity throughout the form and *how we form it/are formed by it* – as we will see in the next chapter(s).

"As a language of convenience we may name discreet areas of the fascia and imply their plural nature by so-doing. However, the wholeness is always and only expressed as ONE fascia".

John Sharkey, Dundee University, 2019.

Much new information about fascia was presented at the first International Fascia Research Congress, in 2007, resulting from the work of pioneers since Andrew Taylor Still and including many curious and committed scientists, clinicians, surgeons, anatomists and bodywork professionals in all fields who constitute our modern day philosophers, with a portfolio of ideas between them. Together, in a collaborative network of communication and scientific research, artistically presented, the Fascia Congress is moving towards its sixth worldwide exhibition at the time of writing. This will take place in 2021. Further information and details of the network of dedicated individuals in every field that come together, from all over the globe, to

Moreover, to some extent we express it uniquely according to use, so, although we have a general pattern within the species, we are working with asymmetries and biologic similarities rather than rigid geometries or machines. In other words, you do it your way and I do it mine. We can share the idea, we can even recreate the process and make new patterns and synchronise and mimic each other, but we are never identical. You already know that in a class we may all do the same yoga pose or athletic feat, but no two will be identical. The science begins to confirm why that might be so.

What this comes down to in general terms for our teaching is that we cannot usefully separate structure from function because they are not separate or architecturally separable – nor do ANY function in isolation. They intimately relate to each other and co-create/respond to forces, via our internal space and *biomotional integrity*. You move and create form as you form shapes by moving. You experience "being moved" on an emotional level and shape accordingly in suitable tissue response. We need to keep an overall sense of the whole as movement teachers, and as yoga teachers we sit at a huge advantage. We bring this work to the rest of the world can be found at www.fasciaresearch.com and www.fasciaresearchsociety.org. They are too numerous to refer-

A New Word

ence individually and no doubt some will challenge specific details here. However, if this does no more than shed light on the need to reconsider anatomy, biomechanics and physiology, and endorse the whole body that yoga and any movement practices are devoted to, it will have ignited curiosity and, therefore, been worthwhile.

are trained in shapes, sensory awareness and kinaesthetic attention to their formation; it's an asset in understanding fascia and realising the Cinderella story in action. *We are pre-disposed to using our understanding of fascia to move better.*

"Biomotional" is a new word that might be easy to grasp on paper but is not easy to "get". We have been brought up on, and reasonably nourished by, a diet of biomechanical function based in separate muscles and individual bones. These then move at the articulating joints between them. Quite why the study of motion is called biomechanics and human bodies are treated as if they are designed as machines first (and human beings second) is not fully answered by our scientific history. In reality, we are not machines; we do not move mechanically and we do not have mechanistic joints. That is the difficult, if obvious, point. Robots have mechanical joints and we have not yet managed to design a robot that moves as fluidly or as intelligently and responsively/adaptably as human beings can.[42] We have underestimated the complexity and genius of the human form, for it does not only behave in a biomechanical way, but also in what we might call a "biomotional" way.

"And that machine thinking comes from the notion that the body is built up from parts. That is the machine-view. That is not true: the embryo shows us loud and clear: First the whole then the parts. First the matrix, next the elements, first the body, then the organs!!!!!!!!!

*A machine is built up from parts. That the system might work LIKE a machine does not prove it IS a machine. That you can replace a joint by a hinge does not prove it is a hinge. It works **like** a hinge and that is a big essential difference!!!"*[43]

There is, technically, no such word as "biomotional". However, the term "biomechanical" somehow implies automation, and the human form, given the fascial matrix, does not really resemble a robotic lever-armed system. Biomechanical is a term that refers to movement methods of the locomotor system as if it is a hard-matter-based physical machinery. We are entirely made of various soft tissues, including relatively compressed, hardened soft tissue (bone and cartilage) and relatively supple or folded and softened *soft tissue* (viscera, muscles, membranes and vessels), enclosing gel-like substances and fluid flows (colloids and emulsions). These may have various properties but do not appear to exhibit purely

Understanding fascia and its fluid medium, the containment of the cells and the extracellular matrix in which they reside, is why robotics is about mechanics and we are about individual grace and guts. Whether in light or clumsy gestures, coordinated or awkward moves, we express our fascial make-up as uniquely as we are shaped. We are not cloned. We do not conform to a rigid plan. Ours is a fluid, self-motivated, sensory kind of geometry, full of choice and personal interpretation that began with our embryonic genesis and remains whole.

We are conscious archetypal beings, developing continuously from our embryonic origins to the best of our abilities at the time, under the circumstances in which we find ourselves. The tissue can and does, with the appropriate dose and degree, respond to new loading patterns, if we understand how they accumulate. The body represents, essentially, time in motion, which we will consider in later chapters. Physically and metaphysically, it doesn't reduce to the component physical parts as if they were formed separately and bolted together.

mechanical characteristics such as a machine might have. In essence they are tension–compression fabrics and tubes, continuously related to each other. That is, soft tetherings of various types, not nuts and bolts. Machines have parts while mammals have continuities. No part can be removed from a living body without affecting the rest because it is originally in an unbroken, continuous matrix. Thus the word "biomotional" is offered here to enhance the sense of soft tissue organisation that we will explore in later chapters. It does not replace the term biomechanical; however, it seeks to expand our sense of movement in nature and the yoga classroom.

Everyone you teach *already has* organised body architecture. They come to you to assist in refining and optimising how they move it, in the context of the particular style of movement or yoga you teach – and their *embodied* story. Once the overall architectural principles are understood, common to every cell, muscle, organ and the whole organism, the pieces begin to fall into place, literally and metaphorically held together by our tissues.

We have to go back to the beginning to ask the embryo (your embryonic origins) how it formed (how you formed yourself). Then, in the light of fascia research, we begin to see how the whole formation remained whole throughout life. This allows us to understand our architecture as a self-contained, self-organising system of something we can call an organic "living tensegrity", also called biotensegrity. We will give this some chapters of its own because it upgrades our understanding of the soft-matter vehicle we live in, to a three-dimensional (multi-dimensional) integrated whole that actually moves independently of gravity and in very intelligent ways.

Yoga could be said to already understand many of these "new" aspects of the science instinctively, by incorporating them into its ancient and holistic practices, much like many of the martial arts. We have to go a little deeper, however, to confirm why the kinaesthetic intelligence we explore on the mat is so multifaceted. This is vital, otherwise we risk segregating and fracturing yoga with reductionist principles, and there is no need to do that.

Yoga is a beautiful medium in which to demonstrate this work because it works this way in practice, demonstrably.

Notes and bibliography

1. Sir Winston Churchill, in a speech to the House of Commons on 28 October 1944.
2. Jaap van der Wal, "The Architecture of the Collagenous Connective Tissue in the Musculoskeletal System – An often overlooked Functional Parameter as to Proprioception in the Locomotor System". This article is published as supplement to a lecture at the Second International Fascia Research Congress, Amsterdam, 27–30 October 2009, with the title "The Architecture of Connective Tissue as a Functional Substrate for Proprioception in the Locomotor System". (Jaap van der Wal MD PhD, University of Maastricht, Faculty of Health, Medicine and Life Sciences, Department of Anatomy and Embryology, P.O. Box 616, 6200 MD Maastricht, Netherlands.) It includes a revised version of part of Van der Wal's doctoral thesis, submitted to the University of Maastricht in 1988, entitled "The Organization of the Substrate of Proprioception in the Elbow Region of the Rat".
3. John Sharkey, Dundee University, 2016, Biotensegrity focused soft-fix Dissection programme; lecture.
4. In August 2019, Clinical Anatomist John Sharkey led a team of Fascia experts presenting a Fascia Symposium to the 19th Congress of the International Federation of Associations of Anatomists (IFAA), which is held every 5 years. In 2019 the Congress was held, for only the second time, in London, England. The IFAA Congress is a unique opportunity for medical professionals to share research and new developments in anatomy and anatomy research. Applications are peer-reviewed; presentations undergo rigorous scientific scrutiny, before being accepted for presentation. In the event, a presentation by John Sharkey, Drs Carla Stecco, Vladimir Cheremnsky, Rafael De Caro, Veronica Macchi and Andrea Porzionato was enthusiastically received by the large number of delegates at this prestigious event. In the same year the professional journal of anatomists, *Clinical Anatomy*, produced a Special Issue journal, (Volume 32, Issue 7. October 2019 Pages 896–902) devoted entirely to the topic and science of Fascia. This is scientific progress with a capital "P" and is referred to in more detail in later chapters in Part A.
5. Ibid.
6. Ibid.
7. Leon Chaitow DO, 1937–2018. https://www.ntc.ie/hdipnmt/ NTC's Higher Diploma in Neuromuscular Therapy was originally written in 2003 by John Sharkey, MSc, Leon Chaitow, DO and Judith DeLany, LMT. *The National Training Centre will continue to honour Leon Chaitow's legacy by passing on the spirit and essence of his work through the world's leading bodywork authorities on the Higher Diploma in Neuromuscular Therapy.*
8. University of Chester, Parkgate Road, Chester CH1 4BJ. The University of Chester is a public university located in Chester, England. The university originated as the first purpose-built teacher training college in the UK.

9. John Sharkey MSc, Clinical Anatomist (BACA), Anatomical Society (Full Member), Exercise Physiologist (BASES)
10. John Sharkey (2019) Can Medical Education be Enhanced by the World's First 3d Printed Fascia Models and Plastinated Specimens of Fascia Superficialis and Profundus? *Biomed J Sci & Tech Res* 15(4):2019. BJSTR. MS.ID.002749.
11. Ch. 2 in Andrew T. Still, *Philosophy of Osteopathy*, A.T. Still, Kirksville, 1899.
12. Jaap van der Wal, private communication, July 2013.
13. See Dr Guimberteau's work. Jean-Claude Guimberteau, MD (http://www.endovivo.com/en/livres.php). His DVD: *Interior Architectures*, is available on the same site. See also *The Architecture of Living Fascia: The Extracellular Matrix and Cells Revealed Through Endoscopy*, Handspring Publishing Ltd., Pencaitland, 2014.
14. Ibid.
15. Ibid.
16. Ibid.
17. The author would like to express profound and reverent gratitude to all donors.
18. Introduction in Robert Schleip, Thomas W. Findley, Leon Chaitow and Peter A. Huijing, *Fascia: The Tensional Network of the Human Body*. Churchill Livingstone/Elsevier, Edinburgh, 2012.
19. Donald Ingber (1998) The Architecture of Life. *Scientific American*, Feature Article, January 1998.
20. Luigi Stecco and Carla Stecco, *Fascial Manipulation: Practical Part*, English edition by Julie Ann Day, foreword by Robert Schleip, Piccin, Padua, 2009.
21. *The Architecture of Living Fascia: The Extracellular Matrix and Cells Revealed Through Endoscopy*, Handspring Publishing Ltd., Pencaitland, 2014. Ch. 6, Adaptations and modifications of the multifibrillar network, p. 159 to 162.
22. Jaap van der Wal, personal communication, July 2013.
23. N.D. Theise et al (2018) Structure and Distribution of an Unrecognized Interstitium in Human Tissue. *Science Reports* March 27– and see Appendix A
24. John Sharkey (2019) Letter to the Editor. *Journal of Bodywork & Movement Therapies* 23 (2019) 6e8.
    Article by Stephen M. Levin - 2018/08/21, SP , Bone is Fascia - published on ResearchGate and as a special contribution within the Introduction of Susan C. Lowell de Solórzano's *Everything Moves: How Biotensegrity Informs Human Movement*. Handspring Publishing Ltd, Pencaitland, 2020.
25. N.D. Theise et al (2018) Structure and Distribution of an Unrecognized Interstitium in Human Tissue. *Science Reports* March 27.
26. "When including intramuscular connective tissues, periosteum and superficial fascia as part of the body wide fascial net as outlined above, fascia can then be seen as one of our richest sensory organs. It is certainly our most important organ for proprioception (Schleip, 2003)." R. Schleip, D.G. Müller (2013) Training Principles for Fascial Connective Tissues: Scientific Foundation and Suggested Practical Applications. *Journal of Bodywork and Movement Therapies* 17:103–115.
27. Jaap van der Wal, private communication, including the following references (notes 28–35):
28. J. Drukker, H. van Mameren, J.C. van der Wal (1983) Connective tissue structures in the cubital region of man and rat. Their role in guidance of forces and their role as a substrate for proprioception. *J Anat* 137:432.
29. H. van Mameren, J. Drukker (1984) A functional anatomical basis of injuries to the ligamentum and other soft tissues around the elbow joint: Transmission of tensile and compressive loads. *Int J Sports Med* 5 (suppl.):88–92.
30. H. van Mameren, J.C. van der Wal (1983) Comparison of the organisation of the connective tissue in relation with muscle and nerve tissue in the cubital region in man and in the rat. *Acta Morphol Neerl-Scand* 21:169.
31. H. van Mameren, W. Groenewegen, H. Rensema (1984) A computerized drawing method to make representations of the collagenous connective tissue structures in situ around the elbow joint. *Acta Morph Neerl-Scand* 22:253.
32. H. van Mameren, A. Lataster, H. Rensema, J. Drukker (1985) The use of modern imaging techniques (CT-scanning and NMR) in the study of the locomotor apparatus. *Acta Morph Neerl-Scand* 23:247–258.
33. J.C. van der Wal (1988). The organization of the morphological substrate of proprioception in the elbow region of the rat. Unpublished thesis, University of Limburg, Netherlands.
34. J.C. van der Wal (2009) The architecture of the connective tissue in the musculoskeletal system – an often overlooked functional parameter as to proprioception in the locomotor apparatus. *Int J Ther Massage Bodywork (IJTMB)* 2(4):9–23.
35. J.C. van der Wal, "Proprioception, Mechanoreception and the Anatomy of the Fascia", Ch. 2.2 in Robert Schleip, Thomas W. Findley, Leon Chaitow and Peter A. Huijing, *Fascia: The Tensional Network of the Human Body*, Churchill Livingstone/Elsevier, Edinburgh, 2012.
36. J.C. Guimberteau, J.P. Delage (2012) The multifibrillar network of the tendon sliding system. *Ann Chir Plast Esthetique* 57:467–481.
37. P.A. Huijing, G.C. Baan (2001) Extramuscular myofascial force transmission within the rat anterior tibial compartment: proximo-distal differences in muscle force. *Acta Physiol Scand* 3:297–311.
38. J. van der Wal (2009) The architecture of the connective tissue in the musculoskeletal system, an often overlooked functional parameter as to proprioception in the locomotor apparatus. *International Journal of Therapeutic Massage & Bodywork* 2(4):9.
39. John Sharkey, Dundee University (2016) Biotensegrity focused soft-fix Dissection programme; lecture.
40. Article by Stephen M. Levin - 2018/08/21, SP , Bone is Fascia - published on ResearchGate and as a special contribution within the Introduction of Susan C. Lowell de Solórzano's *Everything Moves: How Biotensegrity Informs Human Movement*. Handspring Publishing Ltd, Pencaitland, 2020.
41. J. Sharkey (2021) Fascia and tensegrity. The quintessence of a unified systems conception. *Int J Anat Appl Physiol* 07(02):174–178.
42. The relatively new field of Soft Robotics is using the principles of Biotensegrity (Ch. 6) to create a new generation of robots. Vytas SunSpiral (Thomas Willeke to 2005) is a computer scientist and roboticist at NASA who has shared many fruitful discussions and collaborations over the years with Tom Flemons. His website is www.magicalrobot.org/BeingHuman/.
43. Jaap van der Wal, personal communication, July 2013.

4

The Remarkable Human Blueprint

"The body has its own way of fighting illness, readjusting itself to harmony. We all want to survive and be well and will find infinite ways to serve our needs. There are no obstacles to this tremendous urge to live. The body will always strive to overcome the difficulties impeding its existence. To live is one of the greatest miracles."[1]

Vanda Scaravelli

Yoga is about the process of unifying form and the union of all our aspects. This includes the mind, the being and the form of the body through which we express ourselves, in action and in stillness; both are performances of a sort. Embryology is about the process of forming from original unity (one unicellular being) as much as it is about the formation of all aspects of us into one whole multi-cellular being, aspiring to unity. Yoga and embryology are intimately related. Perhaps all we ever needed to know about yoga but were too afraid to ask is there, in the embryo.

It is interesting to consider that we all began as embryos. Like the acorn that somehow "knows" how to become an oak tree, we know what is required to become all that the remarkable human blueprint promises. The embryo essentially self-assembles, motivated by the miraculous ability to animate the codes and patterns it inherits, through the matter of its own architecture – literally and symbolically. Embryology is the study of how we achieve this. In a medical context, this is described as the progressive stages of developmental growth on a somewhat linear and horizontal timeline. In the advanced practices of yoga, it becomes a metaphor for the symbolic growth of our emerging consciousness, in anything but linear patterns. The fundamental question remains: how exactly does the embryo differentiate, in time, to emerge as us?

Whichever lens we look through to explore our origins, embryology is the story of an evolving work in progress. The process could be described as an evolution, a convolution and a revolution, in the sense of its volume, its spiral motion sequences and its incorporation of every performance to form the next "volution" if there is such a word to describe the voluntary nature of that self-directed assembly. It is very complex; however, it describes only one particular period in our development, which is a progression of changes on a continuum throughout our lives. Each of us goes physically from a uni-cellular conceptus to a multi-cellular embryo, from fetus to neonate, newborn to baby, toddler and child. We all undertake a journey to whichever point we reach, through a process of adolescence to arrive at adulthood, and eventually elderhood. We continue to express this in a body that presents "time" or "sensitivity-dependent periodicity[2]" at each cyclical stage to which it has developed, in an invariably unique way.

Yoga is interested in developing our awareness of that process and becoming ever more present to it. The yogic Yantra speaks of a "sacred journey", which might describe the developmental weeks of embryonic forming or the developmental years of a whole life. They are seen in these terms as a microcosm of the macrocosm. The question of scale differentiates them. At this early stage of embryogenesis, yoga views the energetic body as part of the forming process. Medical textbooks, in contrast, identify process in terms confined to physical developments and the genetic codes that authorise them, usually compressed into as linear a timeline as it is possible to reduce them to. It is a difficult task, because every single stroke of embryonic development takes place in the round and impacts the entirety of the form it is in the performance of forming. It is invariably a multi-dimensional metamorphosis, as is the case for the rest of the ensuing life cycle(s), perhaps predicted by that which precedes and predicting what proceeds this transformation-in-progress, we each perform.

Research into the role of the connective tissue offers some interesting invitations that seem to help bridge between these linear and non-linear ideas. Given its unifying nature, the fascia is, perhaps unsurprisingly, evoking a new curiosity around classical explanations of our original formation.

Embryogenesis: the word "embryo" comes from the Greek meaning "young one" and came to mean "fruit of the womb" (literally "that which grows", from *en* "in" + *bryein* "to swell, be full"). "Genesis" means beginning. At the earliest stage, one name for the fertilised egg is the "conceptus", from the Latin "a collecting, gathering, conceiving"; the term can also be used at the metaphysical level to describe the conception of a new idea.

Sensing into Form

When we practise the yoga poses, by exploring the shapes of new forms we develop our physical bodies as well as our mind and being; our inner and outer sensory awareness. We practise to become more articulate, developing our inner sense as we perform the poses while, with our outward attention, we listen to where we are in space, seeking congruency between them, in all the variety of shapes, directions and ways in which we can balance and respond to and from the ground (see Ch. 5). We move in the gravitational field and although we are no longer wrapped in the fluid chambers of our original forming (morphogenesis), we might say we are wrapped in gravity, matched and perfectly balanced by ground reaction force (see Ch. 6). We are managing and exploring the subtle, invisible forces within and around us, all the time.

Much like the forming embryo, we interact with biodynamic forces, rates of change and relationships between the forms. We experiment with the forces in which we are growing and moving, as a whole body, all the time: from the outside in, the inside out, side to side, rotation to counter-rotation, and so on. On the mat, we consciously explore the ways the forms and forces interact as we effectively change them, by moving. That might be very similar to what the embryo does. The earliest cells grow and organise the forms by moving and changing biodynamic forces[3] and genetic patterns; they consequently change each other. Yoga could be said to do the same, since we all express its forms and practices uniquely.

"If you think the adaptability and range of possibilities and complicated interactions in the body of an adult is a beautiful achievement, you can multiply that by a million in the embryo. It appears as a kind of chaos, if you can say that of something that contains and emerges into such exquisite and various order."[4]

Chemistry or Geometry?

The scientific and medical books on embryology tend to take a point of view based mostly around genetics. However, that view is changing. Advanced technology in instrumentation and the new questions arising from research in connective tissue biology are affecting every field of knowledge; the study of the embryonic process seems to include them all. From maths, physics and chemistry to biology and music we can find rhythmical patterns and correlates in the embryonic forming process. Authors such as Richard Grossinger, in a work rich in metaphor,[5] take a phenomenological approach, comparing the embryo to the galaxy, the difference being one of scale. Emeritus associate professor of Anatomy and Embryology, Dr Jaap van der Wal (see Ch. 3) presents the embryo as a sentient being, highlighting the primary role of the fascial matrix and the subtle exchanges that take place as it self-develops, through the medium of that maternal context. Proprioception is presented as our original *sensing* of form and van der Wal[6] describes human beings as multisensory and aware, unified from the beginning. The suggestion is that we learn from the embryo, as distinct from thinking we might explain entirely how it functions from the anatomy of the parts (as if we ever get to tell it how, before it self-assembles!). Understanding living tensegrity extends the point of view further, unifying the science and the symbolism in the geometry that is fundamental to both.

Yoga's most ancient history is richly woven with symbolic geometry (see Ch. 12). It is no coincidence that the earliest pre-embryonic forms can be shown geometrically to present many aspects of Sacred Geometry (see Chs 2 & 12) and the principles of Divine Proportion and the Golden Ratio. More contemporary studies of geodesic geometry[7] are also providing new lenses through which to view embryological forming. The symbolism is rich and rewarding on every level and, depending on what we are looking for, embryology resonates with many people in different ways. The same patterns are original to the yogic Yantra's, so we are constantly learning how the newest science of Body Architecture re-iterates the ancient wisdom that precedes us.

The Scientific Questions

The potential role of the fascia in our bodies is gaining in significance in many fields. Embryological research carried out by Evans (a developmental tissue biologist and anatomist) and colleagues in 2006 refers to the fascia as "the forgotten player".[8] It suggests that connective tissue may be more primary than muscle tissue, essential for the **creation** of the "musculoskeletal unit". Evans' research is endorsed by Sharkey[9] and Levin[10] and van der Wal.[11] As we learn that the fascial matrix cannot be logically excluded from understanding the musculoskeletal system or any of our movements, new ways of examining embryogenesis are emerging.

This point of view suggests the continuity seen in Jean-Claude Guimberteau's films of the living (adult) matrix (see Ch. 3). Guimberteau places great emphasis on the way the connective tissue matrix is organised and omnipresent. It has multiple functions, as is suggested here. The paradigm shift from thinking in terms of muscle and bone units to thinking in terms of continuity of form throughout the tissues *in their variety of texture and density* is highlighted by such research questions as these.

"Connective tissue: the forgotten player? … Skeletal muscle is invested and anchored to a number of specialised connective tissue layers organised as the endo-, peri- and epi-mysium [see Ch. 3]. These layers not only act as a conduit for blood vessels and nerves but because they become continuous with the connective tissues of the tendons and other muscle attachments, they are essential in transmitting the motive force of the muscle to the attached structure (e.g. bone) as appropriate."[12]

*Water is a term of convenience used loosely here, referring to a transparent droplet that is really the "embryonic soup" of mesenchyme that will become the embryo. It describes the major component of this "soup", rather than implying that it is much like the water running in a stream or from a tap/faucet, since it is, essentially, *bound* water. Think egg white, in terms of the more viscous, or gel-like properties of this (mostly water) embryonic medium. It will become important in later chapters in Part A. As an example, the jello or jelly you make for a "jelly and ice-cream" party, is about 98% water, with gelatin or other protein, acting as a binding agent. Squishing that jello/jelly between a child's fingers doesn't leak any water as such – as it expresses the properties of "bound water" (see Ch. 7).

What if muscle protein arises from *within* the fibrous net of the ubiquitous fascial matrix; if fascia is the primary placeholder of our potential form (and all the forms within it)? It would make sense that the integration of growth functions and their forces animate the appropriate changes that bring about the different structures. What we call (variously) tendon, ligament, muscle, bone and cartilage (visceral wrapping and neuro-vascular vessels) are all woven together in an intimately organised morphology. Could bony calcification (that comes so much later in the process) be the result of cartilaginous placeholders in the blank folds of the origami canvas? As we fold, enfold and unfold into forms, could they be a densification response, when *we* are strong enough to balance strong forces moving through the denser connective tissues? In other words, can we pose the question that the fascial matrix *is the primary* structural "*materia biologica*" of embryogenesis, through and with which we feel our way into form? Van der Wal[13] suggests it is the biological fabric, and his formal writings on the subject are eagerly awaited.

The Embryonic Period

At the earliest stage of our development, the moment of conception, the embryo is whole and complete, so let us start from that beginning.

How the embryo essentially forms itself is a complex and exquisitely detailed series of events that take place over a period of just five weeks (from approximately week 3 to week 8 after fertilisation). In that short space of time, a tiny ball of water* just visible to the naked eye becomes a recognisable, if barely, developing baby human, about the size of an acorn. It still has a long way to go to become a newborn; however, the plan (the whole anlage, or rudimentary basis of a particular organ or part) is in place. It has an immature heart and primitive, but nevertheless distinct and functioning, organs: head, spine, body wall and limbs; pulsing lungs, moving fingers, and toes, eyes, ears and nose. They are all ready to grow and develop into the precise features we embody and enjoy exploring on the yoga mat.

The Journey

The embryonic journey is mostly described in books as a number of *quantitative* events, one following after the other in sequence. In fact, many of the events happen at the same time, in one co-creative, *qualitative* process of development; in 360 degrees. Each one relies on the other and the whole is something indefinably and unpredictably greater than the sum of the parts. It is not like building a robot or making a soft toy, with the right amounts of each ingredient. Nothing in the embryo is bolted on or added afterwards or part of a linear time sequence. The entire biomotional orchestration is a symphony of emergent properties (see Ch. 6) expressing an interdependent (and interrelated) global and local performance.

For the yoga practitioner, it is fascinating to discover that the heart descends according to the (reverse) order of the yogic chakras, from the crown, ultimately down to the coccyx (see Ch. 12). The first, pre-embryonic heart cells syncopate the rhythmic growth of the embryo, brain first. They are pushed downward by the growing brain, over the crown, placing the heart opposite the spine. The face folds then unfolds upwardly from there, as the spine grows down the back at the same time; so chakras 5, 6 and 7 (in a very metaphorical sense) grow back up from the heart. The heart is eventually incorporated with the "septum transversum" (which becomes the diaphragm) as the thoracic cavity is formed. The third chakra descends from the fourth (heart) and as the spine grows down towards the tail, the second and first chakra positions arise later in the sequence, completing the base of the torso at the root chakra (Mulhadara) (see Ch. 12). From this point of view our subtle body is formed originally in our physical form, from the crown towards the tail, in the multi-dimensional patterning process of a mobius strip (see margin note).

We could say it is more like folding an exquisitely elaborate origami sculpture, in that the innate geometry of form has a sequence but the whole arises from the folds and interrelating creases and invaginations of the original "*single piece of pape*r". (Which in our case is an *original sphere – which is beyond our standard visualisation ability to interpret.*) All folds come together at the end, they all rely upon each other, and if one fold is inaccurately pleated, it affects the whole finished form. So too with our embryonic developmental folds; uniting to create our basic morphology, or human shape.

Every fold, every enfoldment, every pattern and pulsing rhythm of the embryonic progression happens inside continuously connected pockets. The pockets form within pockets in this multi-dimensional, fluid, biodynamic origami continuum. The folds form tubes and bags, as these are volumes rather than flat paper pleats. Our "one piece of paper" has no edges; it is formed in the round; it is in the round, i.e. tubular. The pockets and apparent spaces are formed such that the folding consequences bring us and all our organs into the shape of an embryonic miniature human being. Each phase takes those

If that is the case, i.e. that a mobius-strip-shaped sequence takes place, then in full 3D, the embryo forms by folding through itself and around itself. It is a sequence called "invagination" that means the embryo "turns itself inside out to form". The mobius, in the round (or 4D), would be a Klein bottle pattern that can move through itself and takes us into the realm of Hyperbolic Geometry (see Note 7, Graham Scarr: in his book *Biotensegrity: The Structural Basis of Life*, Ch. 10 Complex Patterns in Biology, p. 118 onwards, Second Edition). There is an illustrated example of how a Klein bottle pattern may be fundamental to the organisation of human form and forms within the whole. This 4D matriarchal (*meaning of the mother and of the matrix – which comes from mater – Latin for mother*) organisation gradually makes sense once we realise that the entire embryonic structure begins and ends with two spheres meeting and folding (within another one that enfolds them), enfolding and unfolding into form, from within those spheres. That is almost impossible to imagine (and much harder to write about). Suffice to say here, it is anything but linear!!

sacs with it, as it itself folds, and, in less than two months from conception, the emergent creature incorporates all of them, on every scale. It then grows and expands into the fluid sacs (*amniotic and chorionic*) from within which it formed. We discover that the enfoldings and organisations are all from the same original "piece of paper". That is, the single, tiny ball of fluid (somewhat like a dew drop) enclosed in a membrane that is the fertilised egg (wrapped in its adjacent and surrounding soft-tissue containers).

The Embryonic Parts are Whole

In the embryo section of many books on the subject, each tiny enfoldment stage and position has been reduced to a two-dimensional icon, annotated and given a name (which is considerably longer in the writing than the length of the formed embryo), in order that the sequence of metamorphosis can be followed, albeit reduced to a somewhat linear progression, for convenience. In textbooks the embryological sequence is usually presented visually as a series of graphic icons, cut out of the spherical sacs in and around which the actual embryo folds itself. The placenta, which is part of the embryonic self-assembly, is often assigned the status of a separate item, despite the umbilical cord being the result of the enfoldment of the original yolk sac. The embryo self-assembles its own body and that of the placental supply system. At the earliest stages, the placenta holds the functions that the embryo must acquire and incorporate. They must progress together, in a manner that unifies the nutrient supply with the nurturing/nurtured architecture.

The word "yoga" means unifying. The primary, connected chamber of our origin holds our entire remarkable human blueprint in potential as one unified form; the size of that original water* droplet. It multiplies into folds within folds, part of this original uni-cellular being residing in the nucleus of every other cell, each one a "mini-me" (see margin note) capable of all that the others can do, albeit with their own specialisations. Every part of us arises from the one whole unit of us, from which we emerge. It is somewhat like an Escher painting or a Rumi poem. "The embryo is the architect of the architecture that forms the embryo. Indeed, it forms the architecture to express the architect". The reasoning mind comes a considerable time after.

The term "mini-me" comes from John Sharkey, Clinical Anatomist, who describes every cell in the human body as a "mini-me" of the person who effectively self-assembled it.

Depending upon which text you are reading, development can be a literal and prosaic description of stages or a poetic story of transformation. Either way, many people (even those who have studied the basics of embryology as part of a medical degree) can learn the facts without necessarily realising that in three dimensions, the embryo forms from the actual meeting of two tiny water* bags, both inside another surrounding one (Fig. 4.1).

The embryo takes these sacs with it during every fold of the journey to formation. It only sheds them at birth, having structuralised its own outermost layer (skin) inside what becomes the surrounding amniotic sac. The skin itself is formed from the lower continuity of the amniotic membrane. They are not separate entities. This is almost impossible to represent as multi-dimensional form in two-dimensional media, even visually. It is entirely impossible in words, as they are simply an inappropriate medium. The essence of that continuity (and its sentience) is exactly why fascia is raising so many questions

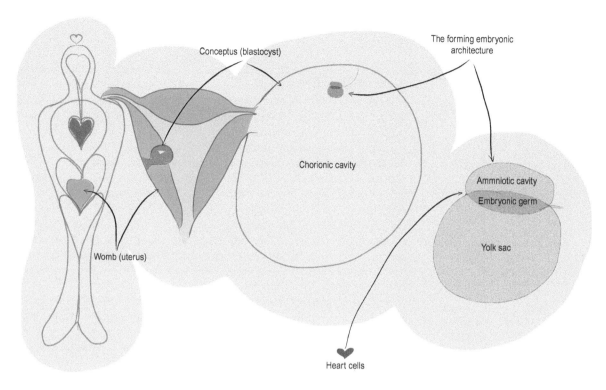

Womb (uterus)

Conceptus (blastocyst)

The forming embryonic architecture

Chorionic cavity

Ammniotic cavity

Embryonic germ

Yolk sac

Heart cells

Figure 4.1

The embryo forms at the meeting place of the upper (future amniotic) sac and the lower (yolk) sac. The heart begins just beyond where they join, above what will become the crown. It is not a seed or a germ between the sacs. It is the sacs.

and inviting different perspectives to account for our anatomy, physiology and biomechanics, at all stages of our development. Fascia seems to play an essential role in every aspect of our formation; perhaps that is how it earns the title "organ of organisation" as it clearly organises and seems to unify the embryological forming processes. It is quite literally mind-blowing and beyond reason, so fitting it into words is at best a reductionist attempt to point to the moon. Even visually, we are reduced to 2D images that, like the cross-section of the orange in Chapter 3, don't tell you much about the morphology or the wholeness.

Heart-felt Beginnings

In Figure 4.1 we see that the inner chambers touch each other, forming the upper and lower sentient membranes that will become the embryo; the future heart starts "above the crown" before the growing brain folds over it. We will also learn that the fluid of these chambers (the "embryonic soup") is the basis of all the building materials[14] and connective tissues from which we form ourselves. The rhythmical beat of the heart begins very early in the process, syncopating the motion of blood to the rapidly growing brain, as we will see in a little more detail below.

Spacialisation

From dot to disc:

Anatomist and embryologist Jaap van der Wal (see Ch. 3) celebrates embryology from a more humanist view of being and becoming. He points out that, at the initial stage of fertilisation, the egg (ovum) is (approximately) 90% cytoplasm and 10% nucleus; it is the largest single cell in the human body, visible (just) without a microscope. When sperm reach the outermost membrane of nutritive cells of the ovum (called the corona radiata; "encircling radiance"), they first rest there and the egg begins to spin within its "radiant crown".

The sperm is the smallest human cell and is made up of (approximately) 90% nucleus and 10% cytoplasm, in other words, the opposite of the egg. These essentially polarised cells enter what van der Wal describes as a "conversation" or subtle exchange. If they merge, the sperm completes the nucleus of the ovum and the ovum completes the cytoplasm of the sperm, and vice versa. Thus, together, they form one whole and complete original unicellular organism; the conceptus, from (and within) which all subsequent multiplications occur. Van der Wal describes the process of spinning as "*a very subtle mutual process of encounter and exchange of signals and substances, which lasts for several hours*".[10] He elevates it from genetic coding reactions to a wondrous

The Sequence of Events

process of recreation at the mutual agreement of the feminine and masculine polarities. A third being, the child, arises when the egg is fertilised and the outer membrane of the egg (zona pellucida; "transparent membrane") shields the conceptus from the outside environment and other sperm.

The entire embryonic process is one of specialisation and *spacialisation,* in that the embryo must form the cavities, tubes, fabrics and membranes, which fold and enfold the organic origami pattern. They all remain connected and continuous, although distinct and differentiated, throughout what Jaap van der Wal calls the "embryonic performance".

Interesting research at Tufts University,[15] in 2011, involved filming the development of a frog embryo using a method that could capture light. The clip shows that what is called "bioelectric signalling" made a holographic light-print in the embryonic tissues. The clip clearly shows a midline and the sensory features of the head, in a moment of illumination. The researchers discovered that if this light-print was interrupted, the tadpole developed abnormally (two heads or two tails, for example). This indicates that the signals interrelate with membrane voltage and pH levels, influencing the forming process of the embryo. Their research suggests this illumination might precede the genetics. Clearly, many questions remain unanswered.

Some geneticists believe this differentiation into form is attributed only to a genetic coding programme, the chemistry of the DNA. Other researchers (epigeneticists) believe that the movements of forces in the forming and growing process create the tension and compression or dynamic fields that participate in shaping the embryo into form. They argue that it is the "movement fields" (kinetic morphology) that initiate which genetic coding patterns get switched on. In other words, what can DNA do without the appropriate cell in which to express itself? Which comes first?

Perhaps we could simplify a little and imagine the genetic codes as "pattern potentials". Since movement is a sign of life, then each vital movement can produce a pattern. Like the colours in a kaleidoscope, there is a limited number of individual, coloured pieces. However, with reflections and shifts of the structure and motion of the kaleidoscope, infinite variety of patterns occur down the viewfinder. Could we imagine that the colours are the genes and the movement of growing presents them in unique patterns, within the blueprint? Perhaps that is a way of seeing how order arises from many different aspects of the apparent chaos of the embryonic forming. We are all unique presentations of our species, which, paradoxically, makes us all the same.

Table 4.1 highlights the key events in the sequence of embryological forming and provides a basic chronological reference for the rate at which changes take place. What is harder to appreciate is that the forming process occurs in 360 degrees and, in fact, many of the processes happen simultaneously. They do not wait for one event to be followed by another in a horizontal timeline. In many of the drawings and schematics of the forming process, the focus is mainly on the actual embryonic germ changing shape (it has to be) within the chambers from which it forms; as it is in continuity with them. What we have to remember is that this is similar to cutting muscles out of their original habitat and placing them separately on the drawing board. Muscles do not function on their own, out of the context of the connecting tissues and fluids they contain and reside in, and nor does the embryo.

"Life makes shapes. These shapes are part of an organising process that embodies emotions, thoughts and experiences into a structure. This structure, in turn, orders the events of existence. Shapes manifest the process of protoplasmic history finding a personal human shape – conception, embryological development and the structures of childhood, adolescence, and adulthood. Molecules, cells, organisms, clusters and colonies are the beginning shapes of life's movement. Later on, a person's shape will be moulded by the internal and external experiences of birth, growth, differentiation, relationships, mating, reproducing, working, problem solving and death. Throughout this process, shape is imprinted by the challenges and stresses of existence. Human shape is marked by love and disappointment."[16]

The Basic Process   The three fundamental principles of the embryonic period are:

- for the cells to flow into the right positions (the first three weeks)
- for the forms to fold and grow the emergent architecture into being (weeks four to eight)
- to orchestrate the organisation of the foundational pattern of the remarkable human blueprint once that form has emerged, from which the development of the neonate can grow and emerge. (It is a continuous process, in continuity.)

Bearing in mind that the wholeness of each stage gives rise to the parts (not the other way around) let us consider each of the eight weeks from conception, including the pre-embryonic period.

Week 1   **Fertilisation** (forming the original unicellular being) takes place in the fallopian tube. The fertilised egg travels to the uterus, as it multiplies within itself, contained by the zona pellucida, into daughter cells (Fig. 4.2).

Cleavage (from uni-cellular to multi-cellular). On the way to the uterus (Fig. 4.2), the uni-cellular chamber (conceptus or zygote) begins to rapidly multiply (from conception) into two identical daughter cells. They will then repeat this process (cleavage) to form eight daughter cells. Each one is whole and complete in itself, with nucleus and cytoplasm, smaller than the cell it multiplied from within (see Ch. 13).

On the fourth multiplication, to sixteen cells, the conceptus forms a ball of cells and is called a blastocyst. The surrounding membrane (zona pellucida) has not expanded in size but encloses the increasing number of smaller and smaller daughter cells (blastomeres). By the seventh or eighth multiplication there are over 100 of these. The blastocyst is called a morula at this stage, meaning "mulberry" shape, although it is in fact still enclosed by the zona pellucida (Fig. 4.3).

Table 4.1
Table of embryonic process showing main features of embryonic development in days

Pre-embryonic Period

Week 1	Day 1	Day 2	Day 3	Day 4	Day 5	Day 6–7
Fertilisation	Fertilised egg; the single-celled conceptus in fallopian tube enclosed by membrane (Zona Pellucida)	1st multiplication into 2 identical cells after (30 hours). More dividing into smaller cells	A ball of over 100 cells in the Zona Pellucida carried along the fallopian tube	A ball made of cells with an outer layer and an inner cell mass (the blastocyst)	Beginning of implantation. The blastocyst must snuggle into the uterine lining	The pre-embryonic journey of the fertilised egg, down the fallopian tube, takes about a week. The cells are dividing within the delicate membrane of the Zona Pellucida until they form into the blastocyst (a ball made of cells), losing the membrane and beginning to implant into the lining of the uterus

Week 2	Day 8	Day 9	Day 10	Day 11–12	Day 13	Day 14
Implantation (the week of twos)	Embedding in uterine lining. This is essential or there is no pregnancy. The outer part of the blastocyst has to establish this direct nourishment to grow	Forming the outer chamber and the cavities that will form the inner chambers	Forming layers and linings of the inner chambers that become the amniotic and primitive yolk sac	Forming connection with the mother through implantation, the blastocyst must send out a tiny root into the uterine lining that will eventually become the placenta. This continues to grow from the structures of the outermost chamber	Chambers within chambers form growing spaces of the amniotic sac that meets the yolk sac, forming inside the outermost chamber	A two-layered disc forms where the upper (amniotic) sac meets the lower (yolk) sac. This interface, where they touch, forms the pre-embryonic disc

Embryonic Period

Week 3	Day 15	Day 16	Day 17	Day 18	Day 19	Day 20	Day 21
Orientation Neurulation, Gastrulation; (the week of threes)	Polarity and orientation arise: head end, tail end and laterality. The primitive streak and node predict the Notochordal axis	Early notochord, predicting future spine, axis for formation and support of the entire embryonic forming process	Growth rates pull the upper and lower layers of the pre-embryonic disc apart. Cells pour into the gap from the upper layer	The upper (ectoderm), the middle (mesoderm) and lower layer (endoderm) form 3-layered embryonic disc and notochord	Central Nervous System is induced where spinal cord will grow	Neural tube formation and the somites begin to form. They are organs of the body wall: 360° forming vertebral organisation and the axial body	The heart starts above the crown of the embryonic disc: so-called at this point for the tri-laminar disc that is formed

Week 4	Day 22	Day 23	Day 17–28	Day 26	Day 27	Day 28	
	Neural tube closure begins. Number of somites increasing from head towards tail	Heart pumps the rapidly growing brain, intimately relating the circulatory and neural growth functions	The Folds; Head Fold, Tail Fold and Lateral Fold shape the form and inner cavities of the head and torso. Meanwhile the outer (chorionic) sac grows and the placenta develops	Pharyngeal arches appear and lung buds begin inside the anlage of the thorax	Somites, important transient features of segmentation, grow the embryo. (Number of pairs denotes age)	Neural tube complete. Primitive anlage of ear and eye structures appear	
Week 5 **2nd Month** **5–8 mm**	Day 29	Day 30	Day 31	Day 32	Day 33	Day 34	Day 35
	Arm buds and (about 2 days later) leg buds forming from body. Lung buds forming inside	Developing gut tube from membrane to membrane that will form the mouth and anus at either end	Embryo in flexion as it expands into growing chambers	Umbilical ring forms. Body stalk grows	The heart grows and body begins to form more recognisable proportions	The eyes appear in the cranial formation, initially oriented more laterally.	The lungs develop further as the anlage of the pleural cavity and bronchial apparatus. Thorax forms a primitive breathing pattern
Week 6 **10–14 mm**	Day 36	Day 37	Day 38	Day 39	Day 40	Day 41	Day 42
	Umbilicus forms	Face develops more detail and organisation	Myofascial development (according to the somitic segments) and differentiation	Visceral development and differentiation: e.g. liver filters blood to heart	Ear structures develop for balance and hearing	Differentiation of the heart. Atrial septum formed	Differentiation of the hand digits then the foot. They begin as paddles and transform via four interspacings
Week 7 **17–22 mm**	Day 43	Day 44	Day 45	Day 46	Day 47	Day 48	Day 49
	Limb differentiation and digital rays of the fingers and toes, more detail	Development of the face and cranial formation	Detail of the heart more developed	Expansion of placenta, as chorionic cavity grows	External genitalia appear	Facial prominences fused	Hands, fingers, feet and toes present, eyelids forming, upper lip forming
Week 8 **28–30 mm**	Day 50–56						
	Limbs lengthen proportionately and fold at knees and elbows. Fingers and toes are free and face becomes more clearly organised and proportioned as recognisably human. Tail disappears and umbilicus forms						

Fetal Period (from 9th week onwards)

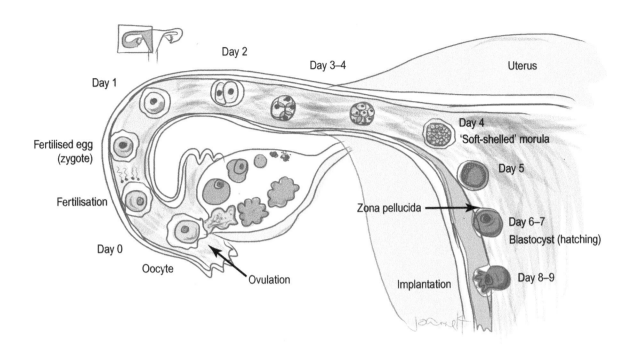

Figure 4.2

The journey of the conceptus (zygote) from fertilisation to implantation (Days 1–9 approximately).

The fact that this is called a morula may be one of the fundamental reasons that embryogenesis is so variously described and confusing in the literature. A morula is a mulberry – an open design, like a raspberry or such fruit, with no surrounding membrane. The surrounding membrane (the zona pellucida) means this structure is not a morula at all. It is a pocket of cells, inside a connective tissue membrane, within which are contained (bound) fluids. That containment creates the "in between stuff" (mesenchyme) of the embryo and is actually the precursor of the circulatory system. Without the membrane, we have no containment for the proliferation of daughter cells to begin the blueprint. For a beautiful presentation of this sequence, albeit in another species, Jan van Ijken[17] has made a film in timelapse photography of a salamander or

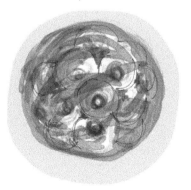

Figure 4.3

The blastocyst, a ball of cells, is still wrapped in its containing membrane (the zona pellucida), a significant aspect of the primitive circulatory processes of fluids between the cells.

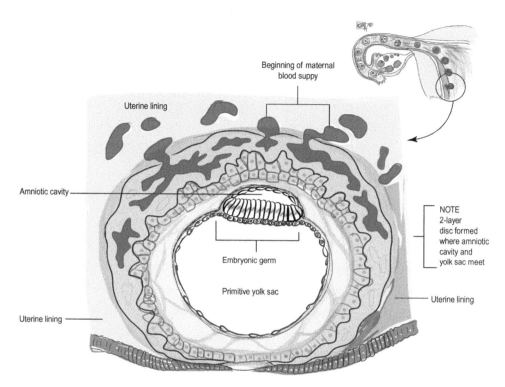

Beginning of maternal
blood suppy

Uterine lining

Amniotic cavity

NOTE
2-layer
disc formed
where amniotic
cavity and
yolk sac meet

Uterine lining

Embryonic germ

Primitive yolk sac

Uterine lining

Figure 4.4

In this sketch the tiny outermost chamber implants within which the sacs of the innermost chambers are forming.

Week 2

newt embryo forming. This will give you a wonderful sense of the massive proliferation of cells, within transparent membranes. It also begins to iterate the rapid, simultaneous multi-dimensional processes of development. Watch and see how impossible this is to describe!

The fertilised egg must snuggle into the uterine lining and literally implant itself. Mother and future embryo respond to each other chemically, kinaesthetically and proprioceptively in multiple subtle exchanges. They form specialised circulations to provide nourishment (including nutrients and oxygen) at the rate the embryo will be able to receive it and send out its own circulatory by-products of metabolism (waste and carbon dioxide).

Implantation. The ball of cells then changes itself into a ball formed of cells with a distinct "outerness" and an inner cell mass around a cavity. It must reach and implant itself in the uterine lining (Fig. 4.4), where it has to suckle its way in to becoming impregnated.

Post-implantation. Implantation confirms the pregnancy. Described as the "week of twos", in this second week the biodynamic origami begins, and folds form into pockets inside the earlier ball, made of cells. An upper cavity forms that will become the amniotic sac and the lower cavity will become the yolk sac, inside the surrounding (chorionic) chamber. This statement grossly over-simplifies a complex sequence in which the embryo forms its own "living accommodation" within (and from) which to grow.

As mentioned earlier, the fascinating aspect of this that is hard to appreciate from two-dimensional schema is that the embryonic germ itself forms from the interface where these two main inner sacs (amnios and yolk) meet. The initial germinating pre-embryo is the in-between – the meeting place where these two "soft bubbles" touch. The embryonic disc actually derives its upper and lower laminae from where the outer membranes (of the amniotic and yolk sacs) contact each other (Fig. 4.5).

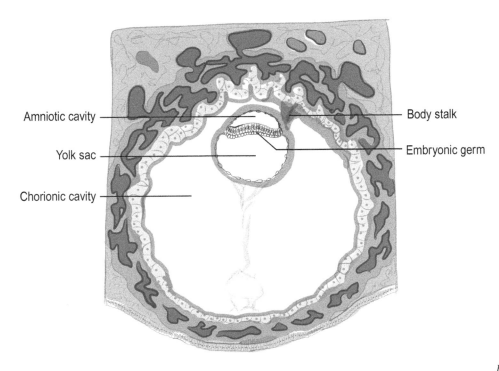

Amniotic cavity

Body stalk

Yolk sac

Embryonic germ

Chorionic cavity

Figure 4.5

Pockets within pockets. The embryo itself is formed where the two main inner sacs meet. It is not a separate seed or a germ between their layers. It is their layers.

Image modified after T.W. Sadler, *Langman's Medical Embryology* (see note 23).

Always in the round: the "embryonic disc" is named in advance of its clarified form. It is not a disc that ends at its edges; it appears two-laminaed where these two sacs touch each other. They remain whole. The embryonic "disc-shape" remains the lower aspect of the upper sphere (amniotic sac) and the upper aspect of the lower sphere (yolk sac) in continuity with each, throughout its growth. They acquire different textures and densities to the amniotic and yolk membrane, incorporating one and being incorporated by the other through the process we will now attempt to describe – however, they never separate from them until birth; they remain in complete continuity.

Membranes will form to "join" them, that will eventually become the mouth and anus at either end of the gut tube, when it has formed in the folding sequences. Once the embryo has grown and folded laterally and longitudinally into tubes within tubes to form the body, it will begin to resemble a developing fetus. At this stage before the folding begins it is *apparently* a two-laminaed disc. When the embryo folds (week 4), it will take these chambers with it, remaining part of them. It folds around the lower one as it is enfolded by the upper one. Thus, it is formed from the continuity of its own architectural continuum. It is self-assembled and self-animated.

Before this embryonic folding sequence can happen, the pre-embryonic disc has to become a volume, by creating a middle. (We might say it "spacialises" into outermost, innermost and in between.) First, however, it has to gather coordinates from which to orientate, in order to organise.

Week 3   **(a) Orientation, (b) gastrulation and (c) neurulation.** Three key processes happen in this third week. The so-called disc also develops orientation with a head end, a tail end and sides (laterality). This predicts an axis, around which the subsequent

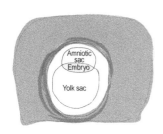

In fact, the different growth rates, mean the outer membrane (from the attached end where the food is closest) grows faster and rounds out over the inner membrane, as they move apart. Between them, an inner "spacialisation" forms, creating a volumetric whole tubular (soft-tissue) architecture. Van der Wal[18] calls this the "innerness" or the "meso" and refutes the term "layer" or "derm" as a misleading way of describing something that isn't layered. In fact, it is more toroidal (donut shaped), the outside and the inside being in continuous continuity; the "meso" describes the volume within the toroidal shape, or morphology.

developmental progress will evolve. It is generally referred to as a "two-laminaed disc becomes a three-laminaed (trilaminar) disc" of the true embryo.

This process is called *gastrulation*. The third process in week three is neurulation, which refers to the formation of the brain and spinal cord.

From a biodynamic point of view, this "enclosure" within a containing membrane is an important distinction because it influences the motion of the internal fluids and shape changes between the cells, in the tension–compression, close packing matrix of the micro-network. It might correlate to a very primitive form of the micro-vacuoles seen in *Interior Architectures*, by Jean-Claude Guimberteau.[19]

Let us consider these stages one at a time:

(a) Orientation. Perhaps we are drawn to the spine in yoga because it is one of our primal and primary features of orientation, present even before the pre-embryonic stage of development is complete. A midline (called the primitive streak) forms in the uppermost membrane of the bilaminar disc identifying axes: a left and a right side, a head and a tail end. (At this time the embryo is about 0.23 mm in length.) We might consider this original organisation as our "null point" (Fig. 4.6)[20]. It remains our movement reference throughout our lives. It is something we consciously explore in yoga practice and recognise in positions of the chakras along the spine (see Ch. 12).

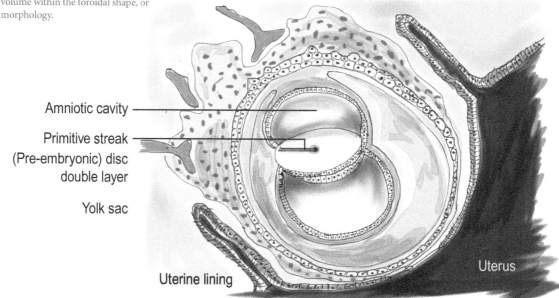

Figure 4.6

The flat embryonic two-layered (bilaminar) disc within its growing chamber. As Blechschmidt describes in The Ontogenetic Basis of Human Anatomy (see note 3): "the apex of the axial process can be considered as the centre or, better, the null point of the developmental movements of the whole [bi-laminar] disc. The apex of the axial process provides a natural reference for interpreting all subsequent biomechanical movements and the action of biodynamic forces."

Modified after images available from the following website, where an excellent chronological visual presentation can be found: www.bionalogy.com/human_embryology.htm

Imagine a blue water* balloon placed on top of a yellow water* balloon. Where the blue balloon touches the yellow balloon, there will be a green-coloured disc, the soft ovoid shape where the two layers come together. Where they meet is going to become the upper and lower membrane of the pre-embryonic disc. Its upper lamina is the lowest part of the blue balloon. Its lower lamina is the upper part of the yellow one; they remain in continuity with the original balloon (amniotic and yolk sacs) throughout the pregnancy.

This delicate structure will eventually include the formation of the placenta, the "other end" of the umbilical cord, where food and oxygen will be supplied for the duration of the pregnancy.

(b) Gastrulation. The upper membrane (lowest "bowl-shape" of the amniotic sac) of the tiny germ grows the most rapidly. It is nearest the source of nourishment. The lower membrane (which in 2D is the upper curve of the yolk sac, in 3D the uppermost "cap-shape") grows more slowly. It is furthest away from the food supply. These differing growth-rates animate cause the formation of volume, as they grow apart from each other and the "middle" or *meso* forms between them:

"as a consequence of rapid differential growth, the ectoblast [upper] glides away from the hypoblast [lower] and an intermediate lamina of loose tissue forms between them. Thus from a biomechanical point of view, the tissue at this depth is strained under tension in a circular and radial direction as the conceptus enlarges. As far as the cells of this intermediate lamina are concerned, they become flatter and this leads to a loss of their intracellular fluid. This fluid collects together in the interstices as intercellular substance. In this way the tissue becomes reticulated or honeycombed. The network is the middle blastocyst form."[21]

It is noteworthy when we consider the self-assembly of the embryonic form that, as van der Wal points out, the embryonic version of us must also assemble the placenta. There is a quality of awareness that must focus outwardly to the primitive "kinesphere" and animate the formation of the placenta *to a point*, where it must return and focus attentively upon the "innersphere" to grow its own architecture. In radial terms we might say *these qualities of attention move centrifugally and centripetally*. These are keys to understanding movement and breath *in the round* that we will explore later; however, they are important *turning points* in our original developmental process. The placenta, initially, does the functioning that the embryo must gradually *incorporate* through the process of self-assembly. According to van der Wal, attention must *approximate* full expansion (outward focus) and then turn towards a counter-balancing inward focus at the appropriate time. If this fails, the issue corresponds to the timing points of miscarriage at 6 and 12 weeks.

The cells from the upper (*ectodermal*) lamina subsequently lose some of their close-packed organisation or structure (de-epithelialise) as that membrane opens out radially (thus *spacialising them*) and cells pour into the space created between the two laminae, through the primitive streak (Figs 4.7 and 4.8). The first to arrive form the *true endoderm* by restructuring their close organisation. Thereafter, they fill the space between the lower membrane (endoderm) and the upper membrane, thus becoming the middle. The upper membrane becomes the definitive ectoderm, while the middle layer is called the mesoderm – which is misleading, because it is never a layer; it is an intermediating volume, essentially, *between* layers; that van der Wal calls "inner-ness".

(c) Neurulation (Fig. 4.9) is the transformation of the neural plate into the neural tube. In concert with the central part of the middle-ness or *meso* (paraxial), the upper (ectodermal) lamina has to fold back on itself along the midline and form the neural tube; a distinct tube, within the longitudinal shape of the forming torso. It does this by invaginating and joining the fold edges (like a zip) along its length. It eventually encloses and forms what will become the spinal cord, longitudinally. The somites, formed from within the paraxial mesoderm, line either side of the neural tube and will form from the base of the cranium position, growing towards the tail, in pairs, dividing the spine into segments. The number of pairs of somites gives rise to the age of the embryo, predicting and incorporating the length and structures of the torso, or (*axial*) body.

This sequence confirms the formation of what are called the "three germ layers" but in fact, in biodynamic terms, the middle part of the embryo represents many aspects of entering three dimensions. The transformation of the two-layered (bilaminar) germ disc into a what is called a "three-layered (trilaminar) disc" is the transition from the pre-embryonic stages to the true

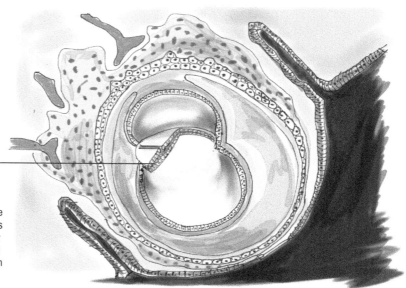

To form mesoderm (middle) cells from the epiblast invade the area between the upper lamina (ectoderm) and lower lamina (endoderm)

Cells pour in through the primitive streak due to different growth rates between the upper and lower laminae pulling them apart and creating a volume between them

There is total dependency upon the mother for nourishment and oxygen. From a structural point of view, there is also a need for containment, with the biodynamic forces of invaginating containers and limiting tissues. The womb, the soft tissue of the abdominal wall and the framework of the pelvis will play a containing role for the growing fetus similar (though on a different scale) to the zona pellucida for the blastocyst. Thus, the balance of forces is maintained in a living tensegrity pattern as the growth function expands and the limiting tissues constrain the growth, offering a reciprocal force transmission, *in the round*. The growth tensions the constraining tissues, while the tissues offer compression (to provide the resistance forces) needed to feed back the biological pattern process. It is relentless, as it will be after the birth, albeit in a different amplitude of forces. *In utero* the embryo is in a fluid, gravity free environment – however the forces of tension and compression are working together to provide the *force transmission pattern* that the embryonic matter (or biomaterial) must learn to incorporate. After birth, the neonate will effectively be "wrapped in gravity".

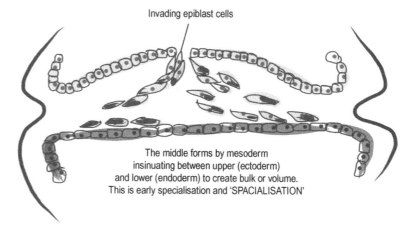

Invading epiblast cells

The middle forms by mesoderm insinuating between upper (ectoderm) and lower (endoderm) to create bulk or volume. This is early specialisation and 'SPACIALISATION'

Figures 4.7 and 4.8

Cells from the upper (epiblast) membrane pour through the primitive streak into the space forming between the upper and lower membranes.

Modified after images available from the following website, where an excellent chronological visual presentation can be found: www.bionalogy.com/human_embryology.htm

embryo. The three main classifications for what the membranes will become are as follows:

- The upper membrane (ECTODERM) becomes the brain, spinal cord, nervous system and skin.

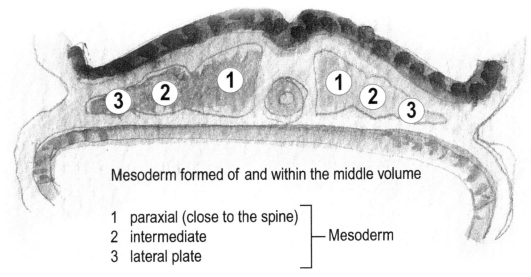

Mesoderm formed of and within the middle volume

1   paraxial (close to the spine) ⎤
2   intermediate   ⎥— Mesoderm
3   lateral plate   ⎦

Figure 4.9

The neural tube forms from the ectodermal membrane folding back upon itself, along its length (C shows how this begins in cross-section). See Fig. 4.15 for a longitudinal view.

The mesoderm. This middle layer (mesoderm) does not form a "derm" (layer) quite like the other two layers, above and below it. The network that the middle layer forms is a loose aggregate (of unstructured, *de-epithelialised* cells) called mesenchyme. It could be thought of as a "mesenchymal milieu" of potential building materials. These include blood cells and other connective tissue and fascia. The cells, such as those producing fascia, muscle, cartilage and bone and "biomaterial" of all the organs and vessels, are contained in and integrated with the connective tissues. They respond to the shapes and forces of the containing forms. These are the architectural components of the forms within and around the forming body walls and cavities. Mesenchymal cells can migrate and move around, serving and mediating the process of formation. This *meso* contains these undifferentiated "forming potentials" that respond kinetically and genetically to various signals, forces of growth and metabolic movement; i.e. responding to the

- The middle aspect (MESODERM) becomes the body wall, cavities, muscles, bones, connective tissues and blood, including the spine and limbs later.
- The lower membrane (ENDODERM) becomes the gut tube, from mouth to anus.

In the process of forming, the embryo can create structure and release it. This means it can close-pack cells together to form a membrane or lining (epithelialise) or release them into a looser aggregate of cells (de-epithelialise). In this way, tissue can respond to changes in genetic chemistry, signals, forces, growth patterns and position by structuralising and destructuralising appropriately. Blechschmidt[22] identifies "metabolic growth fields" that significantly influence our shape-changing movements (kinetic morphology). Fluids and membranes are formed into primitive precursors of networks, systems and structures where some tissues are pulled apart and others are pushed together, folding and expanding, tensioning and compressing, thickening and spiraling, at different rates, but always connected. It is an organic, living tensegrity volume, self-organising its way into form.

The mesoderm subdivides spatially, through its bioorganic origami process of folding (remember nothing separates from the wholeness) either side of the forming central axis into: (1) *paraxial mesoderm* (closest to the central axis), which becomes segmented into somites, predicting the vertebrae (see later); (2) intermediate mesoderm, which will give rise to parts of the shape-changes. This is the pattern of our species, that comes to be uniquely expressed by each one of us in the matter of our fabric; the architecture of our architect self-assembling.

Mesenchyme is defined as "any loosely organised tissue composed of fibroblast-like cells and extracellular matrix regardless of the origin of the cells".[23] It is thought to represent the primitive extracellular matrix of the future adult form. (It is inclusive of the cells in the embryo.) This *meso*, containing the mesenchyme, forms the "connectedness" that holds the

urogenital system; (3) lateral plate mesoderm (outermost), which becomes divided into two parts, mainly due to the excessive growth of the embryo. One membrane becomes associated with the uppermost, ectoderm (*somatic mesoderm*) and the other gets tensioned away from the somatic mesoderm to form in association with the endoderm (*splanchnic mesoderm*). Some lateral plate mesoderm also invades the developing limb buds. These membranes specifically form the shapes, spaces and characteristics of our head, body, viscera and limbs; once the folds are in place the tubes can spiral their way into form, according to the genetic and kinetic patterns of self-assembly.

Within the mesoderm. The mesoderm also divides itself spatially, into three further aspects, either side of the central axis, out to the lateral edges (Fig. 4.10). As it forms, specialised cells move towards the head and form the

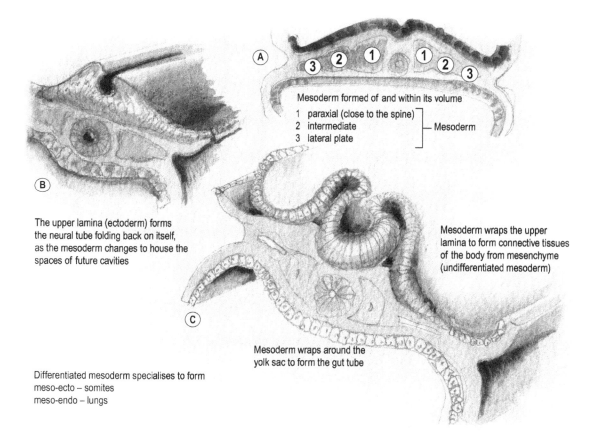

(A)

Mesoderm formed of and within its volume
1 paraxial (close to the spine)
2 intermediate   — Mesoderm
3 lateral plate

(B)

The upper lamina (ectoderm) forms the neural tube folding back on itself, as the mesoderm changes to house the spaces of future cavities

Mesoderm wraps the upper lamina to form connective tissues of the body from mesenchyme (undifferentiated mesoderm)

(C)

Mesoderm wraps around the yolk sac to form the gut tube

Differentiated mesoderm specialises to form
meso-ecto – somites
meso-endo – lungs

Figure 4.10

The other mesoderm cells, which form from the primitive streak, move out from the central axis and form inner (paraxial), in-between (intermediate) and more lateral mesoderm (lateral plate mesoderm).

other two membranes together, forms pockets within them and at the same time keeps them apart. They are not so much separate entities as structuralisations (membranes) around a middle aspect that plays a role in the structure of all our forms.

Week 4

"The primary connective tissue of the body is the embryonic mesoderm. The mesoderm represents the matrix and environment within which the organs and structures of the body have been differentiated and, in fact, are 'embedded' … in harmony with the view that the principal function of mesoderm as 'inner tissue' is 'mediating' in the sense of 'connecting' (binding) and 'disconnecting' (shaping space and enabling movement)."[24]

prechordal plate, which is important in forebrain development, and the notochord. This predicts the spine and acts as a longitudinal support for the early embryo as well as a signalling centre for certain molecules. These play a part in activating and instructing cells in what to do and which specific tissues to form, according to the genetic blueprint. The next stage concerns bringing the basic human form into being, predicting the placement of the human anatomy and physiology.

This week includes the formation of the somites – transient features of the embryo that play a fundamental role in the structure of the spine. It is also the week of folding into form and developing the placenta.

The tiny heart awakens in concert with the somites (Fig. 4.11), orchestrating growth of the spinal structures and body walls, folding and forming in 360 degrees. This in turn causes the whole embryonic disc to fold laterally and longitudinally, growing omnidirectionally from the central axis, wrapping the body form around the heart.

The ectoderm will form the tissues relating to our response to the outside world, that is, our outer skin and our innermost spinal cord, and the nervous system. It is evident that it does not do this separately in layers. Indeed, since all the cells forming the true endoderm and the meso arise from the ectoderm, the embryo invites us to consider that they would all be sensory in nature and provide our inner sense of the outer world. (Perhaps also our outer expression of our inner world?) They may form into specific structures, but the forming materials and processes all arise from the same original membranes, indeed, the one unicellular organism.

With the forming potentials in place as three aspects (so-called *derms*) and three aspects of orientation (on either side of centre in the middle volume), the embryo creates its length (from head to tail), its depth (from back to front) and its roundness of volumetric form by buckling (folding), taking the (upper membrane) amniotic sac with it whilst enfolding the (lower membrane) yolk sac.

The midline of the developing notochord, neural tube and somites stiffen the back orientation (dorsal axis) supporting the embryo as a more densely textured feature of its architecture, still in complete continuity as it is self-assembled from a fold in the ectoderm (lower part of the amnios). The head end, the tail end and the lateral margins all grow around and fold to become the front and sides of the embryonic body. (They bring the whole amniotic sac they are contained within with them, so that the embryo grows inside it, surrounded by it and expanding into it.)

There are three named folds: *head*, *tail* and *lateral*. These attempt to explain this biodynamic origami so that it can be understood in all its three-dimensional (360 degrees) shape-changing patterns.

Embryonic Folding

The **head fold** is first (Fig. 4.12). The embryo grows forwards and gradually buckles underneath, bringing the heart from beyond the crown to the front

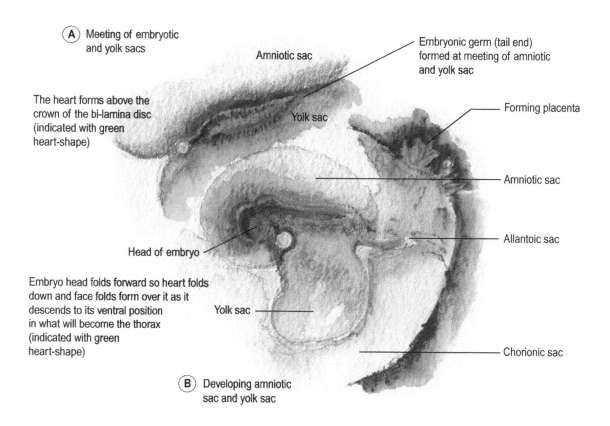

Ⓐ Meeting of embryotic and yolk sacs

Amniotic sac

Embryonic germ (tail end) formed at meeting of amniotic and yolk sac

The heart forms above the crown of the bi-lamina disc (indicated with green heart-shape)

Yolk sac

Forming placenta

Amniotic sac

Head of embryo

Allantoic sac

Embryo head folds forward so heart folds down and face folds form over it as it descends to its ventral position in what will become the thorax (indicated with green heart-shape)

Yolk sac

Chorionic sac

Ⓑ Developing amniotic sac and yolk sac

Figure 4.11

The heart starts above the crown. These two paintings illustrate where the amniotic sac meets the yolk sac, which become the developing embryo.

of the body (ventral); the body walls will form around it. A small portion of the yolk sac becomes enclosed with this fold, incorporating the future foregut (*pharynx*).

Lateral fold. The folding of the lateral sides of the embryo (along its length, making it a lateral fold) comes around the front towards the midline, creating a more cylindrical embryo (Fig. 4.13). As the abdominal wall forms, part of the yolk sac becomes enclosed and incorporated into the embryo as the mid gut (the anlage of the small intestine) and the beginnings of the abdominal (peritoneal) cavity. Mesenchyme and somites form the developing torso segmentally.

Tail fold. The tail region of the embryo is last to fold (Fig. 4.14). It grows backwards, lengthening the axial body and effectively drawing the back of the diaphragm down with it as the somites grow towards the tail. It also buckles under the rest of the embryo, bringing the body stalk onto the ventral surface of the embryo and incorporating the hind gut.

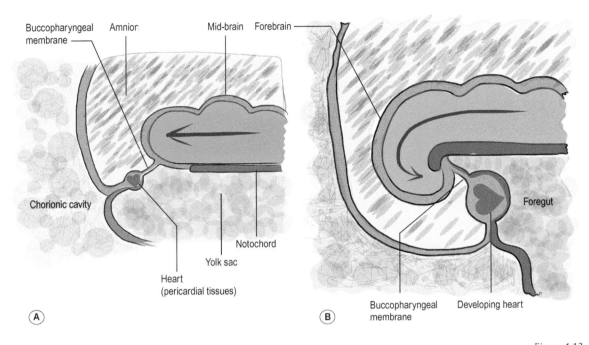

Figure 4.12

The head fold brings the heart to the front of the body.

Folding Consequences

The consequences of this process of folding are that the ectoderm, which was the outer or upper membrane of the embryo, now covers the entire embryo except for the body stalk (Fig. 4.15). The heart and the body stalk are located at the front of the embryonic body because of the head and tail fold. The body stalk will form the umbilicus. Finally during this folding process, parts of the yolk sac become incorporated into the embryo. These gradually form into the gut regions, in concert with the meso (*mesoderm*), the *volume* of the forming torso and future limb buds.

Somites: The Spinal "Spacing"

The growth of the brain, spinal cord and central nervous system is critical for somite development, differentiation and specification (Fig. 4.16). The somites are related to the timing and spacing of how the body walls form (genetically and kinetically) and how the internal spaces, or volumes are enclosed and segmented. They also play a role in limb formation.

Week 5

This developmental week marks the appearance of the limb buds on the outside and growth of the lung buds on the inside.

The lung buds first appear as an outgrowth from the front wall of the foregut, at which stage the anlage of the respiratory organs, the liver bud and the stomach is closely situated around the heart. Remember, they all remain in

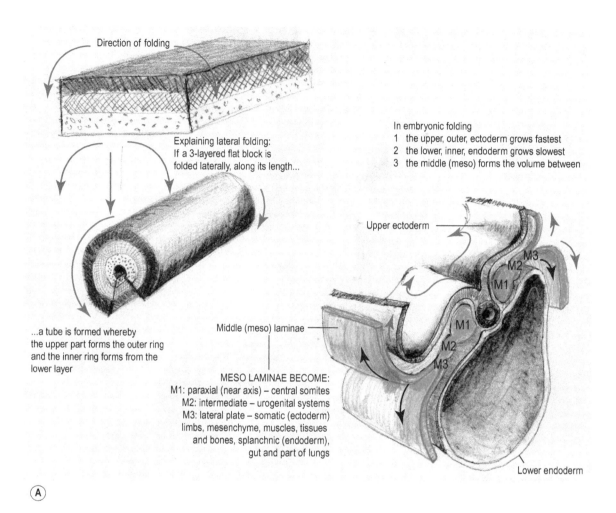

Direction of folding

Explaining lateral folding:
If a 3-layered flat block is
folded laterally, along its length...

In embryonic folding
1 the upper, outer, ectoderm grows fastest
2 the lower, inner, endoderm grows slowest
3 the middle (meso) forms the volume between

Upper ectoderm

M3
M2
M1

M1
M2
M3

...a tube is formed whereby
the upper part forms the outer ring
and the inner ring forms from the
lower layer

Middle (meso) laminae

MESO LAMINAE BECOME:
M1: paraxial (near axis) – central somites
M2: intermediate – urogenital systems
M3: lateral plate – somatic (ectoderm)
limbs, mesenchyme, muscles, tissues
and bones, splanchnic (endoderm),
gut and part of lungs

Lower endoderm

(A)

Figure 4.13 (A)

Explaining the lateral fold.

complete continuity. At no point does anything in this process separate from the original membranous continuum. The cartilage, myofascial and connective tissue components of the lungs are derived from the so-called *mesodermal layer* (see note under *Lateral fold*; margin Fig. 4.13B) – as a continuity of the fabric forming the volume of the torso.

Biodynamic growing forces (tension and compression) are also considered to contribute to the formation of the lungs, *suctioned* outwards into the growing space around the heart that was formed in the folding described. Originating from the endodermal tissues, continuous with them, the meso forms the sacs of the pleural cavities (from mesenchyme) and the lung buds grow

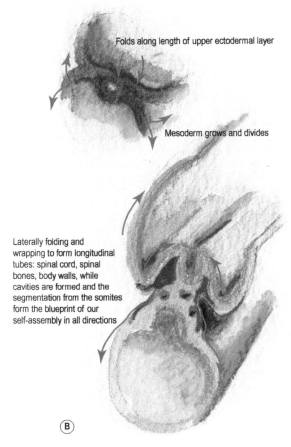

Folds along length of upper ectodermal layer

Mesoderm grows and divides

Laterally folding and
wrapping to form longitudinal
tubes: spinal cord, spinal
bones, body walls, while
cavities are formed and the
segmentation from the somites
form the blueprint of our
self-assembly in all directions

Figure 4.13 (B)

The lateral fold.

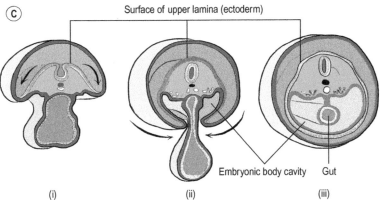

Surface of upper lamina (ectoderm)

Embryonic body cavity   Gut

(i)
Lateral folding begins

(ii)
Shows the connection
between the gut and
the yolk sac

(iii)
Shows the closed (ventral)
abdominal wall; the gut is
suspended from the back
(dorsal) abdominal wall

Figure 4.13 (C)

Image modified after T.W. Sadler,
Langman's Medical Embryology (see
note 23).

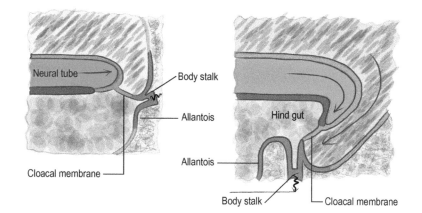

Figure 4.14

The tail fold.

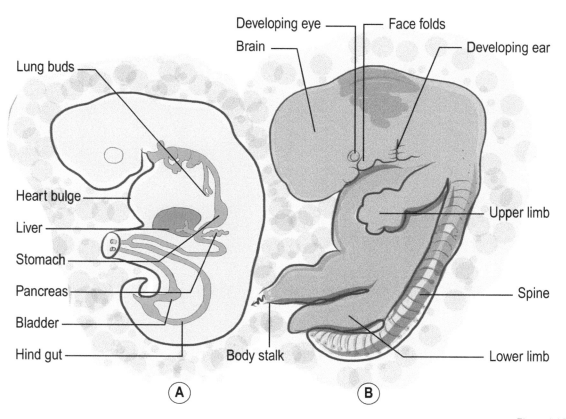

Figure 4.15

The folded embryo showing (A) some of the gut development at approximately Day 31 and (B) the formation of the face folds; developing ear and eye (approximately Day 36). The hand and upper limb are forming before the foot and lower limb.

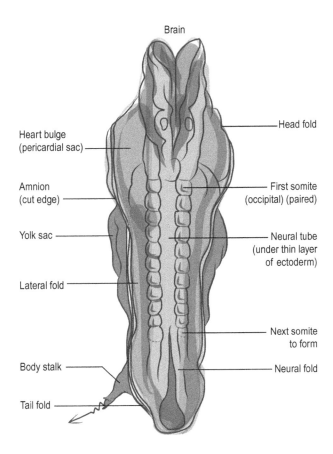

Brain

Head fold

Heart bulge
(pericardial sac)

First somite
(occipital) (paired)

Amnion
(cut edge)

Neural tube
(under thin layer
of ectoderm)

Yolk sac

Lateral fold

Next somite
to form

Body stalk

Neural fold

Tail fold

Figure 4.16

The somites grow from the cranial base towards the tail. Each pair predicts the upper and lower half of subjacent vertebrae, prescribing the spaces between them in the spine. They also grow and form the body wall; tubes within tubes and pockets within pockets. They play a primary role in designating the formation of what we might think of as our "growth rings" as well as their segmental arrangement. It is in 360 degrees.

with the tracheal lining inside their own compartment, or fold or pocket in the fabric. Organised in part by the growing heart, nourished by it, and reciprocally enclosed by the pericardial sac, they will grow to fill the thoracic cavity together, nourished by the blood supply that is also formed from the same living matrix. (It is almost too miraculous to imagine.)

During this folding sequence, there is a "gap" (there are no empty spaces in this process; remember it is a virtual gap or a "preparing pocket") that forms in the outermost part of the middle volume (*lateral plate mesoderm*), within which it subdivides into two more membranes or pockets. This location in the 360-degree volume of continuous membrane becomes an *internal cavity*. This internal cavity then divides again into the primitive heart (*pericardial cavity,* to pericardial sac) and the abdominal (*peritoneal cavity, to peritoneal sac*). They become distinct, although connected to each other by two channels, into which the primitive lung buds form another pocket (*pleural cavity to pleural sac*). Folds form within these biodynamic origamis. They wrap the heart and form between the lung buds and developing mid gut. At the same time they join with a thick membrane (a condensation of meso material) called the septum transversum (meaning "separating across"). This septum transversum will become the respiratory diaphragm through the intricate growth patterns that ensue. *It remains continuous with the abdominal visceral pockets, that form the pockets we name for the viscera.* Thus, what began as a continuous tube-like structure differentiates into three distinct pockets, although they remain continuously connected. They are called cavities as if they are separate from each other, but they never separate – nothing does. The pleural and pericardial cavities become differentiated and divided from the future peritoneal cavity by the textures of the forms, thickenings and densifications, between them. They become the main containers of the upper and lower body cavities. The changing, growing kinetic and genetic signals cause myofascial cells to infiltrate these tissues and the "crossing divider" (the septum transversum) becomes the future diaphragm, forming the roof of the abdominal cavity and the base of the thoracic cavity. They are distinct pockets; the intestines will form in the lower peritoneal pocket, remaining always integrated with the heart and lungs above it, in *their* respective pockets. The diaphragm is then tensioned downward (caudally) at the back by the growth direction of the somites, as they predict the formation of the spine, growing towards the tail, folding under the body as they lengthen. Where this septum transversum is attached to the front of the spine will become the legs (crura) of the diaphragm. In yoga practice we seek to unite breath and motion: the waves of the breath and the movement of the spine. The embryo guides us to recognise that their structures emerge from their original unity and remain continuously organised as such.

"The very development of the respiratory tract and the lung is therefore a remarkably differentiated beginning of the subsequent activity we call breathing. Strictly speaking it is incorrect to talk of the 'first' inspiration after birth. Breathing movements, by which air is sucked in and expelled from the lungs, are late consequences of the most complicated processes that were established and regulated long before birth."[25]

Somites are considered to be transient features of the embryo (they come and go during the embryonic period). They initiate tremendous change and transformation in that time. They form in pairs from the base of the cranium towards the tail, in concert with the mesenchymal meso, into regions. These regions will become the parts of the outermost skin (dermatomes), the inner bones of the spine (sclerotomes) and the muscles and connective tissues between them (myotomes). Between them, there is now research suggesting, they are fasciatomes.[26] Some of the somitic cells also migrate to enter the developing limbs.

Somites are particularly significant for our understanding of the spine. It is a common misunderstanding that a pair of somites gives rise to either side of a single vertebra. They certainly contribute to the length and depth of the spine in sequenced intervals; however, they do not simply predict bony blocks. They prescribe the spaces between the vertebrae, where nerves exit and linking facets form. Each pair of somites represents what will become the lower half of one vertebra and the upper half of the subjacent vertebra.[27] They create the feature of vertebral segmentation, predicting placement of ribs, discs and organising tissues of the body wall. They are "spacialisers" for future forms, rather than structures.

The limbs. As the embryo develops roundness, there is an ectodermal ring all around the outside, like a kind of "side seam" of the embryonic body. As cavities form inside, limb buds appear at the upper and lower points of the torso. At first, they grow as undifferentiated mesenchymal buds, eventually growing away from the torso and forming flat, paddle-like structures (the pre-plan of the hands and feet).

In this fifth week there is further differentiation of the eyes and detail of the beginnings of the mouth and jaw formation.

If you imagine putting your hand into a thick, strong surgical glove while someone holds it, pushing your fingers into the glove-skin, as it is held back (pretend it is attached over your shoulder to the breast bone and spine) – push hard and you will effectively be using your arm and hand as "bones" and the glove as "skin". It will feel something like a trampoline, all around your upper limb. You can readily imagine, then, how the piston-like growth of the "inner tube" of the limb (cartilage that is yet to be compressed

Week 6

By this time, there is more detailed formation of the ear and development of the torso myofascial architecture.

As the young limb buds appear they are fed from the heart, vascularised by circulatory vessels in the tissues (all of which grow from the same original tissue, so it is quite a remarkable orchestration of movement and organisation that the heart rhythm syncopates and accompanies). The anlage of the bone (which is mostly cartilage until suitable forces are put through it, *ex utero*) grows in a piston-like manner outward, while the softer-textured tissue is limited or constrained and tethered by the growth of the blood vessels (from the heart) on the medial side. Blechschmidt[28] suggests that this contributes to the chirality of the limbs; the natural growth pattern of a medially rotated lower arm. Essentially, between them, these forces provide the tension and compression field of natural, spiral patterning of close-packed systems in volume.

into bone) tensions the fabric of the "outer tube" tissues (myofascia and skin), which keeps the inner tube compressed in a reciprocal dance (of a living tensegrity pattern). This also keeps the limbs restrained in a semi-folded *pre-tensioned* architecture. That is the basis of what anatomy refers to as a *pre-stiffened* form. Baby is born in this naturally folded expression that predicts where the cartilage will densify into bone–joint–bone continuity, deep within the limbs and torso, when forces guide it accordingly – it will condense into a variety of textures, all made from the fascial foundation. (See Chapter 6, where we consider these different manifestations of fascial fabrics.)

Also, at this time in the embryonic sequence, the heart becomes more differentiated; also thought to spiral into formation from one "cardio-myofascial" tube, into the complex, four-chambered vessel it becomes. The limbs grow (under tension) and grooves in the hand and foot paddles appear. In the following week, these will become spaces between the digits. (We might call this further differentiation in the process of spacialisation.)

Week 7

The rays of the fingers and toes become apparent (Fig. 4.17), and the eyelids begin to form. The eye primordium is completely embedded in mesenchyme, while fibres of the neural retina converge towards the optic nerve. The face begins to change, as the facial prominences fuse (the meeting of the lateral

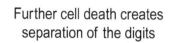

Cell death creates
a ridge for each digit

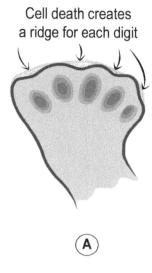

Further cell death creates
separation of the digits

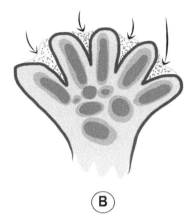

Separation of the
digits is complete

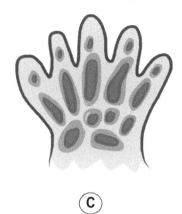

(A)

Developmental week 6
Approximately 48 days

(B)

Approximately 51 days

(C)

Approximately 56 days

Figure 4.17

From a paddle shape, the hand begins to develop as spaces are formed between digits.

folds) and the jaw and nasal swellings form the upper lip. Once again, it is worth noting that nothing has been added or taken away. All this from the original amniotic and yolk sacs, meeting and folding in genetic and kinetic patterns of 360 degrees of roundness.

Week 8 The limbs become longer and bent at the elbows and knees, with fingers and toes free to move individually (Fig. 4.18). In van der Wal's way of seeing, they form the "disjoints" in the continuity of the soft tissue limb growth, in order that movement can be facilitated. This image shows how the anlage of the bones is first formed in cartilage, like a placeholder. However, this style of presentation focuses upon the bone growth, when in fact the soft tissues including the fascia all play a role in the biodynamic kinetics (as well as the chemical genetics) from which the architecture forms itself. It is *all* from the original meeting place of the amniotic sac and yolk sac. It never ceases to present emergent properties from the surrounding context of the mesenchymal milieu in which it resides (see Ch. 6). As such, Figure 4.19 presents it slightly differently from standard text[29] to include the surrounding tissues and growth directions of the whole form.

"Muscles, tendons, ligaments and bones take on identity in concert with arteries, veins, nerves and the organs and life plans they serve. The overall musculoskeletal signature of a bear or walrus is different from that of a mole

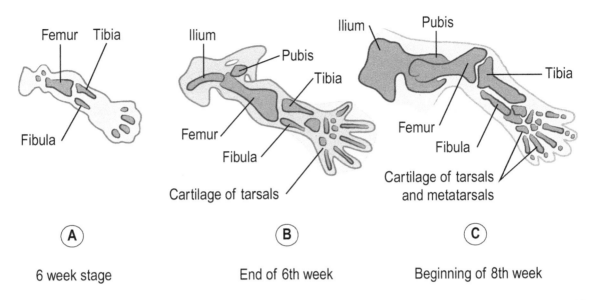

Femur   Tibia

Fibula

A

6 week stage

Ilium

Pubis

Tibia

Femur

Fibula

Cartilage of tarsals

B

End of 6th week

Ilium   Pubis

Tibia

Femur

Fibula

Cartilage of tarsals
and metatarsals

C

Beginning of 8th week

Figure 4.18

Detail of growing limb buds in their metabolic fields, surrounded by the amniotic sac, from which the embryo originally formed in part. The entire development of the embryonic tissues appears as a continuum, which is lost to the limitations of two-dimensional schematic diagrams.

or owl, and that difference is established by small, accumulating embryonic strokes that proceed in waves from the neural tube and somites."[30]

Blechschmidt suggests that all muscles grow into part of a myofascial sling:

"Seen from the perspective of developmental dynamics, muscles cross joints because the muscles develop in segments of various large [connective tissue] sling systems and joint spaces arise within the compass of the same slings. ... the tissue at the periphery of the space becomes stretched forming the joint capsule. Those parts of the joint capsule that are particularly well stretched are called liga-ments."[31]

This is the basis upon which van der Wal considered the tissue-sparing dissec-tion we referred to in Chapter 3. He revealed the continuity of the fascial slings that the muscle cells originally rely upon (see Evans et al.[32]). Indeed, the muscle fibres are made of the essential material in continuity with all that forms. With the muscle element removed, the tissue continuity around the entire joint was clearly revealed. This emphasises the significance of fascial continuity as an essential part of our structure and our original motion. Could it be a kind of soft woven scaffolding in the formation process, a pattern recapitulated on every scale (from organelle to organism) at finer and finer textures (see Ch. 7)? It also endorses ideas of myofascial continuity throughout our form, as pro-posed in the work of Tittel[33] and Myers,[34] among others: "Fundamentally there

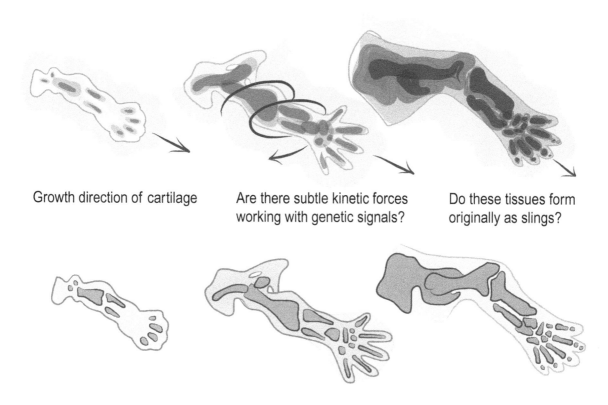

Growth direction of cartilage   Are there subtle kinetic forces working with genetic signals?   Do these tissues form originally as slings?

Figure 4.19

Earlier in this chapter we noted the question about connective tissue, "the forgotten player" (see note 8), and its primary role in providing the motive force for myofascia and osseofascial (bone) formation. If it is indeed such a "keynote speaker" in the story of how our architectural self-assembly finds its way into form, how can the surrounding tissues be presented so that they do not appear to have a role in the scheme of things?

are no differences between the organs of movement in the head, the trunk and the limbs" (Blechschmidt[35]).

Laying down the rest of the remarkable human blueprint. At this point the embryonic period is considered to be complete (Fig. 4.20). There is a great deal more to grow and form; however, the primary purpose of (a) flowing the cells to the right positions, and (b) folding the basic human form into being, so the foundational pattern predicts appropriate placement of the human anatomy and physiology, has been orchestrated. From this point, the embryo becomes a fetus and (c) continues to develop the rest of the pattern of the remarkable human blueprint, once that form *has* emerged, from which the neonate can grow *and* emerge. It doesn't end in the sense that the baby might be said to continue to develop upon these themes, through all the stages from child to elder.

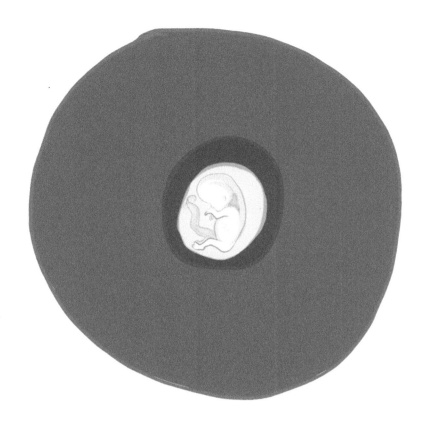

Figure 4.20

The folded embryo at Week 8: approximately Day 49. It is about the size of an acorn (30 mm). The eyelids are forming, the limbs and digits are present. It is still bathed in the fluids of the surrounding amniotic sac, from which it formed and emerged originally, the architect of its own architecture.

Yoga Genesis

In yoga we seek to move and explore being alive in the body's own language, with a quiet mind. We prepare the body for stillness and meditation, another stage rich with embryological symbolism. The meditative practice is designed to heighten our awareness, the involution of our self-sensing senses. Yet it also allows us to absorb and reflect, cocooned in contemplation and conscious of being relatively motionless. We can emerge, nourished and new, reborn after a period of restoration that is part of the cycle of renewal that *Samsara* (meaning "continuous flow") speaks of in yoga. However we describe it, we continue as part of a continuum, stage after stage of ongoing development. Perhaps that is, in itself, the miracle of life.

Notes

1. "The miracle of life", in Part 1 of Vanda Scaravelli, *Awakening the Spine*, 2nd edition, Pinter and Martin, London, 2011.

2. James Gleick, *Theory of Chaos*, The Butterfly Effect, p. 23, regarding the weather, prediction of which is a wonderful example of how tiny changes become exponentially vast shifts in weather patterns. This book is a fabulous read to shed light on cyclical, sensitive processes of emergent properties – something that symbolises the development of the human embryo (or any other developmental story of a non-linear, biological creature). Also: Wikipedia: https://en.wikipedia.org/wiki/Chaos_theory: Sensitivity to initial conditions. Main article: Butterfly Effect.

3. Erich Blechschmidt, *The Ontogenetic Basis of Human Anatomy: A Biodynamic Approach to Development from Conception to Adulthood*, edited and translated by Brian Freeman, North Atlantic Books, Berkeley, CA, 2004. Morphogenetic Metabolic Fields.

4. Darrel J.R. Evans, Vice-Provost (Learning and Teaching), Monash University, Melbourne, Australia.

5. Richard Grossinger, *Embryos, Galaxies and Sentient Beings: How the Universe Makes Life*, North Atlantic Books, Berkeley, CA, 2003.

6. Jaap van der Wal: see www.embryo.nl for papers and courses in which these views are extended and further explained.

7. Graham Scarr, www.tensegrityinbiology.co.uk, article: "Geodesic". See also: *Biotensegrity: The Structural Basis of Life,* Handspring Publishing Ltd., Pencaitland, 2018, 2nd Edition.

8. D.J. Evans, P. Valasek, C. Schmidt and K. Patel (2006) Skeletal muscle translocation in vertebrates. *Anatomy and Embryology (Berlin)* 211 (Suppl 1):43–50.

9. J. Sharkey (2019) Regarding: Update on fascial nomenclature-an additional proposal by John Sharkey MSc, Clinical Anatomist. *Journal of Bodywork & Movement Therapies* 23(1):6–8.

10. Article by Stephen M. Levin - 2018/08/21, SP , Bone is Fascia - published on ResearchGate and as a special contribution within the Introduction of Susan C. Lowell de Solórzano's *Everything Moves: How Biotensegrity Informs Human Movement*. Handspring Publishing Ltd, Pencaitland, 2020.

11. Jaap van der Wal MD PhD, Emeritus Associate Professor Anatomy and Embryology, Maastricht University, The Netherlands.

12. Ibid.

13. Ibid.

14. Deane Juhan, *Job's Body: A Handbook for Bodywork*, Station Hill Press, Barrytown, NY, 1987.

15. Tufts University, 2011 [YouTube: *Morphogenetic fields in the developing frog embryo*]. Video can be seen at: <http://phys.org/news/2011-07-frog-time-lapse-video-reveals-never-before-seen.html>

16. Stanley Keleman, *Emotional Anatomy*; originally published in 1985 by Center Press. Keleman has been the director of Berkeley's Center for Energetic Studies since 1971. He has sought to show "the geometry of somatic consciousness" based on the idea that emotional and psychological reality is expressed in physical human shape. Vincent Perez (anatomist and illustrator) depicts Keleman's concepts of somatic function in strong black.

17. Jan van Ijken; https://www.janvanijken.com/film-projects/becoming/ from his website: *Becoming* is a short time-lapse film about the miraculous genesis of animal life. In great microscopic detail, we see the "making of' a salamander in its transparent egg from fertilization to hatching". https://vimeo.com/316043706

18. Jaap van der Wal: see www.embryo.nl for papers and courses in which these views are extended and further explained.

19. See Dr Guimberteau's work. Jean-Claude Guimberteau, MD (www.endovivo.com/en/dvds.php). His DVD, *Interior Architectures*, is available on the same site. See also *The Architecture of Living Fascia: The Extracellular Matrix and Cells Revealed Through Endoscopy*, Handspring Publishing Ltd., Pencaitland, 2014.

20. Erich Blechschmidt, *The Ontogenetic Basis of Human Anatomy: The Biodynamic Approach to Development from Conception to Adulthood*, edited and translated by Brian Freeman, North Atlantic Books, Berkeley, CA, 2004.

21. Ibid.

22. Ibid.

23. Thomas W. Sadler, *Langman's Medical Embryology*, 11th edition, Lippincott Williams and Wilkins, Baltimore, 2010.

24. Jaap van der Wal, "Proprioception", Ch. 2.2 in Robert Schleip, Thomas W. Findley, Leon Chaitow and Peter A. Huijing, *Fascia: The Tensional Network of the Human Body*, Churchill Livingstone/Elsevier, Edinburgh, 2012.

25. Erich Blechschmidt, *The Ontogenetic Basis of Human Anatomy: The Biodynamic Approach to Development from Conception to Adulthood*, edited and translated by Brian Freeman, North Atlantic Books, Berkeley, CA, 2004.

26. Research re Fasciatomes: Carla Stecco, Carmelo Pirri, Caterina Fede, Chenglei Fan, Federico Giordani, Luigi Stecco, Clogero Foti, Raffaele D Caro (2019) Dermatome and fasciatome. *Clinical Anatomy – Special Issue on Fascia* 32(7):896–902. https://doi.org/10.1002/ca.23408

27. Darrel J.R. Evans (2003) Contribution of somatic cells to the avian ribs. *Developmental Biology* 256:114–126.

28. Erich Blechschmidt, *The Ontogenetic Basis of Human Anatomy: The Biodynamic Approach to Development from Conception to Adulthood*, edited and translated by Brian Freeman, North Atlantic Books, Berkeley, CA, 2004.

29. Thomas W. Sadler, *Langman's Medical Embryology*, 11th edition, Lippincott Williams and Wilkins, Baltimore, 2010.

30. Richard Grossinger, *Embryos, Galaxies and Sentient Beings: How the Universe Makes Life*, North Atlantic Books, Berkeley, CA, 2003.

31. Ibid

32. D.J. Evans, P. Valasek, C. Schmidt and K. Patel (2006) Skeletal muscle translocation in vertebrates. *Anatomy and Embryology (Berlin)* 211 (Suppl 1):43.

33. Kurt Tittel, *Beschreibende und Funktionelle Anatomie des Menschen*, Urban and Fischer, Munich, 1956.

34. Thomas W. Myers, *Anatomy Trains: Myofascial Meridians for Manual and Movement Therapists*, 2nd edition, Churchill Livingstone, Edinburgh, 2009.

35. Erich Blechschmidt, *The Ontogenetic Basis of Human Anatomy: The Biodynamic Approach to Development from Conception to Adulthood*, edited and translated by Brian Freeman, North Atlantic Books, Berkeley, CA, 2004.

5

Sensory Architecture

"Biology textbooks often state that the most important characteristic of organisms is the ability to reproduce, and then proceed to give an account of DNA replication and protein synthesis as though that were the solution to the fundamental problem of life. The ability to reproduce is only one of the properties of living organisms, and it could be argued, not even the most distinguishing one. For there are a number of other characteristics, scientifically speaking, which leave us in no doubt that they are alive; their extreme sensitivity to specific cues from the environment, their extraordinary efficiency and rapidity of energy transduction, their dynamic long range order and coordination, and ultimately, their wholeness and individuality."[1]

Mae-Wan Ho

Sensory refinement is an important quality in all our yoga practices. New discoveries about fascia shift the perspective on many questions. In the last chapter we considered how it arises embryonically. Why do we seek this sensory refinement through the somatic awareness that yoga fosters? How intimately does it relate to our self-sensing regulation and autonomic function?[2] Fascia, in all its richness and variety, provides a new context for exploring these questions about the pattern and matter of human motion and how we move our selves. This fundamental change in context has taken place while, as yet, we have only the classical language to describe it. Fascia research is inviting new and subtle distinctions.

A list of functional or anatomical detail is interesting in terms of mechanics (which is often the bias of technical information about functional movement), but there is an invitation here (particularly for those of us who *teach* any form of movement) to find new terms to describe somatic refinement and sensitivity. Scientific research is discovering new proportions and ratios for assigning senses and sensory responses to the forces that travel through our tissues in motion. The discovery that the fascia is one of the largest and richest sensory organs of the body[3] has made many people start to reconsider and expand on the traditional view of how the nervous system *animates* – as distinct from "functions". As a new context, it is ground-breaking news.

(Notice in Chapter 2, around the time that anatomy emerged as a study, the last women in Europe were convicted and executed for witchcraft (aka convening with the devil). Science was culturally developing out of that era, seeking a kind of neutrality or "truth" that would eventually supersede these superstitions and religious biases.)

Six Senses or More?

We hit semantic difficulties here too. "Touch", "feelings" and "sensing" are all words that have a multitude of possible meanings in the English language. You can be touched physically or emotionally; you can touch something literally or find a sentiment "touching". In using the word "feel" you could be describing a multitude of experiences that provide an even wider mixture of possible meanings, from a literal change in temperature or texture, for example, to a profound emotion. "Feeling" something can be a physical description of a shape, an esoteric response to a poem, or a comment about its non-physical properties. "Sense" can also take many different aspects, and any effort to define its many meanings in scientific language is a little like herding spiders.

Emerging Definitions

The word actually originates from the Greek word *haptein* meaning "to fasten". (This is noteworthy when we consider that the original meaning of fascia is "binding"). "Haptic" later came to mean "able to touch or grasp" from the Greek *haptikos* "able to come into contact with" and since the advent of smart phones, its generalized meaning of "pertaining to the sense of touch" has grown in terms of general usage in the last decade.

Fascia, as the largest sensory organ of the body, does not, however, make the nervous system redundant. Rather, it redefines the qualities, transitions and characteristics of how we sense and organise our responses and what parts of us are actually sensing. We begin to expand our re-cog-nition of the fluidic, breathing, soft-tissue nature of our forms. We are literally and symbolically swimming in (and around) a "sea-change" of how we understand posture, motion and biomotional integrity, personally and professionally.

How would our cultural history have been different if, rather than learning that we are creatures with five senses, able, ideally, to hear, see, touch, taste and smell, we had learned that we had six senses, or more? The phrase "sixth sense" is often used to describe intuitive or inexplicable knowing. It is thought to explain the mysteries of hidden talents in individuals and can sometimes hint at occult domains that may not always be measurable by the physical sciences.

In basic anatomy and physiology, as generally taught, you will find the nervous system described and treated as one distinct system (with a central and a peripheral aspect). Broadly speaking it includes the five senses of sight, sound, smell, taste and touch. The last of these, touch, is usually the hardest to define and the one that accounts for a range of sensory faculties.

Perhaps inherent to the language we use to express ourselves here is a deep knowledge that there is much more to it, certainly when describing human beings.

Is there a place where our primary *sensing* faculty and our feelings actually become one in the body, *unifying* as yoga invites us to explore? Could the new definitions of the fascia unite the physical with the metaphysical, providing a certain psychosomatic congruency, thus honouring the whole purpose of yoga in its ancient wisdom and contemporary values?

Different branches of scientific research (neural science, developmental biology, psychology, embryology, fascia research and so on) are confirming that not only does the fascial "proprioceptive substrate" constitute a sensory organ in and of itself but, given its exceptional surface area throughout the body, it is the largest and richest we have.

Haptic perception is not a new term, however its significance in our efforts to language this sea-change is bringing it forward into general acceptation.

DEFINITION: Haptic; can be used as both an adjective and a noun (meaning it's a "thing" and it's also a word used to emphasise how other things are, such as Haptic Perception).

Meaning: **adjective**: *relating to the sense of touch, in particular relating to the perception and manipulation of objects using the senses of touch and proprioception*; **noun**: *the perception of objects by touch and proprioception, especially as involved in non-verbal communication.*

The question here is "if what we touch (and that which we use *to touch*) are made of fascia – and it is our largest sensory organ – then is Haptic perception the very sense we live in and rely upon, primarily and universally?"

Extensive research, since the first edition of this book, in and around this subject, has been done by Martin Grunwald, presented in his book *Human Haptic Perception*.[4]

So-called "Haptics" are the basis of your smart phone, smart watch or tablet's ability to interact with you through subtle touch forces; one-, two- or three-finger gestures, bringing about different responses, without verbal cues. You may get a "tap" on the wrist to notify you; you slide over your phone's surface to notify your device. These interactive features are known as your smart device's "Haptics" (probably listed in your phone settings, for example, as "Sound & Haptics"). Remember, these functions are essentially designed by human beings; they project from the basis of our own full functioning (whether or not we are intellectually conscious of it). We simply haven't seen it generally applied to the human movement system, in the broader sense of a definition. It is a quantum leap to consider that our entire physical architecture might be based primarily on Haptic Perception skills. Those areas (certainly in the physical domain of medicine, manual and movement therapies) are still steeped in long-held mechanical traditions, seen and classified through the lens of Western medical textbooks. The difficulty resides in how much time has to be carefully taken to introduce new paradigms responsibly, the basic shift being from hard-matter physics to soft-matter, fluid, sensory dynamics. The foundational essence of this paradigm shift is from exactly those two fields of the physical sciences. To put it very simplistically, you are not made of hard matter!! As such, the rules change from linear mechanics to non-linear chaos, which is much harder to navigate, as we will see in Chapter 6. It is inviting new questions and perhaps it is no coincidence that the range of facilities and subtleties we can assign to the fascial matrix is also growing exponentially with the need for new definitions. (As the need for new definitions is growing exponentially with the range of facilities and subtleties we can assign to the fascial matrix!)

Robert Schleip[5] is among several key protagonists, that have contributed to this expansion of our knowledge of the fascia as a sensory signalling system, organising a network of scientists to come together and validate findings from all over the world, under the rigours of scientific research (see Ch. 3).[6] That is by means of practical dissection and via the most authoritative gold-standard, international research laboratories,[7] using advanced techniques to measure and explore the fascia (including, not limited to, the laboratory at Ulm University[8] and various teams of collaborative scientists there). Thanks to notable figures in the field, such as Thomas Findley and Peter Huijing co-facilitating the Fascia Research Congresses, many highly respected scientists and specialists in this area have been able to draw together their extensive bodies of work to bring about this paradigm shift in our understanding.[9]

A Shift in Logic

The point here is the shift in logic. We are seeking to understand the ubiquitous network of fascial tissues, and the fluidic nature of its expressions, that exists throughout the most finely detailed aspects of the living human

In another field entirely, that of robotics (see Grunwald for details on this topic also), these changes in how we view the living body are corresponding to rapid developments in "soft robots". The robotic dogs, for example, mark a departure from previous ways of thinking: rather than just being guided by bigger and better central computers (i.e. a bigger brain). They have been given many more sensory processors in the joints and fabric of the actual model. "BigDog" (Boston Dynamics) is an example of this thinking:

"*BigDog's on-board computer controls locomotion, processes sensors and handles communications with the user. BigDog's control system keeps it balanced, manages locomotion on a wide variety of terrains and does navigation. Sensors for locomotion include joint position, joint force, ground contact, ground load, a gyroscope, LIDAR and a stereo vision system. Other sensors focus on the internal state of BigDog, monitoring the hydraulic pressure, oil temperature, engine functions, battery charge and others.*"[10]

Mechanoreceptors

I use the made-up term "inter-motion" to replace what I believe to be a misused term – that of "shear". Once you understand biotensegrity (see Ch. 6) you begin to discover that there is no such force as "shear" in the human body, unless there is pathology present. That would cause friction, which generates heat. Temperature is a base-line parameter of health (see Ch. 6) and when there *is* shear force operating in the system, it is invariably due to a pathological condition that generates exactly that temperature issue that we call "inflammation". It acts as a warning system of sorts, to alert us to the pathology. Fascia, as a fluid medium, allows for *glide* – and we can sensitively feel where it is inhibited. Shear forces are not a dependable property, despite their common terminology; they occur when other, more subtle, signalling has failed. There is, however, neutral "inter-motion" exchanges between pockets and folds. The entire system depends on them.

body. It is gradually gaining recognition as sensory in nature, in its entirety. It is being described as master of our **sixth sense of proprioception** (see definition).

We arrive whole and complete on our yoga mats, with all our intellectual and instinctive, intuitive and emotional, physical and anatomical aspects intimately interwoven. After all, we are full-bodied animations of our own spirit (or anima/animus), however our individual bodies uniquely express *themselves*; however we choose to describe them. The relatively recent, deeper enquiry into fascia as the very fabric of our form means that our "architecture" is instrumental in holding us all together (literally and symbolically) as a responsive form, informing and transforming and performing every day. The suggestion that it has an intelligence of its own is impacting many fields of somatic study, beyond the physical body, into the realm of psychology, for example.

Further differentiations in how we perceive our inner and outer worlds, and how they respond to us, are encouraging new areas of research and distinction as the understanding of fascia grows and new research emerges. These perceptions include our sense of our inner selves and our autoimmune responses, and, as we will come to see, can address the profoundly integrated practice of yoga at its best and most valuable. These ideas are not so much new as *newly validated* and *newly distinguished* in Western medicine, manual and movement therapies.

Recognising the fascia as a sensory organ makes "sense of the sensing" facility in the human body, even though it may be changing how we attribute certain aspects of the neural system. There are "movement sensors" (*mechanoreceptors*) of different types of sensitivity within the fascial matrix.[11] They are situated in the tissues, particularly at joints, along the fascial interface at the bones (bony periosteum) and between the different depths of the various fascial pockets; wrapping and interfacing the muscles. They can detect the subtlest shifts in motion and "inter-motion" between pockets, pouches and tubes of the body architecture. They detect changes in terrain, through glide (or lack thereof), through shape change and deformation of the tissues. (See Table 5.1 below for specific definitions.) The mechanoreceptors sense, communicate and essentially respond to variations in temperature, tension and torsion, variously distributed throughout the matrix on every scale, even cell to cell. The body you live in really is exquisitely sensitive and interconnected. The sensory attributes of biotensegrity (see Ch. 6) are a new universe for distinguishing motion, conferring a whole new dimension in appreciating these properties of the fascial matrix organisation. The revelation in seeing how wholeness moves around is inspiring once you translate the fascia and begin to appreciate its multiple roles: organising form, transmitting forces and detecting changes and responses at both gross and subtle levels.

What this adds up to, essentially, is similar to *how* the robot dog can walk over different terrains, such as ice and mud, and orientate different loads without being interrupted in its purpose of walking. It begins to explain an adaptive

Table 5.1

Overview of the key mechanoreceptors

Mechanoreceptor	Golgi (Brothers)	Pacini (Brothers)	Ruffini (Brothers)	Interstitial Free Nerve Endings (The Sisters)
CARTOON:	✓	✓	✓	✓
TYPE:	Golgi	Pacini	Ruffini	Interstitial
LOCATION:	Myotendinous junctions, where tendons, tendinous sheets (aponeuroses) attach ligaments and joint capsules.	Myotendinous junctions, deep to the spinal ligaments and a variety of myofascial tissues.	Ruffini corpuscles are found in the peripheral joint ligaments, the dura mater. (Effect may not be limited to their locality.)	Found almost everywhere in the tissues of the body. Highest density in the fascia covering the bones (periosteum).

ARCHETYPE:	Steadiness, balance and sensory refinement. (See notes below table.)	Alertness; excitatory; local awareness.	These receptors seem to enjoy the sense of gentle balance to the overall system and calmness of general focus.	Sensory refinement and variability of local-to-global (and vice versa) balance and homeostasis.
RESPONSE:	Muscular contraction and stronger pressure of touch.	Deep pressure and excitatory stimulus or vibration.	Lateral lengthening of the tissues (in manual therapy). Associated with gentle, yawning stretches (pandiculation).	They are pressure-responsive, half responding to high-pressure and half to low-pressure changes.
INFORMATION:	Pandiculation (yawning stretches, i.e. a lengthening contraction) stimulates the Golgi tendon organs to provide feedback for dynamic changes. Actively loaded stretches, such as those in Hatha Yoga that include stronger holding patterns or rhythmical sequences, can also be beneficial to activate these receptors.	Pacinian mechanoreceptors are thought to be responsive to deep pressure and excitatory, fast or vibratory techniques, increasing local proprioceptive attention. In movement they are used as deep proprioceptive feedback for kinaesthetic control.	Ruffini mechanoreceptors are especially responsive to tangential forces and lateral stretch, and slower, more sustained pressure. They are associated with longer-term changes. Tend to ignore excitable moves, preferring long, slow, deep changes to the tissues. Naturally promote a calming effect on the whole system.	Schleip suggests that a major function of this intricate network of interstitial tissue receptors is to fine-tune the nervous system's regulation of blood flow according to local demands and that this is done via very close connections with the autonomic nervous system, making it even harder to ignore the wholeness of the body-wide network.
BENEFIT:	Practising balancing may develop ever finer distinctions for the Golgi tendon receptors to expand their powerful contribution to body balance, globally.	Thought to increase local proprioceptive attention.	Thought to increase local proprioceptive attention. Stimulating them inhibits sympathetic tonus. We could translate this to mean they are valuable assets in soothing an agitated system.	Free nerve endings are by far the most abundant of all the receptors. Increase vasodilation and rate of respiration. Relate to pain perception; nicknamed "witches and angels" for their ability to switch from proprioception to nociception.[28]

While this cartoon metaphor is useful, these receptors work together in concert. The danger of applying reductionist thinking (to each one) is imagining they separate their roles or work in linear or isolated ways, independently of each other. We are non-linear biologic systems, exquisitely sensitive and coordinated in practice (which is what our practice is designed to foster).

space- and surface-sensing system, that can respond to infinitesimal pressure, friction and vector changes, underfoot. It calibrates joint or locomotion forces to effect a more "sensitive" robot. We "non-robots" can already do all that, we always have been able to; it is built in to our structure. New research is evoking new distinctions about how exactly we manage it and there is much conjecture about how it is described! Nevertheless, it behoves us to remember it isn't new or specialised in us. *We do it anyway*!! We are simply finding new distinctions. (Which may not be simple!)

These mechanoreceptors (which we might also consider as types of motion-sensors, or dare I suggest "*biomotionsensors*") give us all the different faculties described in modern robotics, and more. We are essentially self-motivated, so the notion that our bodies biologically and naturally "self-inform" regardless of what we describe, need not be surprising. The sheer multitude of mechanoreceptors begins to explain the finesse and detail with which we can modify our actions and responses. We do this in very refined ways, adapting to the ground we walk on and the terrain we explore, on or off the yoga mat. They play a role in detecting subtle mechanical changes in local tension to give us not only some of our finer skills of dexterity, but to answer why we can do things (including yoga and dance) the way we can, at the speed and variability we can.

Fascia: a Sensory Organ?

Far from being an inert connecting material that happens to contain the vessels of the nervous system, the fascia is shown to be a sensory architecture that *feels its way into forming and our way into the forms*, as we have seen in Chapter 4. We discover that it is far more than a kind of carpet, over and under which lots of wires (i.e. nerves) are laid down. That would imply that all sensory communication is only attributable to the actual named nerves and tracts of the central and peripheral nervous system. The evidence is rather that the "current" is also in the tissue itself; it is *charged*. This highly responsive matrix does not only have nerves running through it (although it does, and they do). Rather, the fabric itself (or the material of gels, emulsions and colloids our tissues wrap and are formed in) is completely innervated. By its tensional, or more specifically *tensioned*, nature it is also, histologically, extremely sensitive to the slightest movement (or resonance, of vibration). The presence of different types of movement sensors (mechanoreceptors) in every depth and fold of the muscles (including muscle fibres, viscera, vessels, bones, joints and all their wrappings) has revealed variable sensitivities. Throughout the tissues of the entire body there is a refined and sophisticated sensitivity to a variety of subtle movements or forces *on or through* the structure. It merits a great deal of attention if we are to understand more fully how it helps us move better.

The ability to be sensitive to the most miniscule changes is natural and ancient and innate. It is the slightest *deformation* that the mechanoreceptors can detect: a minute change in tension or a shift *between* pockets or membranes in the interfaces of the system. Something like starlings in an airflow; one change fosters many consequences. Some of these subtle detections are in

Examining the tissue cell make-up is called *histological study*, which is the basis upon which the extensive research has been conducted.

response to tensional integrity, which is an essential characteristic of biotensegrity architecture and elasticity (see Chs 6 and 10). Other types of detection are attributed to the different tracts, pathways and organisations of the fascia, i.e. the location and density of the mechanoreceptors and the neural network (which is essentially made of fascia; called the "dura").

The sensitive tissue detects these subtle changes in the internal and external environment (around us and our cells), along the lengths of its tubular networking, to varying amplitudes. Thus, forces can be appropriately distributed (or dissipated) throughout the structure, almost instantly and most economically, to persistently restore the organism to "neutral" in response to gravity. By its architecture (as distinct from only its nervous system), the suggestion is that all tissues can respond biomechanically in very subtle ways via the whole sensory, communicating matrix of the fascia. (That is what I mean by biomotional sensitivity!)

This calls forth new distinctions of "small networks" and expands to an altogether different perspective on the nervous system. Robert Schleip points out:

"Many people think of the nervous system as an old-fashioned telephone switchboard system of the industrial age and therefore incapable of representing finer and more complex processes such as 'life energy' etc. The reader is cordially invited to consider this to be an out-dated model."[12]

Definitions

We have to be cautious here, because Schleip is not saying "we do not have a nervous system" with its central spinal cord and the peripheral nerves emanating from it. The fact remains that if an injury takes place in which the musculocutaneous nerve is cut, then the biceps muscle won't function. However, the new distinctions being referred to here, invite a broader and wider set of definitions for the range of subtle responses we can command. How do we interact with, listen and sense our internal "body communication network" in its most subtle variations? This is a question we often pose in the yoga classroom, particularly regarding the more subtle yoga practices.

Proprioception. This comes from the Latin *proprius*, meaning "one's own", and the word perception, so it translates to our *sense of [our own] self-perception* and relates directly to our positional sensing facility – knowing where we are in space and how we relate to objects around us. A task such as picking up a glass to drink from, for example, involves many refined recognition processes to assess the content, weight, balance and energy required to ensure we do not end up wearing the contents. To sip a drink, as distinct from gulping it, to use and adjust the right amount of effort as the content goes down, are all refinements of our proprioceptive awareness, communicated through our tissues. Children develop this sense gradually, progressing from grabbing wildly at a cup to being able to pick it up by its handle and eventually handling an open glass without tipping it too much or dropping it. These are progressive sensory refinements of proprioception. We use them constantly, if not consciously. They automatically adjust load to threading a needle, or carrying shopping.

Interoception refers to the internal sensing that could be likened to a "gut reaction". It is not new, although relatively recently named. It was originally termed coenaesthesia: "*the neurological model of a mostly unconscious sense of the normal functioning of the body and its organs*".[13] There is much new research around this faculty and proposed correlates with consciousness.[14] The interoceptive centres are distinct from proprioceptive centres in the brain. Interoception includes the sensation of pleasant touch but it refers to a less tangible, but nevertheless aware, instinctive knowing.

Nociception is the perception of various stimuli throughout the body, including the sensation associated with pain recognition. Interstitial free nerve endings are thought to be able to change from nociceptive qualities to proprioception, under certain circumstances.

In 1991, David Butler wrote of the nervous system:

"Arguably, there is no other structure in the body with such connectedness. Stresses imposed upon the peripheral nervous system during movement are transmitted to the central nervous system. Conversely, tension can be conveyed from the central nervous system to the peripheral nervous system.

If the nervous system were to be considered as an organ rather than the multi-segmented structure it is commonly thought to be, it would lead to a far better understanding of the system and of the patho-mechanical and patho-physiological consequences of altering its mechanics. One of the greatest implications of 'organ thinking' is that, if there is some change in part of the system, then it will have repercussions for the whole system. The continuous tissue tract makes this inevitable."[15]

Butler goes on to refer to the distinct aspects of the nervous system that focus on conduction of signals and also defines those others that primarily protect elasticity and mobility of the signaling branches. What is currently happening in research is the discovery of that interconnectivity throughout all the physiological systems, relying as they all do on the fascia for their architecture. There is a collective recognition of the fascial matrix as the connecting organ common to all the systems of the body, including, but not limited to, the nervous system. Effectively, they are redefining each other.

The connectivity (and elasticity) Butler refers to may indeed be considered part of the circulatory and structural systems too. This suggests a more intimate weave with the locomoting system than is portrayed in standard classical explanations. The body-wide architecture effectively forms lattice-like tubing and webbing around muscle fibres, circulatory vessels and neural vessels (neuro-vascular tracts), with cross-links and fluidic, fibrilar structural webs between them. They are not separate systems; although they have distinct characteristics.

Does this mean it is one whole *sensory architecture*? On the gross scale, it also appears to form "rope and ladder-like" structures (tendons) and sheets or planes of tissues (aponeuroses), as well as the looser connective tissue areas (under the skin and between organs, for example). Together these form a *mechanoreceptive substrate* throughout the body, intimately embedded in, or containing, the extracellular matrix. This includes all the structures mentioned above. Also the wrapping of the bones (periost) and (according to many protagonists) the bone itself plays a far from passive role; many consider it to be calcified fascia.[16] It includes the joints van der Wal calls "disjoints". Van der Wal terms the entire matrix a "proprioceptive substrate" and points out that the mechanoreceptors reside *between* the membranes. As subtle movement sensors, they can detect deformation and "inter-motion", that key component of elasticity (see Ch. 8), which includes all the network of parts, orchestrated *together* as one.

What this means is that the fascia detects or senses movement anywhere and everywhere because it is, in fact, sensory. This discovery validates Butler's presentation and expands it somewhat to include the *whole living architecture*. Indeed, the patterns he describes as beneficial to the protection of the nervous system's architecture when the body is mobile are apparently those of the entire fascial matrix throughout the body[17] (Fig. 5.1).

"If one studies a typical muscle nerve (e.g. the tibial nerve), it consists of almost three times more sensory fibers than motor fibers. This points to a fascinating principle that sensory refinement seems to be much more important than the motor organization."[18]

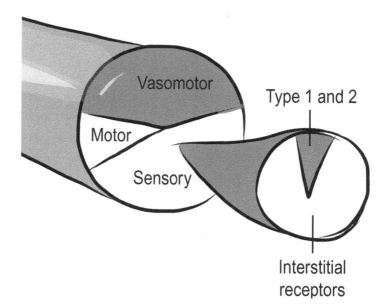

Figure 5.1

A typical muscle nerve (e.g. the tibial nerve) consists of almost three times more sensory fibres than motor fibres.

Sensing the Sensing

We rarely stop to consider how the tendons glide on each other – *unless they don't*. If you invite a participant to do Dog Pose (Adho Mukha Svanasana) and they have a condition such as carpal tunnel syndrome (where the movement of the wrist can be impaired to varying degrees), they might describe in detail what hurts and why they *cannot* do it. That is partly due to restricted gliding in the tendons of the wrist. Consider that the

We practise yoga, we think about the poses and how we change from one to another, while taking it entirely for granted that the lymph, blood, and nerve vessels, the glands, organs, soft tissues and bones will all just participate in our activity. Wherever there is folding, they need to fold with us and restore themselves rapidly after the event (of a pose), by unfolding back the way they came. They usually do! We do not have to check we can bend our elbows. We bend our elbows and find out whether or not they can "do" the pose. The tissue itself feeds back and says "yes" or "no" to the attempt (via sensation "messages") by carrying out the action (or not). It also gradually responds over time to our repeated efforts to train it, cumulatively refining it *temporally*. The invitation is to develop our awareness and ability to distinguish the signals accurately enough to prevent injury to our tissues and to benefit from their aptitude for neck (for example) is not mentioned or even felt, by them, because there is a *lack of* pain. That *absence* of pain is an expression of a healthy body experiencing its own fascial compliance and innate sensory coordination. If the

adaptability. This is the point of being taught, coached and guided. As guides, we seek the optimal way of doing this and communicating suitable feedback for each of the individuals we are invited to train, to help them move better. Bit by bit, day by day, practice by practice. There is a sensory accumulation as the tissues learn new, useful patterns and release or re-organise less useful ones. (See Part C, where we put this into practice).

The Common Denominator

neck begins to hurt too, the participant might begin to experience a connection between the wrist and the neck or upper spine. The point of this example is that the connection is there anyway; it is just silent when it works smoothly. In terms of the fascial matrix, these physical areas are all intimately related, not just because they appear on the

Research suggests that the fascia, including the extracellular matrix (they are not separate, although distinct), becomes the common denominator of all the tissues' connectedness and sensory intercommunication.[20] We are invited to consider it as an important context for mobility and internal motility of all vessels, organs and structures of the body, on every scale. Bear in mind it is *all in a fluid environment*, including the neural network (which we will explore in Ch. 7).

Robert Schleip, in articles for the *Journal of Bodywork and Movement Therapies*, seeks to debunk the traditional notion of the nervous system as a being based upon a dry, electricity wiring diagram; as if that is all it amounts to.

"Current concepts in neurobiology see the brain more as a primarily liquid system in which fluid dynamics of a multitude of liquid and even gaseous neurotransmitters have come to the forefront. Transmission of impulses in our nervous system often happens via messenger substances that travel along neural pathways as well as through the blood, lymph, cerebrospinal fluid or ground substance (Kandel, 1995). This global system for rapid body regulations is inseparably connected with the endocrinal and immune system. Rather than picturing the nervous system as a hard-wired electric cable system ... picture it in your mind's eye as a wet tropical jungle (Schleip, 2000). This jungle is a self-regulatory field with an amazing amount of complexity, continual re-organisation and plasticity, even in adults."[21]

The Speed of Motion

same myofascial meridian.[19] It is also because the tissue connecting them is sensory in nature, is tensioned and responding to elasticity (or the lack of it) through their *whole* tension–compression network (see Ch. 8). The body began as one piece embryologically and it remains that way. We are still one piece, just bigger and more complex. How we describe that, given the research into fascia, is a popular and intriguing question. It's worth the effort, however, as it really supports the subtle aspects of yoga. It provides the web joining and integrating the poses, with the anatomy and the philosophy.

Classically, a lot of work about the neural system focuses on mechanical function and *anatomical* structure. However, those are not necessarily the most helpful resources to explain what happens in an active classroom environment. We need a *language of context* for the felt sense that swiftly translates *at the speed* of classroom activity, or in sport, gym, on track or field. It has to come from the same place as, for example, learning to ride a bike or to swim: discovered and regulated by the participant as their own sensory experience. We might describe the learning process of these events as more "transformational" than "informational". They rely upon the person doing them to discover how they can work. It is a language of participation, spoken in structure and accumulated over time in subtle strokes of adaptation. That is *essentially by the system that perceives them (that we are attempting to perceive and describe). It is a little like trying to look at our own eyeballs. Perhaps this is one reason why we struggle with this new paradigm and the realization that it must have always been this*

The use of the word "field" is something we referred to in Chapter 4 and will revisit in Chapter 6. It takes us from 2D linear maps of the neural network into the multi-dimensional wholeness in which it resides… indeed, in which we reside. (See opening quotation from Rumi in Chapter 1.)

In Dundee, at the Centre for Anatomy & Human Identification in the Life Sciences department, it has been possible since the writing of the first edition to work with John Sharkey, Clinical Anatomist and Exercise

Bridging New Distinctions

Physiologist, annually for the last five years. Even having the intellectual knowledge to appreciate the fascial network as a tensional architecture, I held it in my imagination as a fibrous net. In Dundee, due to the soft-fix Theil nature of the preservation technique, we see the soft-tissue more *like* soft tissue in an anaesthetised living body, which provides a very different view to standard dissection, the usual basis of anatomical study. This facility provides unequivocal evidence for the universal nature of the fascial matrix, just as John Godman described (see Ch. 2). Simply being present to the invariability of tissue continuity, tension and compression-based organisation and relentless "*continuousness*" throughout the whole body (as these are full body cadaveric specimens) changed everything I "thought I knew". The absence of natural "layers" until the scalpel imposes them, is obvious. So is the fluidic, gluey nature of the matrix and the relentless continuity of membranes wrapping **everywhere**, around and through **everything**; regardless of what name you give it, for its location or its relationship to the surrounding structures. I stand in awe and gratitude – to John Sharkey

way. We don't move one segment at a time; we orchestrate motion as a whole.

This local neuro-sensory regulation is an intimate expression and finely detailed feedback system of both the mechanoreceptors and the architecture in which they reside. Analysing those aspects separately is like suggesting we should pick the sand element out of cement, between the bricks of a wall. They ARE it; the very essence of the material in a *living and conscious creature*. We live by the code of our own feedback and we are structured *by* that "feedback fabric". The research reveals a continuity of the nervous system, an expansion that evolves (i.e. includes and transcends) what it was classically considered to be. It is not an alternative argument. It is a complementary and inclusive enquiry. It is not an "opposing definition of a structure", it is an enhanced distinction of *our structure*.

Imagine the central nervous system as represented by the primary colours red, blue and yellow. These colours can appear in many shades and variations to symbolise all that we are familiar with in descriptions of the neural network and its range of sub-branches; the secondary colours, perhaps, moving into the tertiary blends at the peripheries. "Colour" (in this metaphor) is not exclusive to the named wiring diagrams of the central and peripheral nervous system. It brings us to imagining a new, integrated context.

The fascia expands this whole metaphorical realm of "colour" to include all the tonal variations and the subtle hues that are made of various mixtures of pastel shades. These include warm, cool, hot, cold, bright, and the rich variety of the full spectrum of variations we can make on a colour wheel. They all *arise from* the main colours, mixed with varying densities and balances. They are not (ever) separate from the original (primary, secondary and tertiary) basics. Rather they can be seen as a much more refined potential, for finer differentiation: a more subtle palette, so to speak. Fascia expands and deepens our understanding of the nervous system, *including* all its classical annotations of nerves and their branches, rather than replacing them. It is, however, essential to appreciate the new logic that considering the fascia this way can facilitate.

"The human body is one heart, one muscle, one nerve, one net"

John Sharkey[22]

This logic invites us to recognise a distinction between *histological neural feedback* (the electro-magnetic neural impulse the actual tissue emits) and the *signalling* that occurs as a *resonance response* which relies upon the structure of the instrument. They are distinct. The architecture of the neural network has to be tensioned to function as such. (Thus providing the elasticity that Butler refers to.)

The simplest example of this is putting out a washing line, across your garden, to hang out wet, washed clothes (something we do in the English countryside and so far I have seen it in every city around the world that I have visited). If you unravel that line and hang (attach) it between two posts, you have to tension it. If it is too stiff or over-tensioned, it can snap. If it is too slack, it will let your washing drape on the ground. (Not cool.) To be fit for purpose, you have to find a tensional "balance" we might call homeostasis.

There are a couple of keys here: one is that you don't want your washing draped on the ground, because it will get dirty again. *That's a structural issue of suitable tension in the line.* The other is that you don't want your washing to be spoiled, snagged or damaged by the line itself, when you peg out your favourite linen t-shirts. *That's what we would call a histological issue of the material the line itself is made of.* Consider then, that you have strung that washing line suitably across the posts. You now have an issue of weight-bearing or load. Too much and the line might sag, or worse, the angle of the posts might change and that will stretch or sag the line (depending upon which direction they go in – likely towards each other), because the line is attached to the posts. What we are saying here is that the *tissue itself [the line]* in your body can both sense the changes directly upon it and resonate with the changes of the surrounding structures and the forces moving through them all. That is from the clothing hanging on it and the angle of the posts it hangs from. The "line" in our metaphor is conducting neural impulses, facilitating a sensory feed-back system for the resonance field created *in conjunction with the posts,* the ground and the sufficient tension of the whole "washing line" apparatus (or "architecture"). The latter (washing line apparatus) is all about geometry, which is explained in living tensegrity structures (Ch. 6). The former (nature of the line, as a conductor) is being discussed here. They are inseparably whole – but while we consider the nervous system as distinct from the fascia, we would need two separate chapters under two separate sections of the book. In us, they may be inseparable features of our haptic awareness, our sensory refinement and our exquisite sensitivity and ability to adapt.

and to the diligent and respectful staff at Dundee University and to the generous donors that donate their tissues to scientific investigation, that leaves those of us witnessing, in awe.

A New Way of Seeing an Old Way of Being

It is possible to dissect the entire human nervous system (as per the standard annotation of central nervous system (CNS) and peripheral nervous system (PNS)) as one continuous piece; it will resemble a tree. Inside the body matrix it is a continuous tissue tract, under

I have been challenged with the statement "just because there are nerves in the fascia, doesn't make it sensory". That is inaccurate and the journey to finding out why, has been a fascinating one. Peter Huijing's answer to that question provided a segue into the scale of the spell we operate under, while we seek to understand fascia from the outmoded context of classical anatomy. (The challenge mentioned here was based upon precisely such outmoded beliefs.) New understanding requires new language and Huijing invited me into that domain with another question: *"Have you ever heard the sound of a neuron firing?"* I have not (or if I have, I do not *know* that I have). Peter Huijing took the trouble to explain to me that the degree and quality of sensitivity in the human body is such that if every signal it translates had to go via the brain the internal noise of neurons firing would be unbearable:

"Many things can work, function and operate in self-regulation in the context of a sensory matrix. The sound of a neuron firing is very loud. Actually, you couldn't stand the noise if every little thing you did to function every day wasn't self-regulating to an appropriate extent."[23]

tension, as Butler describes. What we are writing about is that which we would have to cut through, in order to cut *to* and dissect this continuous, tree-like network. It is in complete continuity with the tissues *within which it resides*, along every branch, *in vivo*. That is, all that we remove it *from* is in continuity with it (and everything else in the body). We are also discovering that the neural vessels are fascia (dura), and the connections we would have to dissect them *from* are also sensory in nature. This bears repeating, because as many times as you read it, it takes more to realise.

It is marvelously complex. He suggested that how this body-wide sensory system works, from periphery to core and back again, could be likened to a kind of hierarchy in a walled city, where everyday details of the housekeeping do not bother the "head office" of the central nervous system, i.e. the brain. In this metaphor there are gatekeepers, regulating at various levels of management, throughout the whole connected sensory architecture. Not every subtle move we make is a major "call" to the main cables, firing a neuron that goes direct to the brain and then waiting for the brain to direct proceedings. Even at the level of individual cells, there is a biomechanical response or self-regulatory facility, as Ingber has shown through his extensive studies in tensegrity architecture as a principle of living micro-organisms[24] (see Ch. 6).

"Ingber (1993) and his co-workers elegantly provided evidence that the entire cell behaves as one tensegrity system. They devised ingenious ways to apply precise, local mechanical forces to the cell membranes. For example, specific receptor-proteins in the membrane are individually tagged with a microscopic ferromagnet, which, when twisted in a magnetic field, caused the entire cell to stiffen up to resist the twisting. These and other experiments have shown that mechanical signals are involved in regulating many cellular functions."[25]

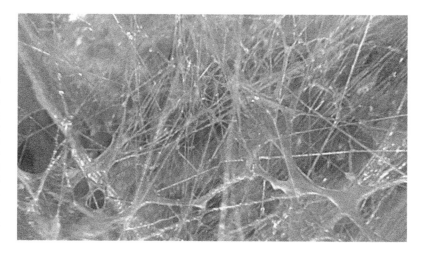

Figure 5.2

The web. This image shows the tensional tensegrity system of the superficial fascia through an endoscope (see Ch. 6). This is the nature of a tensegrity system which is essentially scale free; at the scale of the organelles to the cell, and the cells within the organism itself.

Reproduced with kind permission from J-C Guimberteau; Endovivo Productions.

The impact of this revelatory information is not only in the science itself. It also resides in the scientific confirmation of the **sentient nature of the human architecture**. This is an important statement. When you make it clear to people that they are feeling in this level of detail, they often light up with the validation of their personal experience. It can confirm that feelings sometimes treated (or dismissed) as metaphysical might be based more than we think, on physical sensations and sensory feedback. Moreover, there is both a hierarchical and a heterarchical basis for the *ordering* of these haptic perceptions (see Ch. 6).

If we regard the nervous system as merely an electrical circuit, we treat signals to and from the limbs, for example, as singular messages that travel to the brain (central fuse box) and back, meaning everything goes via the "Head Office". What is meant by a "mechanical response" in the context of a living, tensegral architecture is that the shape resists naturally, it responds automatically, and much faster than the time it takes for an impulse to go to the brain and back. (In other words, you will pull your hand away from a hot-plate, or blink when a fly comes towards your eye, much faster than your nerves can conduct.)[26] The *tissue itself* is responsive, via the various mechanoreceptors found in it, that respond very rapidly to shape change. They form part of the pathway *that can convert* a stimulus to a nerve impulse or a chemical response, making the range, complexity and subtlety of our sensory nature much greater than historically presented by a relatively 2D telephone cable wiring system. The implication is that our sensory vocation is considerably more sensitive and articulate than we realise – it has a broader vocabulary and qualitative nature than is often accounted for in scientific reasoning. In short "it beats us to it" sometimes; we might say it knows more about what's going on than we do!

What we do on the yoga mat is invite exactly this inner sensing, in a healthy way – an "instinctive awareness way" – rather than an "intellectually analytical way". It is a subtle response to the outer forces and an equally subtle influence over/response to them. We are already doing it. The development of this sense of sensing and sensitivity, and the ability to purposefully manage, move and expand it, is the basis of healthy practice. We will look into optimal ways to prepare a class with this idea (of our innate "already listening" state) in mind (see Chs 14 & 15). First, let us look into some of the science behind the sensory nature of the fascial matrix and then explore how we can find appropriate and useful language for this in class.

Manual and Movement Therapy

Scientists and practitioners (especially those with anatomical, movement and manual experience) like Robert Schleip and John Sharkey have devoted much time and research to exploring the neural dynamics of fascial plasticity. This translates into making the practical implications known to manual practitioners and movement instructors in every field of endeavour.[27] Such practitioners – along with many others – are bringing fascia research to the attention of the world at a new level of accessibility. Medical practice is gradually changing too because this one piece of information, that the fascia is the

This whole area calls for new distinctions of sensation, now that fascia is recognised as a sensory organ. How we communicate different *qualities* of pain and nociception requires a somewhat different vocabulary. For example, let's say you stub your toe. The "pain" is one that seems to have a promise of random increase and rising amplitude of discomfort. However, in the structural integration clinic (as one example among many), the sensation of "unsticking" stuck tissues (associated with so-called "myofascial release") is very different: it stops as soon as the practitioner and you stop. These are very distinct types of sensation and each has its own hallmark. One is that of outright, unwanted pain resulting from an injured or insulted part of the body. The other is more a sensation of relieving something (although it can *feel* quite intensely), it usually has a sense of relief with it, somewhere in the story. It may not bring relief immediately, however it has a very distinct intention and quality, unlike the random, unintended, out-of-control nature of an accident.

My father was a regular participant in my weekly yoga class. He began a gentle restorative yoga practice at 75 years of age and was 89 when he passed away, doing yoga up until the month before he passed. He commented one day, when he was in his mid-eighties, that he frequently stood in Tree Pose (Vriksasana) while cleaning his teeth, just to test his balance. In the morning he said, he did it standing on his left leg, at night the right leg. (He felt safe because he had the sink for support if needed.) Perhaps unsurprisingly, he walked easily for some distance daily and claimed throughout his eighties to be growing younger by the day. Upon falling flat on his back, on a muddy slope at 86, he laughed it off and showed no more ill effects than might be expected of a man half his age. He survived a heart condition (that technically should have seen him off two years earlier) by doing his "yoga breathing" every time he had

richest sensory organ of the body, transforms the way we perceive our clients, students and patients. It has implications in every field of medicine, from pain management and surgical intervention to recuperation and recovery: both physiological and psychological therapeutics. It goes beyond pathology to performance relative to any individual. It is key to yoga teaching and therapy.

Pathology is outside the scope of this book; however, it is noteworthy that research includes the discovery that *proprioceptive input strongly inhibits* spinal cord processing of myofascial nociception. (Nociceptors respond to a variety of stimuli in different parts of the body. They also carry pain signals from the peripheral to the central nervous system.)[28] This is a complex area of study and any brief summary greatly oversimplifies it. However, what "proprioceptive inhibition" means fundamentally is that *if someone can consciously develop their own body awareness (interoception and proprioception), they begin to lay a powerful foundation, upon which therapeutic intervention can result in improved movement and experiencing lowered intensity myofascial pain.* (Which effectively means the body can prefer moving to hurting.) In practice, this points to the value of yoga as a pursuit that deliberately seeks to bring us into more conscious awareness of our body (in motion and stillness), both internally and externally, by improving proprioception and interoception, supported by this biofeedback mechanism. By so doing, there is an active possibility of reducing myofascial pain, or even preventing it through practising conscious and appropriate movements in a cumulative way, building both (interoception and proprioception) gradually over time. Structural integrity appears as an asset for body, mind and being – for scientific (not just esoteric) reasons.

We often tend to stop moving in order to avoid pain. Research into non-specific low back pain, for example, suggests that such immobility can result in matted tissues and patients show *decreased* proprioception.[29] Thus, the further implication is that improved proprioception, and the fostering of appropriate movement and awareness of it, can decrease the overall experience of pain. This does not necessarily refer to gross movements, involving huge effort and range, of the type that might exacerbate an injury. It includes tiny micro-movements that encourage and foster subtle proprioceptive awareness *in and of the tissues*. Certain neurological disorders, such as Parkinson's disease for example, provide another instance wherein movement ability can appear to be transformed, through a fuller understanding of the neural network. Understanding its integration with a wider tissue matrix than is usually considered in classical ideas of a "wiring system" leads to quite unexpected changes and possibilities.

When you are happy, you access a different part of the system to direct the brain. This is considered to be stimulated in part by sound, as in music for example. Musical sounds have an influence on re-ordering the neurological signals (or signaling pathways), for motion, via the lateral or medial lemniscus system (which describes neurological pathways that travel via the inner ear mechanism).[30] The movement to music, such as dance (especially with rhythm and sound), changes the standard pathways that, in classical anatomy, are an angina attack. Perhaps our sensory calibration is cumulative to an extent? For sure, the weekly yoga classes built what he called his "bounce" and he always used his breathing techniques to sleep beautifully. (Case presented with his prior permission.)

usually assigned directly to limb movements. This allows for what appears to be a temporary, but nonetheless transformational, change in movement ability for such patients. They can express greater range of motion, neuro-muscular co-ordination and haptic perception and responsiveness. (By following these references it is possible to see how patients expressing these complex neurological conditions can appear completely transformed in a movement-to-music class.)

Yoga knows how to deepen our self-sensing of conscious and autonomic functions. It is, arguably, an important part of its purpose. That is not necessarily intellectually, but through instinctive practice on the mat. However, it is fascinating to see how science is revealing the subtleties of exactly what works, and why. There is a great deal of compelling evidence to show that the more we explore our proprioceptive and interoceptive qualities of subtle movement, the more value this awareness can accumulate for our whole body and being; far beyond the day we do the practice.

"Mechanoreceptors have been found abundantly in visceral ligaments as well as in the Dura mater of the spinal cord and cranium. It seems quite plausible that most of the effects of visceral or cranio-sacral osteopathy could be sufficiently explained by a stimulation of mechanoreceptors with resulting profound autonomic changes and might therefore not need to rely on more esoteric assumptions (Arbuckle 1994)."[31]

It is reasonable to suppose that the subtle movements and quiet aspects of certain yoga practices replicate the effect of some gentle treatment modalities in manual therapy. Self-sensing the cranial rhythm through subtle breathing techniques and meditation has also been shown to have a beneficial effect on the autonomic nervous system. Realising the connecting tissues of our form are sensory brings together the reasons why understanding fascia can have such far-reaching and valuable effects. In some ways it validates the experience of a congruent yoga practice.

The Mechanoreceptors

In a series of articles for the *Journal of Bodywork and Movement Therapies*,[32] Robert Schleip discussed in detail the suggestions that fascial tissue has many and various properties beyond the purely mechanical. Some examples of the different mechanoreceptors are provided here (see Table 5.1) to indicate the breadth of detail the nervous system can include. This is only a very small aspect to indicate the vast orchestration of sensory response that we can consider under this heading of Sensory Architecture. However, it assists us in recognising some of the deep and more valuable, hidden assets of thoughtful movements in the yoga classroom. It also includes the light-hearted cartoon-like images to help us remember at least four of the protagonists in this complex field of neuro-myofascial integration. To give direct examples of the value in appreciating the mechanoreceptors in yoga practice:

"Balance work has a close relationship to developing suitable reflexes: Studies of the fine antigravity regulation in bipedal stance have also revealed a new functional role for Golgi receptors. In order to handle the extreme antigravity balancing challenges as a biped, our central nervous system can reset the Golgi tendon receptors and related reflex arcs so that they function as very delicate antigravity receptors."[33]

According to Levin,[34] we might consider ourselves to be "unipedal". Since we practise developing one-legged yoga postures, it may be a valuable resource in pursuit of sensory refinement.

We could, perhaps, consider the nervous system to activate via a kind of volume control – orchestrating body-wide sensations according to a symphonic range of different variations in sensation. Each symphony depends on the purpose (what is being played) at the time. You (the conductor) get to modify multiple aspects of the whole orchestra.

In seeking metaphors to describe this complexity in a new context, Schleip likens the tissues to schools of fish, changing direction *en masse*. According to Professor Darrell Evans,[35] the starlings in an airflow (or "murmuration" as it is collectively called) are also a fitting description of how the embryonic cells flow and form in what we might call "crowd control patterns", where the fluid flows induced by the kinetic changes, change the kinetic patterns and the influences of the movements in concert (which in turn influences the movement).

Bodies are not linear systems and do not respond in a linear manner. A yoga practice invites us to take the tissues into different directions and, over time, they respond by gradually accumulating some changes and releasing others. This builds the local and global loading responses in the fabric of the body and so we are able to respond to the cumulative effect of training or teaching the body (see Ch. 7 and Part C), gradually over time.

"An attitudinal shift is suggested, from a mechanical body concept towards a cybernetic model, in which the practitioner's interventions are seen as stimulation for self-regulatory processes within the client's organism."[36]

The mechanoreceptors have been found to proliferate at joints and interfaces where the various fascial membranes move over each other.[37] The reason they are called "mechanoreceptors" is because they sense mechanical changes. This means effectively that they can respond "instinctively", adding to the list of faculties of the fascia. Mechanoreceptors contribute to its role as a sensory organ that is supremely sensitive to changes in movement perception and able to adjust to them, in self-regulation. The tissue will respond sensitively and instinctively to meet (and adapt to) demand and this is why it is so important to ensure that we provide suitable loading patterns. They can become habitual or repetitive strain patterns if the same planes of movement are repeated too frequently or undertaken for too long at a time. Used wisely, however, they can expand our range and become more refined and resilient as we mature. We are designed for variability and adaptability and we can train the body to optimise those assets as we age. Having said that, however, (it bears repeating) "conscious movement" doesn't necessarily mean gross or forceful movement.

Sthiram Sukham (The Steady and the Sweet): Neural Integration

One of the points of the physical yoga practice is to become more readily and relatively steady and balanced in a variety of directions, to find that "sweet steady" place (of Sthiram Sukham) from moment to moment. Another is to develop the ability to be still, as a matter of choice and counterbalance. That is, effectively, an *appropriate inhibition* by the nervous system, guiding the muscles to be still. When inhibition is adversely affected, muscles default to their basic function, which is to contract (see Appendix B). This is a fundamental (and fundamentally misunderstood) aspect of the neuro-myo-fascial system. Neural integration means we can be still when we choose. It means we can move one part of the body, while the rest is less involved (see Part C, Ch. 15), designed to foster this innate facet of biomotional integrity. The practice focuses on that which is not moving as much as it does upon that which is. Stillness is a skill, a dynamic ability to find equilibrium that seems to become a distinct asset to neural integration.

This research validates many of the suggestions of established yogic practices in that they enhance balance and calm the body, by working on the nervous system and accumulating the ability to respond appropriately (a word that has the same root as "proprioception" – the name of the sense

Table 5.2	
Fiction vs. Function – some fun facts to bear in mind in practice:	
Muscle Fiction	**Neuro-muscular Function**
Muscles work in antagonistic pairs.	Muscles work in concert, like the keys that tune a guitar or harp. They may seem to tune one specific string, but because of the next point, they inevitably affect the tuning of the entire instrument.
Muscle are attached to bones.	Muscle fascia (myofascia) is attached to bony fascia (periosteum); both the bone (which is arguably calcified fascia[38]) and the muscle (which is protein within the myofascial fibres) are in continuity.
Muscles are only attached at their origin and insertion (or distal and proximal attachments)	Muscles are attached entirely in 360 degrees of everywhere to their surrounding architecture and the proprioceptive substrate in which they arise.
Muscles can contract and relax.	Muscles contract. That's it. That's all they can do. (See detail below[39]).
Muscles act on bones, via the joints as levers.	There are no levers in non-linear biologic forms. Anywhere. Ever.
Muscles are each activated by one nerve that serves that muscle exclusively.	The myofascial matrix is sensory to varying degrees of differentiation, along with the neurological tracts of the central and peripheral nervous system that mark their specific enervation.
Muscles can be isolated functionally.	It may feel as if the focus of attention is on one area of the body, but nothing works in isolation as it is one continuous web.

that the fascia gives us). "... *asanas are designed to have specific effects on the glands and internal organs, and to alter electrochemical activity in the nervous system*" (from the teaching of Swami Sathananda Saraswati).[40] Yoga originally incorporated more than making shapes on a mat, and fascial research into new distinctions of this "biomotional intelligence system" endorses many aspects of its most ancient rituals.

Sixth or First Sense?

Research implies that we actually have at least six senses, including the proprioceptive sense associated with the fascia. If we go back to embryogenesis, in the light of our forming blueprint this might not be so surprising. Given that the mesenchyme and so-called mesodermal layer arise originally from neural crest cells, one might be forgiven for asking the most naïve of questions, which is "Why wouldn't our connective tissues all be sensory?" Until relatively recently, however, there has been no context for that question to be examined, let alone answered, on quite such a global scale.

Could it be that the sense provided by this tissue of organisation is not so much our sixth sense but rather our primary or formative sense, one that arises within our most original architecture? Could the fascia provide the context in which the generally accepted five senses occur? Some epigeneticists suggest that the embryo forms and senses chemically and mechanically as it grows.[41] It certainly seems feasible that we continue to do that as we grow up.

The fascial matrix transforms proprioception and its distinct aspects into THE common sense of our organising matrix. It changes how we see not only the "musculoskeletal" function but also the neuro-muscular system and the categorisations assigned to physiological systems in general.

Not only does the fascia act as a body-wide sensory organ, but it would also appear that there are different qualities of sensory orchestration from different organs. While research suggests that we have specific interoceptive awareness, like a "gut brain", other areas of science suggest we have a specific ability or sensory awareness in the "heart brain".[42]

Heart-felt Becoming

In the embryo, the heart begins its development just beyond what will become the crown, where the upper and lower layers of the embryonic germ disc are formed (see Ch. 4). Thus, the heart takes neurological tissues with it as it develops, forming, folding and feeding them as it, itself, is moved, formed and surrounded by them. It grows itself, at the same time as it provides food for the brain and spinal cord to grow, deepening its own faculty as it is called on to provide the nourishment for the rest of the body and organs to deepen theirs. The sensory, fluid, forming matrix is "**one**" at the outset. Needless to say, the architecture of the heart is entirely formed in fascia.[43]

"The heart is not a solo player in the quantum jazz of life. Instead it is in symphony with all other players, intermeshing and syncopating with their varied rhythms ... it is the complex rhythm of the organism dancing life into being, in which every single player is freely improvising and yet keeping in tune and in step with the whole."[44]

The last 20 years have also seen considerable advances made in heart research. The HeartMath® Institute (in Boulder Creek, California), for example, has shown that key information about how the heart functions lies in understanding the variability of the spaces in its rhythms. Heart rate variability is an important non-invasive tool for the assessment of well-being as it correlates with health and a sense of happiness on a number of measurable levels.[45]

Although we generally do not consider the heart to be a component of the nervous system but rather to be part of the cardiovascular system, a growing understanding of fascial architecture may be changing this view:

"The heart has an extensive communicative network with the brain. Input from the heart not only affects the homeostatic regulatory centres in the brain but also influences higher brain centres involved in perceptual, cognitive and emotional processing."[46]

"HeartMath® researchers propose that the heart's electromagnetic waves may interact with the fields of organs and other structures to create hologram-like interference patterns that 'inform the activity of all bodily functions'. The other half of the process is that the heart is also informed by the activity of all bodily functions, which is reflected in its rhythmic variation from moment to moment."[47]

We are building a picture here of why segregating yoga into the classical construct of reductionist thinking *does not serve us*. Yoga only ever espoused the heart-felt wholeness of body, mind and being. This makes sense of a practice that centres on self-awareness to honour the source (you) in order to serve and become a resource to others. Contemporary science is endorsing yoga, at its most intelligent, deeply invested as it is with ancient Vedic wisdom. There is no need to break it down into component parts that suggest a far less sophisticated organism than the one we move around in and sense ourselves to be. If we are going to break down the parts, then we must remember that in the classroom they present themselves as whole beings that are back together again!

Yoga practice lives right here, encompassing many aspects of exploring our form, via our felt sense and our sense of self, so that we can welcome this expansion of the basis of our personal anatomy and physiology. Yoga is certainly not comfortable if it is restricted to the biomechanical analysis of the postures on a one-size-fits-all basis. If anything, this containment and time spent in moving on our mat is designed to bring us into the present sense of our presence, or even "pre-sense", to become more aware and more attentive to the experience of being-in-a-body, for the sake of it. It can also enhance our ability to anticipate.

We do not necessarily divide our practice into an inner world and an outer world, but we do accumulate very subtle levels of distinctions for ourselves. Rather we seek to be a conscious interface, or a kind of conduit, that can make sense of the difference between, say, a feeling of poise and a sense of being still: being ready to dance and enjoying being present to being. We become the balance between inner and outer forces, developing sensory refinement as the membrane between them, moment by moment.

*"...It is within this network of intermediary neurons, arranged end-to-end and side-by-side between our sensory nerve endings and our motor units, that all of our tone levels, reflexes, gestures, **responses, expressions, memories,** habits, tendencies, feelings, attitudes, postures, **attributes and** styles have their genesis. It is called the* internuncial net, *and it has come into its fullest flower in the human being. (Internuncios were official messengers for the Pope taking information and bringing back responses from the various courts of Europe.) This net composes roundly ninety percent of our nervous systems, including the entire spinal cord and brain*[48]*."*

Deane Juhan, *Job's Body*

Further reading

Pathology is outside the scope of this book. However, yoga is becoming as interested in the therapeutic effects of its science as it is in the performing of the art. We are inevitably working with the fascia and, if we are able to improve its resilience, adaptability and health, it could naturally have profound overall effects on well-being. The following interesting excerpt from an interview between Dr Robert Schleip and Professor Stuabesand may be indicative:

"*Another aspect is the innervation and direct connection of fascia with the autonomic nervous system. It now appears that the fascial tonus might be influenced and regulated by the state of the autonomic nervous system. Plus – and this should have ramifications for your work – any intervention in the fascia system may have an effect on the autonomic nervous system in general and on all the organs which are directly affected by the autonomic nervous system. To put it more simply: any intervention on the fascia is also an intervention on the autonomic system*". Excerpt from the second part of Robert Schleip's articles: Fascial plasticity – a new neurobiological explanation: Part 2. *Journal of Bodywork and Movement Therapies*, April 2003.[49]

The Concise Book of Neuromuscular Therapy: A Trigger Point Manual by John Sharkey. This book provides an excellent concise overview of the nervous system and integrated application inclusive of the fascia.[50] (See Appendix B.)

Notes

1. Mae-Wan Ho, *The Rainbow and the Worm: The Physics of Organisms*, 3rd edition, World Scientific Publishing, Singapore, 2008.
2. The autonomic nervous system is the section of the nervous system that controls the involuntary actions of the smooth muscles, heart, and glands.
3. Robert Schleip and Heike Jäger, Ch. 2.3, "Interoception: A New Correlate for Intricate Connections Between Fascial Receptors, Emotion and Self Recognition", in Robert Schleip, Thomas W. Findley, Leon Chaitow and Peter A. Huijing, *Fascia: The Tensional Network of the Human Body*. Churchill Livingstone/Elsevier, Edinburgh, 2012. Ulrich Hoheisel, Toru Taguchi and Siegfried Mense, "Nociception: The Thoracolumbar Fascia as a Sensory Organ", Ch. 2.4.
4. Martin Grunwald (2008) *Human Haptic Perception: Basics and Applications*. 10.1007/978-3-7643-7612-3.
5. See www.fasciaresearch.de (Ulm University) for detailed information and various articles for both scientists and clinicians; Robert Schleip, Thomas W. Findley, Leon Chaitow and Peter A. Huijing, *Fascia: The Tensional Network of the Human Body*, Churchill Livingstone/Elsevier, Edinburgh, 2012; Robert Schleip and Amanda Baker, Fascia in Sport and Movement, Handspring Publishing Ltd., Pencaitland, 2014.
6. In August 2019, Clinical Anatomist John Sharkey led a team of Fascia experts presenting a Fascia Symposium to the19th Congress of the International Federation of Associations of Anatomists (IFAA) which is held every 5 years. In 2019 the Congress was held, for only the second time, in London, England. The IFAA Congress is a unique opportunity for medical professionals to share research and new developments in anatomy and anatomy research. Applications are peer-reviewed; presentations undergo rigorous scientific scrutiny, before being accepted for presentation. In the event, a presentation by John Sharkey, Drs Carla Stecco, Vladimir Cheremnsky, Rafael De Caro, Veronica Macchi and Andrea Porzionato was enthusiastically received by the large number of delegates at this prestigious event. In the same year the professional journal of anatomists, *Clinical Anatomy*, produced a Special Issue journal (Volume 32, Issue 7. October 2019, pp. 896–902) devoted entirely to the topic and science of Fascia.
7. See www.fasciaresearch.de (Ulm University) for detailed information and various articles for both scientists and clinicians; Robert Schleip, Thomas W. Findley, Leon Chaitow and Peter A. Huijing, *Fascia: The Tensional Network of the Human Body*, Churchill Livingstone/Elsevier, Edinburgh, 2012; Robert Schleip and Amanda Baker, Fascia in Sport and Movement, Handspring Publishing Ltd., Pencaitland, 2014.
8. See www.fasciaresearch.de (Ulm University) for further details. P. Barlas, D.M. Walsh, G.D. Baxter and J.M. Allen (2000) Delayed onset muscle soreness: effect of an ischaemic block upon mechanical allodynia in humans. *Pain* 87(2):221–225. R. Schleip, A. Zorn and W. Klingler (2010) Biomechanical properties of fascial tissues and their role as pain generators. *Journal of Musculoskeletal Pain* 18(4):393–395. Robert Schleip, Adjo Zorn, Fascia Research Project, Institute of Applied Physiology, Ulm University, Ulm, Germany. Werner Klingler, Department of Anesthesiology, Ulm University, Germany.
9. See www.fasciaresearch.de (Ulm University) for detailed information and various articles for both scientists and clinicians; Robert Schleip, Thomas W. Findley, Leon Chaitow and Peter A. Huijing, *Fascia: The Tensional Network of the Human Body*, Churchill Livingstone/Elsevier, Edinburgh, 2012; Robert Sleip and Amanda Baker, Fascia in Sport and Movement, Handspring Publishing Ltd., Pencaitland, 2014.
10. See https://www.bostondynamics.com/legacy - Big Dog (2004).
11. Robert Schleip (2003) Fascial plasticity: a new neurobiological explanation, parts 1 and 2. *Journal of Bodywork and Movement Therapies* 7(1):11–19; 7(2):104–116.
12. Ibid.

13. Robert Schleip and Heike Jäger, Ch. 2.3, "Interoception: A New Correlate for Intricate Connections Between Fascial Receptors, Emotion and Self Recognition", in Robert Schleip, Thomas W. Findley, Leon Chaitow and Peter A. Huijing, *Fascia: The Tensional Network of the Human Body*. Churchill Livingstone/Elsevier, Edinburgh, 2012.
14. A.D. Craig (2009) How do you feel – now? The anterior insula and human awareness. *Nature Reviews Neuroscience* 10:59–70.
15. David S. Butler, *Mobilisation of the Nervous System*, Churchill Livingston, Edinburgh, 1991.
16. John Sharkey (2019) Letter to the Editor. *Journal of Bodywork & Movement Therapies* 23:6–8.
    Article by Stephen M. Levin - 2018/08/21, SP , Bone is Fascia - published on ResearchGate and as a special contribution within the Introduction of Susan C. Lowell de Solórzano's *Everything Moves: How Biotensegrity Informs Human Movement*. Handspring Publishing Ltd, Pencaitland, 2020.
17. See Dr Guimberteau's work. Jean-Claude Guimberteau, MD (www.endovivo.com/en/dvds.php). His DVD, *Interior Architectures*, is available on the same site. See also *The Architecture of Living Fascia: The Extracellular Matrix and Cells Revealed Through Endoscopy*, Handspring Publishing Ltd., Pencaitland, 2014.
18. Robert Schleip (2003) Fascial plasticity: a new neurobiological explanation, parts 1 and 2. *Journal of Bodywork and Movement Therapies* 7(1):11–19; 7(2):104–116.
19. See the Arm Lines in Thomas W. Myers, *Anatomy Trains: Myofascial Meridians for Manual and Movement Therapists*, 2nd edition, Churchill Livingstone, Edinburgh, 2009.
20. H.M. Langevin (2006) Connective tissue: a body-wide signalling network? *Medical Hypotheses* 66(6):1074–1077.
21. Robert Schleip (2003) Fascial plasticity: a new neurobiological explanation, parts 1 and 2. *Journal of Bodywork and Movement Therapies* 7(1):11–19; 7(2):104–116.
22. John Sharkey is co-author of the One Series, in 2016, at NLSSM, London, UK.
23. Personal conversation at the Belgian Fascia Research Conference in 2012, Brussels.
24. Donald Ingber (1998) The Architecture of Life. *Scientific American*, Feature Article, January 1998. Ingber's research has since advanced considerably; see his webpage at https://wyss.harvard.edu/team/executive-team/donald-ingber/. An article on Ingber is available in full on http://www.scribd.com/doc/35190367/Architecture-of-Life-Scientific-American-by-Ingber.
25. Mae-Wan Ho, *The Rainbow and the Worm: The Physics of Organisms*, 3rd edition, World Scientific Publishing, Singapore, 2008.
26. A.W. Goodwin (2005) Paradoxes in tactile adaptation. Focus on "vibratory adaptation in cutaneous mechanoreceptive afferents" and "time-course of vibratory adaptation and recovery in cutaneous mechanoreceptive afferents". *J Neurophysiol* 94(5):2995–6.
27. Robert Schleip – see www.fasciaresearch.de, www.somatics.de for detailed articles and Robert Schleip, *Fascia in Sport and Movement*. Handspring Publishing, Ltd., Pencaitland, 2014.
28. Robert Schleip (2003) Fascial plasticity: a new neurobiological explanation, parts 1 and 2. *Journal of Bodywork and Movement Therapies* 7(1):11–19; 7(2):104–116.
29. H.M. Langevin (2006) Connective tissue: a body-wide signalling network? *Medical Hypotheses* 66(6):1074–1077.
30. Eckart Altenmüller, Gottfried Schlaug (2015) Chapter 12 – Apollo's gift: new aspects of neurologic music therapy. Edited by: Eckart Altenmüller, Stanley Finger, François Boller. *Progress in Brain Research*, Elsevier, 217:237–252
    ISSN 0079-6123, http://www.sciencedirect.com/science/article/pii/S0079612314000302
    ISBN 9780444635518, https://doi.org/10.1016/bs.pbr.2014.11.029.
    Further reading and presentations, TedX: Kathleen Howland, PhD, http://www.kathleenhowland.com
31. Robert Schleip (2003) Fascial plasticity: a new neurobiological explanation, part 1 and part 2. *Journal of Bodywork and Movement Therapies* 7(1):11–19; 7(2):104–116.
32. Ibid.
33. Ibid.
34. Stephen Levin, "The Tensegrity-Truss as a Model for Spine Mechanics: Biotensegrity". This paper was first presented at the 12th International Conference on Mechanics in Medicine and Biology, Lemnos, Greece, September 2002.
35. See Ch. 4
36. Robert Schleip (2003) Fascial plasticity: a new neurobiological explanation, parts 1 and 2, *Journal of Bodywork and Movement Therapies* 7(1):11–19; 7(2):104–116.
37. Ibid.
38. See Reference Note 16 above
39. See Appendix B: by John Sharkey
40. Quote from teachings of Swami Sathananda Saraswati: Asana Pranayama Mudra Bandha: Yoga Publications Trust, Munger, Bihar, India.
41. Donna Jeanne Haraway, *Crystals, Fabrics, and Fields: Metaphors that Shape Embryos*, North Atlantic Books, Berkeley, CA, 1976, 2004. Foreword By Scott F. Gilbert, another epigeneticist.
42. Mae-Wan Ho, *The Rainbow and the Worm: The Physics of Organisms*, 3rd edition, World Scientific Publishing, Singapore, 2008.
43. Doris Taylor, PhD, Director, Regenerative Medicine Research at Texas Heart Institute, http://texasheart.org/Research/RegenerativeMedicine/.
44. Mae-Wan Ho, *The Rainbow and the Worm: The Physics of Organisms*, 3rd edition, World Scientific Publishing, Singapore, 2008.
45. Christopher-Marc Gordon, Physiotherapeut PT.hcpc. UK Heilpraktiker Osteopathie Naturheilmedizin; research at Ulm University.
46. Mae-Wan Ho, *The Rainbow and the Worm: The Physics of Organisms*, 3rd edition, World Scientific Publishing, Singapore, 2008.
47. Ibid
48. This quote is taken from Deane Juhan's book, *Job's Body*. The bold type is further emphasis added by John Sharkey to endorse and expand the point. It has been sanctioned by Deane Juhan in private correspondence; June 2020
49. Robert Schleip MA: Cert. Rolfing Instructor & Feldenkrais Practitioner, Rolfing Faculty, European Rolfing Association e.V., Kapuzinerstr. 25, D-80337 Munich, Germany. *Journal of Bodywork and Movement Therapies* (2003) 7(2),104–116.
50. John Sharkey, *The Concise Book of Neuromuscular Therapy – a trigger point manual*. Lotus Publishing, Chichester, England and North Atlantic Books, Berkeley, California, 2008.

6

Living Tensegrity Structures

"Engineers make structures for specific uses, to support something, to hold something, to do something. My sculptures serve only to stand up by themselves, and to reveal a particular form such as a tower or a cantilever or a geometrical order probably never seen before; all of this because of a desire to unveil, in whatever ways I can, the wondrous essence of elementary structure."[1]

Kenneth Duane Snelson, 1927–2016.

Kenneth Snelson's structures serve "only to stand up by themselves" which is something we already do. It is the question of *how* we (already) do that, and what biomechanical properties we assign to the answer, that is so profoundly challenged by fully understanding fascia.

What Exactly Does "Tensegrity" Have to Do with It?

At the most elementary expression of ourselves as living structures, we are already demonstrating a balance of internal and external, of "equal and opposite" forces. Just by being alive and "standing (or sitting) up by ourselves" doing yoga on our mats, we demonstrate that. By breathing and taking up space, as a volume, we are expressing a homeostatic balance of forces in all dimensions, still or in motion. Those are the balance of gravity and *ground reaction* force.

The question for us in a yoga context is, how *do we stand up and do inversions* without our heads falling off, *if they are upright inverted pendulums* as classical biomechanics would have us believe. Our heads don't tend to fall off, yet *if we were made of stacked bones* (as we are also told in classical biomechanics) they would routinely roll off the spinal "column" as soon as we tilt the top of our vertebral "stack" (along with any other vertebral bodies balanced there). That is *if* the spine *really* was a column and the bones were *really* stacked. (They're not – and neither are we!)

We integrally *sustain* our wholeness on the yoga mat; bits of us don't break off, even when we are balancing our whole body on one foot. By the same token, we can climb cliffs and climbing walls, holding on by fingertips and toes (Fig. 6.2C), yet we don't routinely expect to break bits off or watch them topple

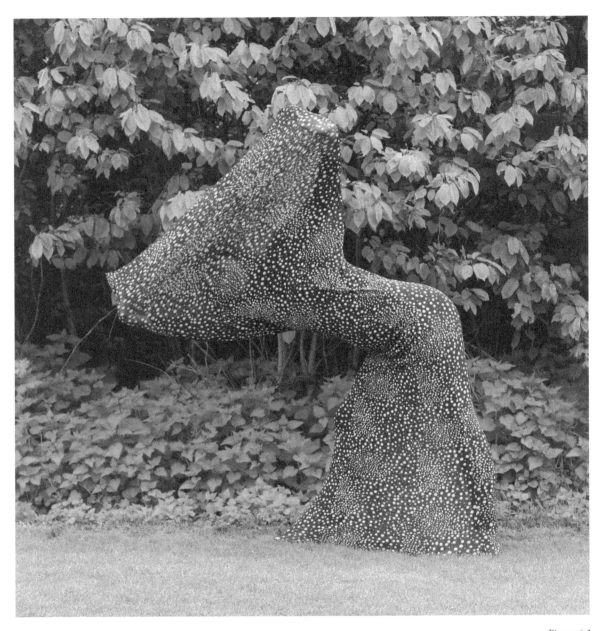

Figure 6.1

This is a visual metaphor for the tensional nature of the fascia matrix. It is body-wide and scale-free. We are a pre-tensioned architecture; everywhere in the healthy body is under appropriate tension.

Image: Amy Very; model: Helen Eadie. Reproduced with kind permission of Art of Contemporary Yoga Ltd. With loving gratitude to Trudy Austin (at TrudyAustin.com) for this gorgeous tube to play in.

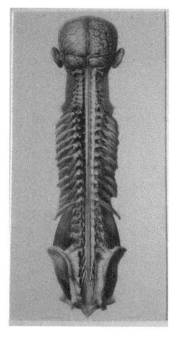

Figure 6.2A

This classical painting of the spinal column in early anatomy studies, shows the posterior view precisely as if it is a column and comprised of stacked vertebrae. It ignores the implications of the curvature, by showing only this view.

away! If you weigh 80–90 kg, then how does a part of your body that weighs less than one to five percent of that support all the rest of you? If the smallest parts of the furthest extremities (fingers and toes) are the only contact with the ground, or the rock wall, how do we do that? Indeed, in a handstand, or in side-plank, or even headstand, the least of you is attached or supported and the rest is in a position wider than the hand-, head- or footprint – where do columns fit into it? (They don't).

It transpires that tensegrity structures *model the forces* that actually explain what we do and how we are enabled to do it. Your living biological, pre-stressed architecture[2] is integrally designed to do what it does; which is balance, shift, shuffle, tilt, bend, straighten, spring and spiral. *Levers have nothing to do with it.*

This is an essential piece in the puzzle about fascia and how understanding its organisation can enhance our appreciation of how essential *tension-compression* forces are to every aspect of yoga, in motion and stillness. Not just compression (as in columns), not just tension (as in string nets), but an exquisitely detailed expression of nature's geometry *as a unified* tension-compression architecture.[3] It is invariably one that has its frame on the inside, *entirely enclosed in the round*. It is a valuable exploration, because it allows us to find a congruent reflection of the unifying nature of the yogic journey for the body, the mind and the being, as we will see. The forms and their patterns are universal – and so too are the geometries they express. That even suggests unifying yogic philosophy and anatomy – however let's consider the body first.

Fascia and Tensegrity

"Synergy refers to the observation made first by R. Buckminster Fuller that in any system the whole is always greater than the sum of its parts. The behaviour of tensegrities is a visual demonstration of this"

Tom Flemons[4]

We have established that our form is self-assembled as a sensitive fabric (see Chs 4 & 5) out of one piece. That fabric senses the shifts in forces moving through the form in all directions, *constantly*. It also senses the forms shifting in response to each other *with the forces*. It is a profoundly complex, interrelated management system of exchange from outside in and the inside out, constantly oscillating its living responsiveness. In a way that could be described as the *animation of our animated form*. We are already doing it. It is our integral kinematic blueprint – *always and only EVER in the round as a volume.*

Gravity is a radial force and we occupy 360 degrees of the space around us, in a way, defying the gravitational forces pressing us to earth. We animate *ground reaction force* in order to stand up and do the postures, breathe and move, naturally resisting gravity's pressure. That is *already what is happening*; it is what we might call "a given pre-disposition". It essentially describes how we are/move. The climber (see Fig. 6.2C) is literally hanging upside down in the picture, with the potential to spring up and outward (around the overhang) in his spring-loaded architecture. It has nothing to do with levers or stacked columns of bones. This body architecture is defying gravity in a naturally self-contained way, internally generating the forces he requires to animate such a movement. The spell under which lever-based biomechanics continue to mesmerize us is broken, right there. It is the wrong logos.

Snelson's "unveiling of the wondrous essence of elementary structures" describes, in models, these tension-compression **forces,** working together to sustain their volume *without stacking*. They **form** what Buckminster Fuller called "tensegrity[5]" and applied to architecture, in the form of geodesic domes (more on that later). Decades after Fuller, Donald Ingber[6] discovered that similar logic makes sense of how individual cells move around and maintain their volume within the body, at the level of the **microcosm**; particularly sensitive to biochemical and "mechanobiological"[7] responses. Stephen Levin[8] applies research to the living **macrocosm,** coining the term *biotensegrity* to explain how our bodies and movements correspond to these founding principles – *on every scale*. Tensegrity models may explain how our cells move and organise inside of us: as a reflection of how the whole body moves in our environment, remaining self-contained. That is to explain the way we move into and out of the yoga postures; *all of them – in all positions - at all times.*

In other words, living tensegrity provides a global explanation of how our form is performing and responding to internal and external forces constantly seeking balance (homeostasis and allostasis – see margin) between them, on *every* scale. That is the balance between the *innersphere* and *kinesphere* (see Ch. 17), the compression and the tension between gravity all around us, relentlessly pressing us to the ground (compression). The equal and opposite *ground reaction force* naturally (and precisely) resists it (tension), to maintain our volume as a biologic form, in all positions. Together, these two forces (tension and compression) are within and behind our every move, as a living tensegrity system, essentially made of soft matter (that abides by the same rules on the inside as the outside). That is the key reason why we can't readily apply the more classical biomechanical models, which are derived from hard matter forms. **We are made of soft matter and the rules are different**. We are based in geometry, which circles us back to the ancient yogic philosophies as well as making sense of how we practise the asanas, bandhas, mudras and meditations – indeed, it describes how we

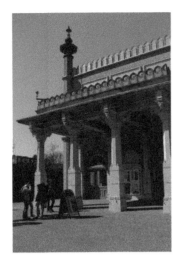

Figure 6.2B

Columns in architecture are stacked compression structures at 90 degrees to the ground; designed to support all that is above them, in precise, right-angled geometry.

Image reproduced with kind permission from the photographer, Bex Hawkins.

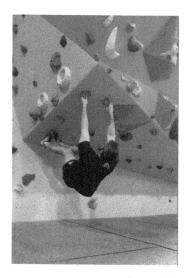

Figure 6.2C

This climber weighs 87 kg. The entire body weight is almost entirely held in place by his fingertips and the toes of one foot. (The next sequence in the video shows a swing outward and upward, from this triangulated position.) That is an indication of how the body uses internal and external forces to balance itself in ways that classical biomechanical leverage does not account for.

Image reproduced with kind permission from Ben Avison (model).

live *as self-regulating, breathing volumes*. (Breath-motion being the signal that we are alive!) Yoga, as a "unifying principle" honours this unifying expression of life force; it is unifying the rules of soft matter, as they apply to all living things.

We could say that biological or living tensegrity (Levin's *biotensegrity*)[9] is the algorithm[10] that explains our volume and the forming of it, into the shape we hold ourselves to be, *whatever shape we are in*. We are always a volume and we need *volumetric* rules (of geometry) to explain how we move into stillness and out of it. Levers fail that qualification, since they are two-dimensional structures, moving around a pin-joint in one plane (see Part B). (Levers describe hard-matter physical structures and we live under a different subset – *soft-matter physics*.) We may contain some pretty "hard" bones, which on the spectrum of our soft tissues are the most crystallised (approximately 30% of them are; the rest of the inner bone material is more like porridge than wood or solid crystal in the living body) (Fig. 6.3). Yet they are nonetheless part of the soft tissue matrix, including the superficial fascia, which we might consider at the other end of that "harder to softer" spectrum. It is "all us", "all in us" and all developed *from and by* us, as embryos[11] (see Ch. 4).

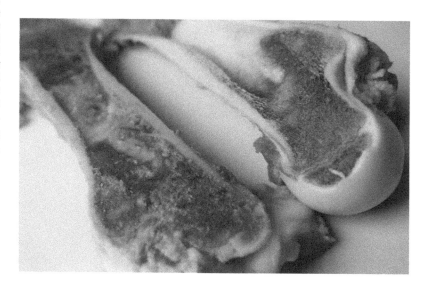

Figure 6.3

This is cross-section of mammalian bone, showing the crystalline pattern of the internal mass and how narrow the stronger, harder margins are. The texture inside is mostly like the consistency of thick porridge, except at the ends where you see the cartilage (white).

Photograph by Bex Hawkins. Reproduced with kind permission from Art of Contemporary Yoga Ltd.

Biologic Forms

Biological creatures are, by definition, non-linear and they behave according to the rules of soft-matter, *non-linear* forms, naturally and *invariably*. There are no "partial" aspects of this. The weave of the fluid, sensory matrix can alter, the fabric can change, thicken, stiffen, soften; the folds can manifest all kinds of different shapes and patterns inside to outside and outside to inside. The thickness of the containing fabric can vary the shapes of the forms (see Ch. 7), which are always whole and contained *as a volume in space*. However, they *don't behave* in a linear manner, because they are not straight, or flat, or organised in lines, with a beginning a middle and an end, a starting point and an ending point. From conception to death, we live in (and as) a *continuum*, a *volume that is complete in itself*. Non-linear biologic forms don't have exact fronts, backs, sides, tops and bases like flat-packed kitchens (see Ch. 9). Living creatures respond to forces *in the round*.

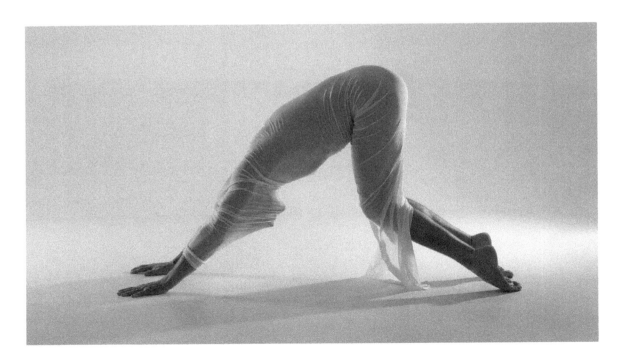

Figure 6.4

Barely on his feet, weight on hands, in this image the model is "the right way up" – however his spine still isn't stacked – obviously. His weight is contained – notice how lightly he balances on his forefeet.

Model: Wibbs Coulson; photographer: Amy Very. Reproduced with kind permission from Art of Contemporary Yoga Ltd.

Embracing Paradox

"In creating this mathematics, Newton embraced a paradox. He believed in atoms, small but ultimately indivisible – not infinitesimal. Yet he built a mathematical framework that was not discrete but continuous, based on a geometry of lines and smoothly changing curves. 'All is flux, nothing stays still,' Heraclitus had said two millennia before. 'Nothing endures but change.' But this state of being – in flow, in change – defied mathematics then and afterwards. Philosophers could barely observe continuous change, much less classify it and gauge it, until now. It was nature's destiny now to be mathematised. Henceforth space would have dimension and measure; motion would be subject to geometry."[12]

In the absence of computer-generated graphics and 3D printing, this was hitherto a feat of the imagination and adequate description, which makes da Vinci's geometric drawings quite astounding for their day (Fig. 6.5 and see Ch. 1). *Leonardo da Vinci saw architecture when he studied human form. The weave of the myofascial matrix, taken globally, expands the possibilities of how we define form.*

Looking back into the history reveals that Newton (see Ch. 2), besides distinguishing a profound understanding of gravity, also **invented calculus**. Before that time, geometry was the dominant lens through which three-dimensional forms were studied and discussed, how they occupy space and move around. (Recall from Chapter 2, that Newton was socially ridiculed as the "great geometer" by Blake.) With the advent of calculus, there was a way to *symbolise* (in letters and numbers on paper) how forms move, at various rates, *calculating* the variabilities and "mathematising them".

Thanks to Newtonian calculus, it was possible (for the educated elite) to describe how volumes move around in (and occupy) space (including the variations and possibilities), through a system of symbols, in equations that were far removed from the forms they described. Symbolic mathematics developed complex themes and calculations, presented in a universally recognised system as a valuable kind of "short-hand". It was akin (in its day) to the programming language behind the workings of your computer. It creates the platforms for the programmes to run, within which are the algorithms that organise them. Understanding that short-hand was a specialised skill, a tool to explain the organisation of the celestial bodies as well as things moving on earth.

This represented significant progress, so long as everyone remembers that the algebra is *symbolising* the original form *as an abstract equation* to imply its wholeness as a volume occupying space (Fig. 6.6). In and of itself, the equation is not the whole volume in space – it is a string of symbols *representing it*.

Equations Do Not Equal Experience

"Newton was eager, as the Greeks had not been, to extend the harmony and abstraction of mathematics to the crude sub-lunary world in which he lived. An apple was no sphere, but he understood it to be flying through space along with the rest of the earth's contents, spinning across 25,000 miles

each day. Why then, did it hang gently downward, instead of being flung outward like a stone whirled around on a string? The same question applied to the moon: what pushed it or pulled it away from a straight path?"[13] *(see Fig. 6.7.)*

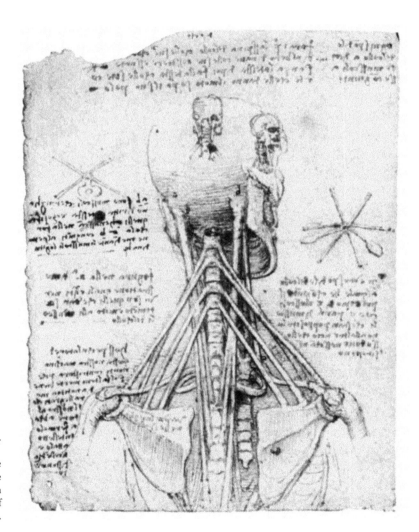

Figure 6.5

Leonardo da Vinci saw architecture when he studied human form. The weave of the myofascial matrix, taken globally, expands the possibilities of how we define form.

The algebraic equation *symbolically* describes why the apple hangs *down* from the tree, igniting the growing understanding of gravity that hallmarked Newton's genius.[14] Regardless of the apple's shape, what matters in the algebraic equation describing its fall are its *centre of mass* and the rate (*velocity*) at which it drops (when it does), via the shortest path, towards the centre of the earth, interrupted by the orchard floor on its way.

THE LOVE FORMULA

$$x^2 + (y - \sqrt[3]{x^2})^2 = 1$$

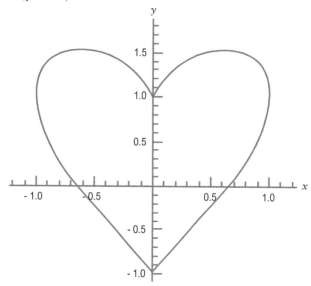

Figure 6.6

This is the algebraic equation for the shape of a valentine heart. It doesn't have quite the feel of even a heart-shaped, red emoji – let alone a loving feeling. Mathematics wasn't about love, however, it was about calculating accurately to describe nature; so calculus was an essential tool of progress.

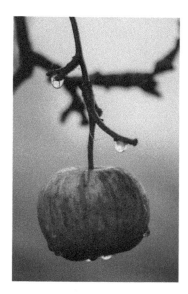

Figure 6.7A

The single apple.

Photo by Moritz Kindler on Unsplash.

How Round Things Organise: Rules Of Close-Packing

At the time, calculus provided an essential means to confirm the new distinctions of gravitational force as physical laws of nature, a phenomenon that influences *everything*. The symbolic apple (although not precisely spherical) remains rounded; it only *falls* in a linear pathway. Like us, in every moment and movement, it is obliged by the rules of physics to take the shortest route towards the earth's centre. The *equation explaining* how the apple falls to earth tells you little about the apple, or how it grows (itself), looks, tastes or self-assembles. The laws of gravity tell you much more about the *forces acting upon it* than the form they are interacting with (however intimately related they may be).

The apple grows itself, while it is connected to the tree (Fig. 6.7A), which is connected to the earth while the apple is a *living* growing, organic fruit. When all the apples have fallen or been picked, they may technically be dead apples, however they are still rounded and pack together in particular patterns of "close-packing", with spaces in between them. If they were inside a sealed bag, you would have a model of "a bag enclosing round things" much like any membrane enclosing cells (think embryo and pericardium enclosing heart cells and pleura enclosing lung cells). The **forces** between

Gluick points out "Newton did not need an apple to remind him that objects fell to earth", explaining how the intricate history of the times (inclusive of Descartes' philosophies), developed Newton's understanding of gravity over decades. Gravitational force transmission didn't arrive

Forces through Forms

as a flash of inspiration one sunlit afternoon in 1666. The growing distinctions of forces – and their impact on form – are often collapsed in our understanding and application of classical biomechanics and living anatomy today. It is echoed centuries later in the growing understanding of tensegrity as a natural explanation of force transmission in the human body. While we show caution around collapsing the distinctions of functional movement theories and human experience, tensegrity emerges as a compelling model of force-transmission through forms; whatever we feel.

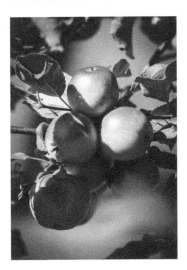

Figure 6.7B

Close-packed apples naturally abiding by the laws of close-packing, as a growth pattern.

Photo by Jon Sailer on Unsplash.

those close-packed apples are what the tensegrity models are representing. The bag represents the enclosing membrane: just as the apple skin represents the enclosing membrane of the apple-cells inside it; they grew inside it – expanding the skin as they did so. (They never stack together like a Rubik's Cube, packing in cubes; that is not how soft-matter things work, as we will see; they close-pack as round things; which are actually icosahedral. It is the founding law of nature.)

From apples close-packed together inside a bag, think organelles inside any cell, or cells to organs, organs to organisms and so on. Living things are close-packed systems in and of themselves; they are made of round things, essentially organised by fascia (if we are talking animals and humans – cellulose if we are talking flowers and plants). Fascia/cellulose act as the connective "in-between" and the membrane surrounding it. Living forms manifest collectively as tubes and pockets and pouches that are never anything other than continuously inter-connected, in the body, or form, they express. That is how they close-pack, as organic forms (see Fig. 6.7B). As soon as this is applied to an organism that can *move itself*, the pattern (constantly) phase changes (or you could also say, as there is phase change, the organism constantly moves) – *that movement denotes the mother of all forces, Prana, which is life force.* Trees do it too; just considerably slower than we do.

Historically, after calculus was invented to explain volumes, geometry tended to be considered a supplementary study, until it was dropped altogether from most curriculums, today. This was happening when the "aesthetic aspect" of art was being cut out of anatomy (see Ch. 2), to reveal the anaesthetic reductionist parts; explained as mechanics while the industrial age was cultivated. Calculus became the default to describe volumes moving in space because it didn't require (unreliable) imagination to envisage the shapes in 3D that the equation could represent "more accurately". On the yoga mat, however, back here on earth, we live as, at least, 3D volumes. We simply don't reduce to algebraic equations (or lines, levers or flat planes), we are not cartoons, or deducible as algebraic equations, even if they can provide accurate calculations of the vectors we move through. *They never deliver the experience in present time*; that is *our* job, as we engage in performance, expressing our vitality, as "ourself", as best we can. **Mechanical equations do not help us move better**.

Behind our vital (multi-dimensional life) cycle, with all its patterns and geometry, we could say there is an algorithm that applies to all living things. That algorithm represents our constant responsiveness to gravity and ground reaction force: it is *biological tension–compression integrity* – something Dr Stephen Levin refers to as *biotensegrity*.[15] The biology is relentless, the balance of tension and compression forces ubiquitous and the expression of homeostasis **is** the balance between those forces, transmitted through the (pre-stiffened) fascial matrix. It gives rise to structural integrity of the life of the form(s): you, me and the rest of this animated collective of living beings on earth, breathing together on the earth we are bound to. Gravity keeps pushing/pulling us

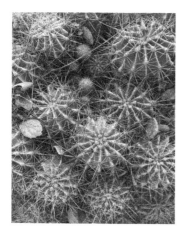

Figure 6.8

Cactus geometry pattern; these are the patterns of nature, in what is known as "4-fold" or "6-fold" and so on, patterns. These cacti have a 12-fold pattern. Such patterns are innate to the nature of self-assembling formations everywhere, if we look for them. (Image author's own.)

Figure 6.9

A conundrum: always in the round, whether it is the cells of the tree or the seed it grew from: the bud it grew, the flower it manifested; the pollen it displayed, the bees that cross-pollinated it (so that it became the fruit [apple] that contained the seed that contains the cells of the tree that grows the apples). The whole cycle of life is based in specific patterns and numerical geometries that self-organise naturally into the geometric patterns of the volumes interacting. Volumes inside membranes that close-pack as round things. They invariably default to the flower of life and tree of life organisations, described in geometric formulae (see Ch. 12) and more easily "seen" in those 2D patterns. As we said in Ch. 1, that is only a way of seeing them "on paper". It becomes less obvious in living form – nevertheless, it is the foundation of its structural integrity as a living, biologic (non-linear) architecture. We don't do squares and cubes. We do round things and tubes.

towards the earth's centre and we keep pushing/pulling back in 360 degrees of volumetric, tubular networks. That's just how it is.

We might call it *living tensegrity*, to distinguish it from the *models* of tensegrity. Models (like the Manhattan Toy Company Tensegritoy, designed by Tom Flemons; Fig. 6.9) model the geometry and the tension–compression **forces.** Together those two forces co-create the third (volume), as a result of their interactive balance and pattern of organisation. As such, tensegrity models are *triangulated forms.* (Tension and compression co-create tension–compression unity. There are three forces in the Whole Trinity and three struts in the most minimal model.[16]) That is another way of saying, we are round things in membranous bags, not square or cube-like stacks in blocks and columns. We hold ourselves up in space; columns stack themselves upon the ground; movement of the structure is usually detrimental to its upright integrity.

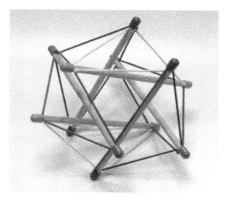

A useful definition from Leonid Blyum is as follows: "…biotensegrity is based on a high mathematical level definition of tensegrity that refers to the architecture of tensioned frameworks/networks at different size scales and NOT on a narrow specific embodiment of struts and cables that are 'palpable' in the tensegrity toys."

Calculus had an impact upon the study and *appreciation* of volumes. It may serve us to re-establish the original geometry (see Ch. 12) to describe the original wholeness it sought to explain and represent (and biotensegrity seeks to do that). If we have the idea that we can reduce human formation to formulae (and performance to the genetic coding of our species – see Ch. 4), we limit our qualitative appreciation of our form, as well as our experience of it. We don't reduce easily – however long-held the spell of reductionism is.

Our *natural* forms are *unique and individual, self-assembled, self-motivated* volumes-in-process. We are forming, deforming and reforming, from moment-to-moment, as a soft-matter container, occupying space, contained by our outermost sleeve, *all the time,* wrapped in gravity, in time. Living or biological tensegrity provides the algorithm behind that performance in time, *all the time.* It is a scale-free algorithm, so it can account for the changes in a

Close-Packed Soft Matter

When you see people packed together in a crowd, inside a subway train, for example, they abide by the same formulas of tension and compression. The difference in such an example is that the train is made of hard matter, which is highly resistant to shape change (unlike the bark of the tree or the skin of the fruit, that expands as its internal volume swells). The people in the train are all made of soft matter, so they jostle and push and get pushed together (to a tipping point of being crushed) inside the "cell" of the train carriage. We prefer space around us, in a yoga class, so we can explore our shapes "in our own space" – nevertheless, we are simply behaving as loosely packed soft matter beings, moving inside a "cell", provided by the walls of the room. Yoga in the park and on the beach has a feeling of freedom to it, but we are still wrapped in gravity. In a way, we could say, we are simply moving as a loosely packed "close-packed" collective on the planet! Humans being are still connected, albeit metaphorically, by our common intention and attention, just with a wider "in-between" volume. When we are scrunched together on a train, we are still inside a volume, with similar close-packing issues; but the train doesn't expand and in-draw, like the sac around an organ for example, or our breathing torso around our visceral organs. The train isn't made of soft matter. Unlike us, it is mechanical hard-matter.

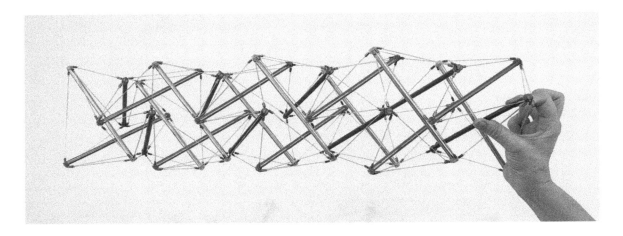

Figure 6.10A

A tensegrity mast. It begins as continuous strings, which are not elastic, joined together, without tension, at specific points, into which the metal tubes are inserted. As the whole mast tightens, the stiffer spacers take up their roles. It assumes this shape which, when dropped on its end, bounces several inches off the ground and maintains its tensional integrity and innate elasticity.

Reproduced in kind acknowledgement of Bruce Hamilton, designer of this mast. http://www.tensiondesigns.com.

(1) **Homeostasis** is a popular word denoting healthy balance (see definition). John Sharkey suggests another term that better describes the fact that, as living soft-matter forms, we seek balance in constant motion, in direct response to various forces.

cell nucleus within its cytoplasm and cell walls, just as it can account for the behaviour of that cell within the organ[19] (and the organ within the organism) – and it is metaphorically recreated by the body-in-a-tube (see Fig. 6.1) here and on the cover. No surprise, it is the same forces in microcosm reflecting the macrocosm (and the cosmos). It is the physical description or (at least)

(2) **Allostasis** is the term he suggests and both are offered here for consideration.

1. the tendency towards a relatively stable equilibrium between interdependent elements, especially as maintained by physiological processes.

2. the process by which a state of internal, physiological equilibrium is maintained by an organism in response to actual or perceived environmental and psychological stressors. Therefore, *allostasis* is the process that keeps the organism alive and functioning, i.e. maintaining homeostasis or "maintaining stability through change" and promoting adaptation and coping, at least in the short run" (Bruce S. McEwen, *Neurobiology of Aging*, 2002).

Tensegrity models come in all shapes and sizes. The integrity of the model is of course based upon hard matter materials – the sticks and string of the model *constructed to demonstrate* the **forces**. Our bodies, representing the **forms** in which tensegrity works *in vivo*, incorporate and express tension and compression *forces* into far more complex soft-matter geometries than most models demonstrate, organised by the organising matrix of us – the fascia (the form). The tensegrities based upon living things move as self-contained, liquid-crystalline (see Ch. 7), self-authorising matrices that can stiffen and soften and change *themselves*. We are, as John Sharkey points out, "made of one thing" (we could call it the "materia biologica" of our living tensegral organisation) – fascia.[17] The toys do not represent forms of muscles and bones. They symbolise forces that move through them, which are scale-free. Moreover, they are in constant flux – as we will consider in the next chapter. Movement is an asset to our structural integrity; it is not detrimental, as it is to columns.

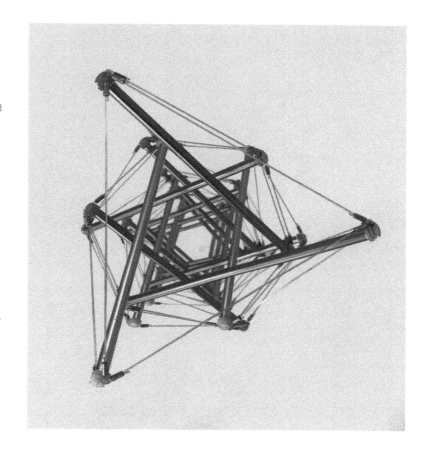

Figure 6.10B

End shot of the mast in Fig 6.10A, showing the triangulated basis revealed in the pattern of Solomon's Seal or the Star of David. As in Snelson's Needle Tower, the end elevation of the mast appears in cross-section, at any point, as a plan view of the star tetrahedron (see Ch. 12).

3D map of spacing (the *spacialisation*) we encountered in Chapter 4, in the embryonic journey into form. We continue to develop on the same principles, every move we make, on or off the mat.[20]

Whatever we call it, round things behave in certain ways, as collectives. Be they cells in an organ, people in a classroom or planets in a cosmos, the round things don't care (see Ch. 5 for murmurations of starlings and shoals of fish). Nature expresses all of them, through all of them, via assigned and recognisable (bio-tensegral) behaviours that make sense of their form(s) *anyway*. Better still, like the apple, they are self-assembling and can retain their shape independently of gravity, which implies the rules they abide by are *already present within them*. They are the rules of our original self-assembly

The picture of "Helen in a tube" (see Fig 6.1) symbolises cellular containment, the next level of her whole body, pushing out toward a containing "cell wall" which the fabric is mimicking, as a visual metaphor. It resists deformation,

at conception (see Ch. 4). Nature *already* organises round things together in collectives. She always has; this isn't new. Every living thing on this planet has been doing it since the planet began; indeed that is *how* the planet began. The issue with this idea might be its scale – and its scale-free-ness. It is great, big, huge. It rewrites the books.

"....biotechnologists have developed a very intriguing discipline, termed: mechanobiology (pioneered by Professor Donald E. Ingber), that focuses on the key role of mechanical forces and their responsibilities, in matters relating to biological structures and their functioning regardless of the size. This mechanobiology discipline, however, calls upon several approaches that cut across all scientific disciplines, namely: mathematics and physics, medical sciences and chemistry. Nonetheless, much in this new discipline has been borrowed from the cellular tensegrity theory, which dictates that living systems use principles of tensegrity architecture to govern how molecules self-assemble to create multi-molecular structures, organelles, cells, tissues, organs and living organisms."[21]

just as she does. Her limbs are long, tubular shapes that fold at the "dis-joints"[18] (unlike the more spherical apples). Nevertheless, they are rounded, volumetric containers being contained (and close-packed) by the tubing fabric. Her body is containing the cylindrical pattern of her bones and muscles inside their skin. Each of those is inside its own "pocket" or "fold" of the fascial matrix, like a skin-within-a-skin. The pattern continues, evident in the tube-like shapes of the muscle fibres and fibrils within the limbs and body, to the tiniest bilaminar wrapping of every cell, close-packed in the organ "pocket" on the same basis of a tension–compression structure. It goes on, in what is called a "heterarchical arrangement" that is omni-directional, throughout the form (see Chs 7 and 12). It is also hierarchi-

As we discussed in Chapter 4, *the architect self-assembles the architecture, through which to express the architect, as the architecture.* Every living thing is its own architect and its own architecture, expressing itself as such.

This is how living shapes organise themselves; the patterns of the forms invariably respond to the patterns of the forces (of tension and compression). They interact with each other to express themselves; we express them uniquely *as* life force. Indeed, that is how we become us – by moving the forms and growing and changing the forms, with the physical, mental, emotional life forces that animate through us all the time. Those forces in yoga are symbolised by Ida and Pingala, the principle of masculine and feminine, or negative and positive, attraction and repulsion,[22] tension and compression. In every case they combine to create a third, co-creative balancing force. One that spontaneously arises as a result of their co-creative pattern and balance. In yoga that force is called *Shushumna*, the neutral, the stillness, the tension–compression *allostasis* (see margin note). We are made of the tissue of expression of these forces, structured and sensed by the same matter, expressing its universal patterns within the matrix, as the matrix itself.

The Fruit

cal, in that the body self-organises with specific priorities as we move and adjust the metabolism to do so, in space–time.

How does it serve to explain human motion via lever-based mathematics that apply to hard-matter stick figures in 2D (bolted together with pin-joints), that conform to linear equations and move in flat planes? It makes sense of Pinocchio, who

The orange (see Ch. 3) close-packs its juice droplets more obviously than we can see the apple close-packing its apple droplets (or bone or muscle or any tissue close-packing its fibres or "muscle droplets" for example – see Ch. 7). They are nevertheless bound together by the proteins, minerals and compounds of the fluids and fabrics of their architecture, just like the bits of orange-ness that close-pack to form a whole orange. There are different densities, but the principle *forming forces* are, nonetheless, tension and compression (see discussion of bound fluids, Ch. 7), attraction and repulsion within their fluidic matrix. This applies to us, as much as the fruit. We too are made entirely of pockets of bound-together cells. *Our basic fabric is fascia; theirs is called cellulose. Same, same but different.*

"Tensegrity is the model that binds – and it binds all the other models"

John Sharkey

requires a puppeteer to activate the *semblance* of motion in 3D, but the self-motivated experience is present as missing. We shape-shift and restore ourselves *as volumes* by ourselves. It matters, when we want to understand how the living matrix works *its own tension–compression integrity,* **with no strings.** Those of us fortunate enough to have healthy bodies are our own puppeteers, **operating from within.**

The word "matter" (and matrix) come from Mater, Latin for mother. The word "pattern" comes from Pater, Latin for father.[23] They combine, or unite, to form the third incorporation (child), arising from their co-creative expression of life force. These are sacred principles at the foundation of the cycle of life.

Floating in a Sea of Tension

What is immediate and obvious in experience can be hidden from a two-dimensional format presented on paper. In architecture, for example, you take a leap from looking at the plan view or side elevation on the drawing board to experiencing the actual building. When you physically experience occupying the space that the drawing is designed to *represent,* it is almost beyond imagination. Even virtual, three-dimensional images cannot recapitulate your sense in space of relative relationships between the parts. We have to make that leap to explode

Fascia means "binding" or "bandage" and haptic means "to fasten"; we are bound together by the tensegrity of the fascial structure and its continuity. The haptic sensory response seems to ensure and foster connectedness and continuity in the most sensitive and exquisite detail, *throughout our architecture.* That sensitivity *is* the matrix of the form, responding to the forces. (We will explore this in practice in Part C.) The structural impact of that is *distributed throughout the form* by the geodesic rules of geometric force transmission,[24] by which all living things have to abide, entirely, as volumes moving in space. Otherwise referred to as a "tensegrity" model, aka Levin's "biotensegrity" when applied to living forms.[25]

Yoga already expresses itself in some of the most beautiful slow, soft and fluid sequences of Vinyasa to explore this interrelated, biomotional integration, in active movement sequences. Yoga makes sense of why preparing the body to sit, eventually for many hours at a time, in complete stillness, would be considered a powerful asset of self-awareness and self-regulation. It would be a simple (but not easy) state of deep listening, of profound balance between forces, as an expression of self-organising authority and refined haptic perception (see Ch. 5) *as a volume,* self-regulating its structure, form and function.

We *grow* our limbs and body *into* a pre-tensioned form. The potential bone tissue of the embryo (think "cartilaginous placeholder") grows considerably faster than the surrounding tissues, so we are already pre-stressed into form from the outset.[26] We are in a kind of "Babygro" body suit, the dense, inner (bony) part of which grows faster than the materials in between it and the skin. That causes it to take on what is called a "pre-stiffened" architecture. It means the bones act somewhat like self-developing poles inside a self-assembled tent-pole pocket, to tension the canvas (tissues), so that it holds its shape (see Ch. 4).

How this "tent-pole" idea of a pre-stiffened architecture came to be known as a "tensegrity" is a beautiful story, told in all its detail by Graham Scarr[27] in his book *Biotensegrity: The Structural Basis of Life.* Kenneth Snelson was the sculptor who designed one of the first floating compression structures, in 1948, known as his "early X-piece".[28] The architect Buckminster Fuller (Snelson's teacher at the time) recognised the model as a keystone presentation of how the *forces* operate in round things.

"…This fact was invisible to and unthought of by historical man up to yesterday. Before this mid-twentieth century fact discovery, there was naught to disturb, challenge or dissolve his "solid-rock," and other "solid things" thinking. "Solid thinking" is as yet comprehensively popular and is even dominant over the practical considerations of scientists in general and even over the everyday

logic of many otherwise elegantly self-disciplined nuclear physicists. Tension and compression are inseparable and coordinate functions of [all] structural systems..."[29]

out of linear theories of biomechanical levers and feel how tensegrity principles might be innate to our structure. From a diagram (meaning two [dimensional]) to a hologram (meaning whole) requires a sensory leap of awareness and attention. As soon as you hold a tensegrity structure this makes immediate sense; its volume and resilience resonate with your own *through the proprioceptive experience* of holding it.

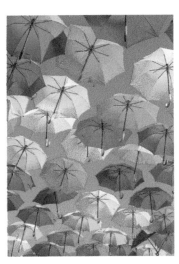

Figure 6.11

Umbrellas show an example of a tensioned structure; it is not a tensegrity as such, however, it is an example of how a harder tissue and a softer tissue can combine in a tension–compression-type organisation to co-facilitate structure; and fold into a different shape, without changing length. (This is such an important issue, when we apply tensegrity principles to yoga. See Appendix B).

Image reproduced with grateful thanks to Unsplash: Guy Stevens guy-stevens-dEGu-oCuB1Y-unsplash.

Fuller had already been studying geodesic domes on the basis that (to over-simplify very complex vectors) round things close-pack in geometries relating to the 60-degree angles of triangulation (think apples in a bag). Linear and square things close pack in 90-degree angles (think Rubik's Cube). The square things form compression structures (and stack) while the round things form tension–compression arrangements and tend toward self-organising non-linear forms.

Fuller recognised the essential importance of Snelson's sculpture and coined the term "tensegrity" from a compressing and joining of "tension" and "integrity". Snelson maintained the importance of recognising that the compression struts "float in a sea of tension".

In the studies of the human body, many anatomical icons (fondly known as cartoons among anatomists) present images of the body as if the bones somehow overlap, or stack one upon the other. Unless there is a pathology present, bones do not touch each other, however close together they may appear. Anatomically speaking, it is not healthy when bones do anything *other than* reside in their "sea of surrounding tissues". Those tissues are variations on the theme of fascia (we will consider this more in Chapter 7). However, they are all – by virtue of their forming process – under tension at all angles, in all directions of force – because they are inside a rounded structure (see Ch. 3, Jaap van der Wal).

Once again, where art meets science, alchemy occurs! Like da Vinci in the Renaissance, drawing the first S-shaped spine, Snelson (an artist) re-presents form for the anatomists. Snelson may have identified something about the spine and all its vertebrae (along with all the rest of the bones) that anatomists didn't consider significant. The overall organisation of the body, as a "floating compression system" makes perfect sense of its whole structure (which is destroyed anatomically, if the bones and muscles are cut up and away from each other and the fascia connecting them is discarded – see Ch. 3). *In situ*, the tissues form (and are formed in) a tension–compression network.[31] Nothing is excluded and everything is included, especially when we consider bone as calcified or mineralised fascia (see Ch. 1) and blood as a form of connective tissue. The difficulty that arises here is that the tensegrity models have to be made (manufactured) by someone, using two materials. It therefore appears that they represent the fascia as a continuous (tensioned) network and the bones as the discontinuous (compression) network. That would be inaccurate on three counts:

1. The tensegrity models demonstrate how the forces move – in and through a cell, or body.
2. What, inside your body, is not continuous?
3. Where in the body does the fascia stop (to be described as *dis*continuous)?

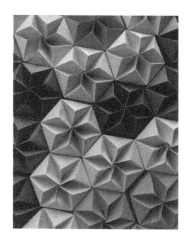

Figure 6.12

This origami image shows each hexagonal origami model, made out of one piece of paper. Imagine your structure formed *as one piece* in a variety of shapes (including but not limited to these patterns) and it can fold in and unfold out; without ever changing the amount of material. Only the configuration changes. (See Appendix B.)

Image reproduced with grateful thanks to Faris Mohammed on Unsplash: faris-mohammed-z0UfETjRl0g-unsplash.

Kenneth Snelson (1927–2016) was an artist, sculptor and geometer. His profound understanding of how nature shapes form in space can be seen applied to many aspects of science and art. He wrote: "My art is concerned with nature in its primary aspect, the patterns of physical forces in three-dimensional space."[30] I had the great privilege of speaking to Kenneth Snelson in his studio in New York City in 2015. It was an inspiring conversation in which he warned me to consider "tensegrity"

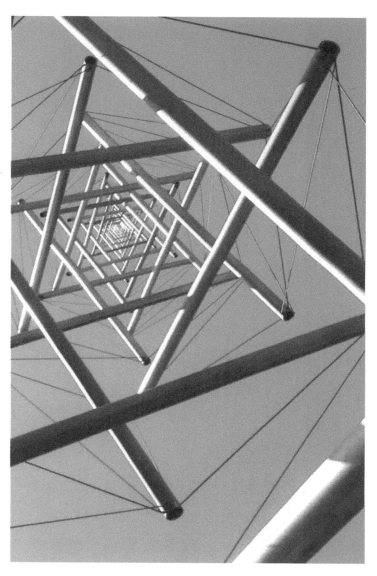

Figure 6.13

Snelson's Needle Tower relies on two forces arising: those of tension and compression, based upon the 60-degree angles of triangulated forms and abiding by the laws of round things in nature and their innate geometries relating to spheres.

"We are made only of one foundational, fundamental material expressing a multitude of specialities dictated by the addition of various components such as cells, myosin's, piezo2, hydroxyapatite and so on".[32]

Snelson's work on *Weaving, the Mother of Tensegrity*[33] is also beautiful in terms of making sense of how fascial tissue spirals itself into a lattice-like carefully for its nature as a "floating compression system; that floats in a sea of tension". He saw it, I believe, as an artist with a profound respect for Nature and how She paints and sculpts so many versions of emergent properties in everything. Everything that abides by fundamental cosmic laws. He wanted me to be intrigued with the "floating" part and the "sea of tension" – never disconnected from each other, in wholeness. *As we chatted, a white dove flew into his studio and he had to pause the conversation to let it out. It felt like a gift to me, with such a beautiful symbolic and spontaneous gesture of nature, to highlight the conversation – as one might mark an important line in a book that you want to remember forever.*

Tensegrity is a beautiful term, because within "integrity" is the "integer" which means "intact" and arises from the Latin meaning "whole or complete". It shares a root with "integrate" and "integral". In the modern dictionary, even under the medical use of the term integrity, it is described as a "state of being"!

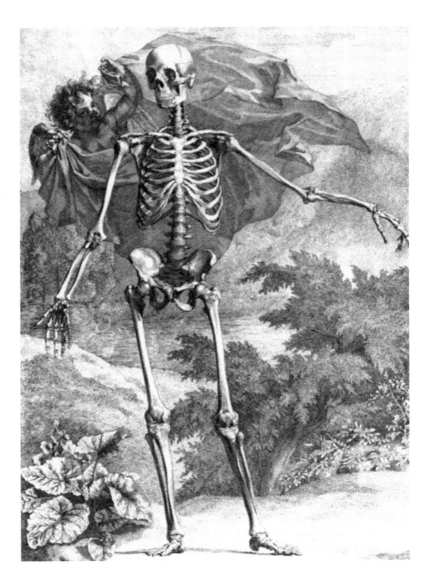

Figure 6.14

This beautiful image from Albinus on Anatomy[46], drawn by Jan Vandelaar, shows the human skeleton. This is the classical model. However, it cannot stand up like this without the connective tissues that are missing from the drawing.

weave, to facilitate so many variations in thickness, arrangement and forms and earn its poetic name as our *materia biologica*. It is extraordinary, especially if you accept that bone can really only be starched (calcified) and crystalline fascia[34] (see Ch. 7). We will look at how the shapes of tensegrity structures can be so various, after the early story of applying these forms to biology is told.

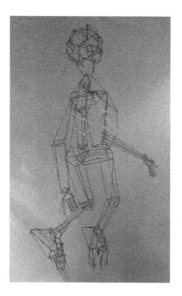 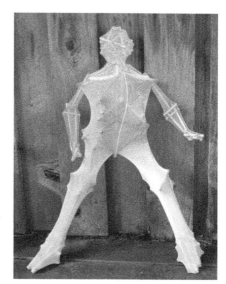

Figure 6.15

This model of the human form as a biotensegrity architecture, by Tom Flemons
(reproduced with his kind permission), does stand up on its own.

Our heads and limbs don't fall off – *therefore nothing can be stacked*. It is tensioned together (and very tightly bound) and compressed by the tensional forces. It is compressed together (and very tightly bound) and tensioned by the compressional forces *at the same time*. Levin (as an orthopaedic surgeon/ spine specialist) had his work cut out, but his patients kept being able to move better.

The rules of living tensegrity explain more than the overall form. The same algorithm lies behind the forming process of our first moment as a unicellular being, self-assembling (as we did) into the form we are now in, whatever that is. It is a performance we could say we do all day, every day, whether we are injured or not. We still abide by the "fasciategrity" rules of formation into forms.

Exercising our biological tensegrity is essentially *what we already do*. No self-respecting cell has a clue what a lever is, or how to behave like one. Your arm or leg may *look a bit like a lever* when its shadow is reflected as a silhouette (2D) on the wall. It is, however, a volume – which requires more than a flat-plane 2-bar system to explain it. That is just accurate. Your physics are not based solely on compression, but tension–compression as a combined, mutual, co-creative force transmission system.

Yoga and Living Tensegrity – the Perfect Training System?

The implications of understanding fasciategrity are exceptionally valuable for yoga teaching. This is largely because it is relatively easy to see tension–compression balance globally in the body once you know what you are looking at (see Ch. 17).

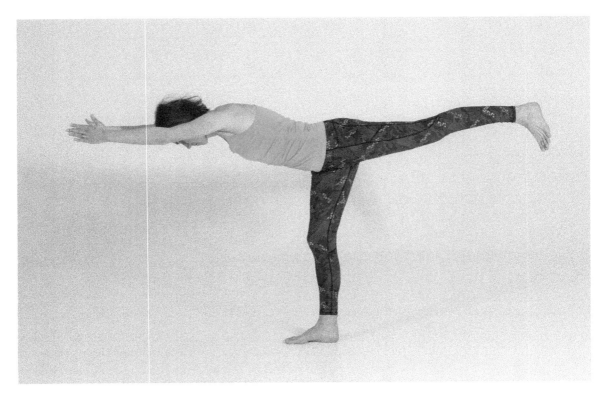

Figure 6.16

If the spine were a column, this pose would not be possible.

Model: Helen Eadie; photography: Amy Very. Reproduced with kind permission from Art of Contemporary Yoga Ltd.

Fasciategrity is a term created to explain how fascia abides relentlessly by the rules of self-assembly under tension–compression organisation. Just as Fuller created a syntactic of Tensional and Integrity, so John Sharkey and I answered many questions asking how fascia and biotensegrity relate to each other, with another syntactic. Thus, the term (somewhat tongue-in-cheek) "fasciategrity". Since we used it, other terms have arisen, such as "fascinteg-rity" but it doesn't have quite the same originality or ring to it!!

Once you develop a clear sense of how a living tensegrity structure is defined and expressed, it simplifies what you are looking for and amplifies the difference a small adjustment can make (see Ch. 17). What can be developed as a skill is the recognition of how the parts of us can be integrated and united by these principles, then translated usefully into movement management and precision and poise. Here, we will attempt to define the logic, and in Part C we will apply it to a number of postures and reveal its relative simplicity in practice. This does not mean fasciategrity is the answer to everything, but research that comes *from movement* and describes what we can already do, is intriguing. It makes sense of us as self-motivated and self-stabilising creatures. It is quite different to taking abstract biomechanical theories and trying to make the movements fit them. All research relies, to some extent, on the way the question is posed. The force transmission principles of tensegrity as the algorithm behind our motion patterns invite new questions about how we move as closed

The seeing lens of Fasciategrity distinguishes the balance between stiffness and elasticity (see Ch. 10) and this can provide a direct path to enhance body-reading skills. Adjustment cues become more relevant and accurate

The Gravity Line in Cueing

(see Ch. 17, Part C), *at the speed of a movement class.* Eventually we can develop our own (internal) sense of tensional balance, largely because it becomes a resonance that we see and sense by learning to read the shadows – a skill worth developing. It is unique to each of us. The practices in Part C are designed to enhance this haptic awareness of the fascial matrix, particularly for yoga teaching.

We are aligning with a different theory of movement that accounts for all of our range and makes sense of what we readily do in a yoga classroom, regardless of angle, position or speed. Trees, flowers, mammals, birds, insects, fish, all fauna and flora do this. They fold and unfold and move their volume as a contained but constantly changing morphology in perfect balance with the gravitational field around them, never in straight lines! (See Ch. 4 – it is a forming principle in embryology.) It is a system of coordinated resistance and surrender, stability and mobility, so fundamental to yoga practice. It is the growing, forming embodiment of "Sthiram Sukham" expressed as life. It invites us to re-evaluate a new context for some of the Sanskrit terms with which yoga is described, endorsing them. They can appear less literal and more naturally symbolic of our full, dynamic, geometric architecture (see Part C).

kinematic chains (Ch. 8). (According to Scarr,[35] this is key to understanding the basic organisation around specific joints.) Our volume, woven together by the fascial matrix of our forms, can be described geometrically. We will find out in Chapter 12 how eloquently those patterns are reiterated in some of the ancient wisdom behind yoga.

Yoga teachers often talk about the "gravity line" and a sense of being centred in the standing postures in particular: the idea of imagining a plumb line passing through the exact centre of the body, from the crown to a space between the feet, or the sitting bones if you are seated. This cue allows the body to sense itself sitting or standing "tall and straight", aligned in gravity.

There is, however, a fundamental problem with this visual idea, which is that gravity does not work in lines any more than people do (and the spine is curved – see Ch. 9). It is not simply a linear force and the idea that it is keeps certain awkward biomechanical arguments alive. Gravity is a radial force. We might imagine the opposite direction of a radiant light beaming out from the centre of the earth; gravity draws everything towards that centre. The ground interrupts us. It also gives us something to resist, in order to stand up or make adjustments. (We rely on it so completely that we can take it for granted.) As Leonid Blyum[36] points out: you can't adjust someone doing yoga in outer space, there is nothing to resist.

This is how we all live on a globe without being crushed or floating off; it is what we already do anyway. With such a radial force operating upon our contained architecture, the body is originally and ideally designed to respond morphologically to tension and compression forces throughout its network. We live in constant counterbalance: the ground reaction force (see Ch. 7) in response to gravity in *multi-directional* expressions.

Tension and compression are paired elements of our force transmission system, i.e. a network through which those forces are transmitted and, we might say, translated into movements congruent with our intentions. **Yoga is about unifying forces, multiplying up to the whole, rather than dividing down to the parts.** Together, tension and compression facilitate the "third force of *equilibre*", at any moment in time (of tension–compression combined). *It is what we already do.* Biotensegrity, once understood, is a superb explanation of *how we already do it!*

The difficulty in describing this lies in the limitations of theory versus experience. The first is restricted to words on a page while the second occurs in living experience of our form (i.e. the difference between the apple vs the calculus describing how it moves!).

How does the gravity "line" work, when the overall form of the human spine is a nonlinear "S" curve? It ideally has to be S-shaped, in order to be able to manage the range of positions, loads and movements human beings can do and facilitate natural rebound. It is designed to manage all the different internal and external changes while remaining spring-loaded, as a whole, *as we breathe*. When the human spine is not in an

S-shape, the person living around it is often impaired in their range and quality of motion (see Ch. 9). (Monkeys, for example, have relatively straight lumbar spines, and they move very differently from us over the ground and through the trees. They sit a lot and use their arms to swing through, or swing from, in very different movement signature to most humans.)

We do not move around the gravity line; rather, we occupy the contained space that works constantly to oppose its radial force on every aspect of us. In Figures 6.17 and 6.18 Wibbs is demonstrating this.

These, like any other fluid sequences or expressions of movement, are whole body postures, orchestrated by the organ of organisation – the fascia (in multiple expressions – managing tension/compression forces from within. That is centrifugally and centripetally in the round, volumetric

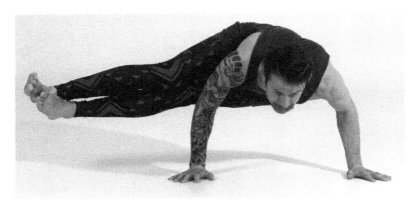

Figure 6.17

Where is this a compression-based structure?

Model: Wibbs Coulson; photography: Amy Very. Reproduced with kind permission from Art of Contemporary Yoga Ltd.

system that obviously is not stacked in vertical or horizontal planes. Such movements (and the above postures) abide by the rules of living tensegrity structures:

First Rule. A tensegrity structure is a continuously connected tension–compression network supporting, containing (and tensioned by) floating compression struts.

Second Rule. A living tensegrity structure is an essentially self-supporting structure that is pre-stressed under tension, which means it can maintain its shape independently of gravity.

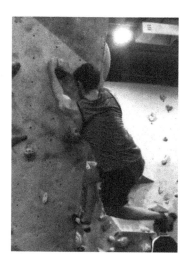

Figure 6.19

It is impossible to reasonably assign compression-based structural rules to this posture when 87 kg of living body are relying upon only 3 points of contact from the most distal parts of the body (fingers and toes essentially) from which to spring (upwards, defying gravity) from this position. The distance is almost the whole body-span, landing safely on three points of contact. That cannot be explained using classical biomechanical principles.

Reproduced with kind permission from Ben Avison.

The image of the climber is a still from a video clip. Ben has just completed an upward, diagonal leap, the full length of his body to grab the rock under his fingers, in this still image. His full body weight now hangs from his finger-tips (having been propelled from his toes), swinging back (using the right big toe as a pivot/brake). The biomechanics involved here cannot be explained by compression columns, levers or flat planes, if that is how the movements are to be attributed. They vividly demonstrate organised closed-kinematic chain variations, including but not limited to spirals, contained from within and success-fully defying gravity.

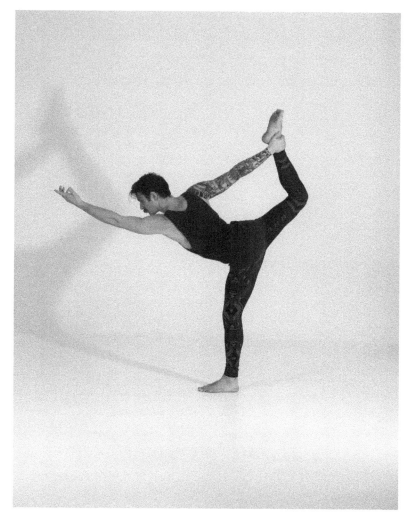

Figure 6.18

Wibb's spine is balancing and managing force and counter-force from multiple angles that challenge any idea that it is a stacked compression column.

Model: Wibbs Coulson; photography: Amy Very. Reproduced with kind permission from Art of Contemporary Yoga Ltd.

Third Rule. A living tensegrity system is a self-contained, non-redundant whole system. All components are dynamically linked so that a force exerted on any part of the system (i.e. a change) is reflected throughout the structure: "forces are translated instantly everywhere".[37]

"How does the fascia assist in distributing the loads? The thoracolumbar fascia wraps the vertebral bodies in diagonal and lateral strands like a woven sleeve with multiple attachments to the vertebrae. Pre-stress maintains the integrity of the spine and slight contractions laterally or even diagonally can extend it, ameliorating compressive loading, separating the vertebrae and sparing the discs."[38]

The actual living tensegrity architecture is so balanced and tuned that it innately resists any force applied by counteracting it and transmitting it throughout the form (see Figs 6.2C and 6.19 of the climber and Figs 6.17 and 6.18 of the Chakrasana pose). What this means is that when we do a twist, for example, the "body" touches a point of natural resistance (a sort of "fasciategral limit") and stops; it tightens or stiffens (*resists deformation*) (see Ch. 10 on elasticity). This is an important feature of our sensory feedback system, preventing us from tearing or damaging our bodies. The Haptic Sense is operating relentlessly and ubiquitously, if we are listening to its subtlety. In the yoga practitioner's body on the mat this is so fast and instinctive, s/he doesn't stop to think about it. The moving geometry, in this instance, includes the ground/mat forming a multi-bar chain mechanism from moment to moment (as does the climbing wall with the climber's body and whichever hand/foot is in touch with it) (see Chs 14 and 15).

Nature's Natural Energy-Saving Design

"Tensegrity systems (when talking of robotic platform design for example) have multiple paths to failure. Tensegrity meshes [think network or lattice] redirect forces such that redundancy is built in [in the sense that, for example,] an injury to a leg or an arm can be accommodated by redirecting the forces along slightly different pathways that don't engage the injured part directly."[39]

A living or *bio*tensegrity system is also extremely economical because the same architecture of force transmission manages the compression and the tension at the same time, at all times; if one area is not functioning ideally, it can find alternative pathways. This also makes sense of what happens in our classrooms. We know that different people do things different ways, depending upon their body type and state of mobility, health and movement patterns. Biotensegrity is a compelling explanation of our adaptability, which yoga seeks to foster.

"After all, both organic and inorganic matter are made of the same building blocks – atoms of carbon, hydrogen, oxygen, nitrogen and phosphorus. The only difference is how the atoms are arranged in three-dimensional space."[40]

"Tensegrity icosahedrons are used to model biologic organisms from viruses to vertebrates, their cells, systems and subsystems. There are only tension and compression elements in tensegrity systems.

There are no shears, bending moments or levers, just simple tension and compression, in a self organ-ising, hierarchical, load distributing, low energy consuming structure."[41]

What This Means in Application and Simple Terms

"We can now look at how and why natural patterns and shapes develop as they do – first principles – with tensegrity models emerging out of this and describing the behaviour of living organisms (and human movement particular)."[42]

Tensegrity icosahedrons are "round things" – which fundamentally means that a sphere is not really a purely 3D smooth curve, but in fact a reflected geo-desic dome; the smoother it looks, the higher the frequency of icosahedron. This is a gross simplification of the work that Graham Scarr has explained very thoroughly and clearly in his book.[43]

The three biggest stumbling blocks I come across in teaching this super-valu-able resource to yoga and movement teachers, are:

1. Looking for obvious tensegrity icosahedrons in the body (which are not there!).

2. How tensegrity principles work in all the shapes we can create as soft-mat-ter forms.

3. In seeking to see ourselves, it is a little like looking at our own eye-balls – it takes a sensory awareness into consideration to "get it". (That might sound unscientific, but intellectual quantitative science doesn't need to divorce us from sensory, qualitative instinct. They can endorse each other if we can move to the next level of awareness.)

The brief answers to these three stumbling blocks can help turn them into stepping stones:

1. Tensegrity icosahedrons (T-icosas) represent *invisible* forces that shape forms! (The biological algorithm behind them.) Think of Buckminster Fuller's geodesic domes, which are basically hemispheres. A sphere is a shape that nature loves for its efficiency. What looks like a sphere, or cell, is actually a variation on an icosahedral arrangement (Fig. 6.20). The smaller the triangles, the higher the *frequency* of that "sphere" – its geometry, when packed with other spheres (cells), is icosahedral.

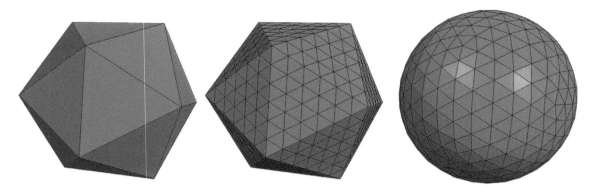

Figure 6.20

This image explains visually the frequency of icosahedrons. The more divisions between the triangles (the smaller each one is), the higher the frequency of icosahedron – which is actually what spheres are. They look like smooth spheres, but they are in fact structurally organised icosahedrons. When they press against each other, as contained cells, these form the foundational geometries that explain their forms.

2.   Tensegrity matrices form other shapes. They are not confined to spheres or icosahedrons. The models can be made to show how their arrangements, as lattices and spirals, can connect to represent tubes (tunicae, dura, fibrils, fibres) and wrap in counter-chiral manners to define thicker or thinner vessels – still adhering to the rules of tensegral tension–compression geometry (Fig. 6.21).

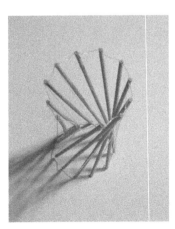
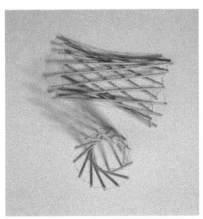
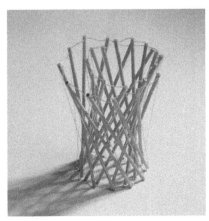

Figure 6.21A–C

These are tensegrity models of tubular lattices. Tensegrity tubes have a direction of spiral. That is "chirality". Each tube is counter-chiral to the one inside it; a growing principle in nature of blood vessels (tunicae) and trees (growth rings). It is the principle upon which peristalsis is based. There are no lever mechanisms in the human body, not viscerally or musculo-skeletally. Every system relies upon the spiral nature of tensegrity-based architectures to move intelligently.

3. This becomes a sensory orchestration in practice! The nearest on paper is the metaphor of Helen in the tube, demonstrating the tensional response of the fabric, tensioned by the compression forces her body is offering, compressed by the fabric. It is self-perpetuating (see Fig. 6.1) and the fabric is tensioned/folded accordingly.

Wholeness in the Yoga Classroom

It is difficult to think in whole terms, biomotionally, when we are used to seeing joints anatomically and biomechanically, via cartoons referencing only the specific muscles that cross them. In yoga, even if we are emphasising a pose for one part of the body, we are counterbalancing that part with the rest, instinctively. Biotensegrity invites us to think globally, although we can express movement locally; it integrates both.

When you press on a floating compression (tensegrity) structure, it presses back at you. When you twist a tensegrity mast, it counter-twists in your hands. The architecture itself responds by bringing balance to the force applied, even if the structure is inert. That is what our sensory bodies do, instinctively, on yoga mats; sensing the force/counter-force sequence from within. Whether we are exploring yoga techniques, or sitting in meditation, breathing in (expanding the whole structure) or breathing out (in-drawing the whole structure), the principle applies literally, symbolically and universally. We go down to go up, rotate and counter-rotate; we go out to go in, and vice versa, as a whole, taking our whole cells with us.

Fascia incorporates both opposing forces and by enclosing, binds them into unity and distinction. It becomes so essential in adjustment to offer a subtle force, to be equally subtly met by the person being adjusted (see Ch. 17).

The various styles of poses do not just rely on muscular forces to place them; like the climber, we spring and bound, soften and release into various postures at different points in our practice, in a continuum. Our bodies travel through space and maintain their integrity. We use our tension–compression network, which is very efficient energetically at its innate force transmission skills. We can organise in a refined and relaxed manner facilitating all kinds of movements at will, from the fluid to the robotic. Relative to our own capacity, we develop range and choice. We can choose how to train this sensitive, responsive material that is the form of our soft body architecture. It allows for an exploration into different types of yoga (or any other movement protocol from martial arts to mime). We do what we want the body to be *able to do,* in order to practise doing it! Then we counter that by the opposite (rest and meditation). It sounds so obvious, but that's how the tissue works.

It is one thing to analyse the variety of postures in the classroom from the point of view of particular antagonistic muscle pairs, levers and fulcrums, but quite another to make sense of them in action. Given that every pose is designed to affect our whole body, local analysis can fail the test of universal application. We are essentially nonlinear biologic systems, not only from the point of view of where our limbs are in relation to our torso. It also applies to our physiology, for example how the breath actually moves us and how we move the breath, throughout the changing duration of a pose. It includes the visceral organs and the gliding internal pockets of our whole tissue matrix; the transitions to and from the pose. The body and limbs, breath and thoughts, feelings and containment occur at once. We experience our spines and our senses before, during and after any one whole asana, at that moment in time, in a continuum to the next. The whole body participates, even that which is required to hold still. We incorporate these paradoxical opposites, as a whole.

As we explore the yoga poses, slowly and therapeutically or fast and athletically, we do so at one with our instinctive style, shape and form. These are whole-body expressions and the more refined (and appropriately balanced in tension–compression equilibrium) they become, the more we can be in command of our poise and balance. We begin to find congruency between structure, function and self-expression of our own unique form.

Living tensegrity, or biotensegrity, is gaining traction in the field of biomechanics as an explanation of global (and local) organic organisation. However, it is an emerging field and not yet fully understood in terms of the organisation of joints and articulations, although research is changing that.[44,45]

When we achieve the beauty of poise and grace in the postures, we become so "full" of the sense of balance within and without that we take it into our lives. It becomes relevant, like a hallmark, in everything we do. It becomes an instinctive way of moving and of being.

Yoga explores our entire soft tissue form at many levels, including but not limited to the shapes we seek to express in the asanas. It does so in the physical realm, on the mat, exploring the body for its ability to glide, balance and make shapes *with and from* the shape it is in. It goes further into the realms of the subtle body, using the power of stillness (on the outside) to explore less obvious motion and motility (on the inside). Yantras (visual resonance) (see Fig. 12.18) and Mantras (audial resonance) are used to vibrate the inner body and focus more on the internal forms, eventually through even more subtle depths of nuanced self-sensing awareness and meditation.

These are gradual processes of exploring what we might call our "outward attention" through the kinesphere, transferring to our "inward attention" through the innersphere.

It is a journey through different *scales of the same biologic patterns of forces through form*, however subtle the forms might appear to the witness witnessing. Ultimately, perhaps we could say that through yogic practice, we seek to attain awareness of the *formless*, and the ability to move easily through the different densities of each level of manifestation. Whichever way we describe the more esoteric practices of yoga, however, there is something extremely valuable about recognising nature's common patterns of energy moving through forms, *on every scale*. They are deep to all aspects of yoga, as we will explore further.

Whatever the questions and discussions about the laws of tensegrity structures, you cannot fully "get" a practical sense of why it is so compelling unless you handle or make one yourself. The easiest is the T-icosa, the icosahedron behind the geodesic domes that Fuller designed. However, tensegrity structures can be made to mimic tubes, bony rings and all sorts of aspects of the body, if the respect for the different *types of biological materials* the fascia can be expressed as, are taken into consideration.

Notes

1. Kenneth Duane Snelson: 1927–2016; Eleanor Heartney, *Kenneth Snelson: Forces Made Visible*, Hudson Hills Press Inc., 2009.

2. John Sharkey (2018) Biotensegrity-Anatomy for the 21st Century Informing Yoga and Physiotherapy Concerning New Findings in Fascia Research. *J Yoga & Physio* 6(1):555680.

3. Graham Scarr, www.tensegrityinbiology.co.uk, article: "Geodesic". See also: *Biotensegrity: The Structural Basis of Life*, Handspring Publishing Ltd., Pencaitland, 2018, 2nd Edition.

4. A note sent via email in private correspondence with the late Tom Flemons, from *The Geometry of Anatomy*, copyright T. E. Flemons 2006; Fuller, R. Buckminster, 1975, Synergetics, Macmillan, pp 372.

5. *Tensegrity*, by R. Buckminster Fuller. Copyright 1961 R. Buckminster Fuller: http://www.rwgrayprojects.com/rbfnotes/fpapers/tensegrity/tenseg01.html
   For more information about the work of Buckminster Fuller contact: The Buckminster Fuller Institute, 2040 Alameda Padre Serra, Suite 224, Santa Barbara, CA 93103. PH: (805) 962-0022.

6. Donald Ingber (1998) The Architecture of Life. *Scientific American*, Feature Article, January 1998.
   Further information: Donald E. Ingber (2003) Tensegrity I. Cell structure and hierarchical systems biology. *Journal of Cell Science* 116:1397–1408 © 2003 The Company of Biologists Ltd.

7. Charles B. Reilly, Donald E. Ingber (2018) Multi-scale modeling reveals use of hierarchical tensegrity principles at the molecular, multi-molecular, and cellular levels. *Extreme Mechanics Letters* 20:21–28.

8. Stephen Levin, www.biotensegrity.com. Stephen Levin and Danièle-Claude Martin (2012) Biotensegrity: the mechanics of fascia. In Robert Schleip, Thomas W Findley, Leon Chaitow, Peter Huijing: *Fascia: The Tensional Network of the Human Body*. Edinburgh, Elsevier 137–141.

9. Stephen Levin, www.biotensegrity.com. Graham Scarr, *Biotensegrity: The Structural Basis of Life*, Handspring Publishing Ltd., Pencaitland, 2018, 2nd edition in collaboration with Stephen Levin.

10. Merriam-Webster definition: a procedure for solving a mathematical problem (as of finding the greatest common divisor) in a finite number of steps that frequently involves repetition of an operation; *broadly*: a step-by-step procedure for solving a problem or accomplishing some end.

11. Jaap van der Wal: see www.embryo.nl for papers and courses in which these views are extended and further explained. See Chapters 3 and 4 for detailed references.

12. James Gleick, *Isaac Newton*, Ch 3, p. 47, To Resolve Problems by Motion, Harper Perennial (Imprint of Harper Collins Publishers), 2004, ISBN 978000716318 2.

13. Ibid.

14. Ibid. Ch 4, Two great orbs.

15. Graham Scarr, *Biotensegrity: The Structural Basis of Life*, Handspring Publishing Ltd., Pencaitland, 2018, 2nd Edition: Foreword, P. xiii, The biotensegrity algorithm. Stephen Levin.

16. Danièle-Claude Martin, *Living Biotensegrity*, Kiener, Munich, 2016. Tensegrity Tripod, p. 5.

17. John Sharkey (2018) Biotensegrity-Anatomy for the 21st Century Informing Yoga and Physiotherapy Concerning New Findings in Fascia Research. *J Yoga & Physio* 6(1):555680.

18. Jaap van der Wal, private communication, July 2013.
    Further Reference: Jaap van der Wal, "The Architecture of the Collagenous Connective Tissue in the Musculoskeletal System – An often overlooked Functional Parameter as to Proprioception in the Locomotor System". This article is published as supplement to a lecture at the Second International Fascia Research Congress, Amsterdam, 27–30 October 2009, with the title "The Architecture of Connective Tissue as a Functional Substrate for Proprioception in the Locomotor System". (Jaap van der Wal MD PhD, University of Maastricht, Faculty of Health, Medicine and Life Sciences, Department of Anatomy and Embryology, P.O. Box 616, 6200 MD Maastricht, Netherlands.) It includes a revised version of part of Van der Wal's doctoral thesis, submitted to the University of Maastricht in 1988, entitled *The Organization of the Substrate of Proprioception in the Elbow Region of the Rat*.

19. Donald Ingber (1998) "The Architecture of Life", *Scientific American*, Feature Article, January 1998.

20. Danièle-Claude Martin, *Living Biotensegrity*, Kiener, Munich, 2016.

21. Charles B. Reilly, Donald E. Ingber (2018) Multi-scale modeling reveals use of hierarchical tensegrity principles at the molecular, multi-molecular, and cellular levels. *Extreme Mechanics Letters* 20:21–28.

22. Graham Scarr, *Biotensegrity: The Structural Basis of Life*, Handspring Publishing Ltd., Pencaitland, 2018, 2nd Edition: Ch. 11, Biotensegrity: a rational approach to biomechanics, p. 129: Therapeutics.

23. Michael S. Schneider, *A Beginner's Guide to Constructing the Universe: The Mathematical Archetypes of Nature, Art, and Science*, HarperCollins, New York, 1994.

24. S.A. Edwards, J. Wagner and F Gräter (2012) Dynamic prestress in a globular protein. *PloS Cmputational Biology* 8(5) e1002509. "A tensegrity structure is one composed of members that are permanently under either tension or compression, and the balance of these tensile and compressive forces provides the structure with its mechanical stability. Macroscale tensegrity structures, which include Buckminster Fuller's geodesic domes, achieve exceptional structural integrity with a minimal use of resources. The question we address in this work is whether nature makes use of molecular-scale tensegrity in the design of proteins."

25. Charles B. Reilly, Donald E. Ingber (2018) Multi-scale modeling reveals use of hierarchical tensegrity principles at the molecular, multi-molecular, and cellular levels. *Extreme Mechanics Letters* 20:21–28.

26. Eric Blechschmidt, 2004, *The Ontogenetic Basis of Human Anatomy*; Ch. 3, Metabolic Fields, Distusion fields. North Atlantic Books

27. Graham Scarr, *Biotensegrity: The Structural Basis of Life*, Handspring Publishing Ltd., Pencaitland, 2018, 2nd Edition: Ch. 11, Biotensegrity: a rational approach to biomechanics, p 129: Therapeutics.

28. Ibid. (Ch. 1, Page 1: Tensegrity, figure 1.1) Also: Danièle-Claude Martin, *Living Biotensegrity*, KIENER, Munich 2016, Ch I, Introduction. Figure 1.1)
29. Portfolio and Art News Annual, No.4, 1961. In addition to this article there is an accompanying Introduction by John McHale. Only the Tensegrity article is reproduced [see link] by permission of the Estate of R. Buckminster Fuller. Link: http://www.rwgrayprojects.com/rbfnotes/fpapers/tensegrity/tenseg01.html [February 2nd 2020]
30. Kenneth Snelson: http://kennethsnelson.net/.
31. Tom Flemons: http://intensiondesigns.ca/bones-of-tensegrity/
32. John Sharkey, private correspondence.
33. Kenneth Snelson: http://kennethsnelson.net/.
34. Stephen Levin, *Bone is Fascia* (See Appendix A), John Sharkey (2019) Letter to the Editor, *Journal of Bodywork & Movement Therapies* 23:6–8.
35. Graham Scarr, *Biotensegrity: The Structural Basis of Life*, Handspring Publishing Ltd., Pencaitland, 2018, 2nd Edition: Ch. 7, The Ease of Motion, p. 73–86; Appendix 5: Closed-chain kinematics and embryological development, p. 159.
36. Leonid Blyum: www.abrtherapy.com/team-member/leonid-blyum/
37. Leonard Dubovoy: see www.biotensegrity.com.
38. Tom Flemons, *The Bones of Tensegrity*, ©T. Flemons 2012, www.intensiondesigns.com/bones_of_tensegrity.html.
39. Tom Flemons, private correspondence, 2013.
40. Donald Ingber (1998) "The Architecture of Life", *Scientific American*, Feature Article, January 1998.
41. Stephen Levin, www.biotensegrity.com: "Tensegrity: The New Biomechanics".
42. Graham Scarr, *Biotensegrity: The Structural Basis of Life*, Handspring Publishing Ltd., Pencaitland, 2018, 2nd Edition: Ch. 2, Simple Geometry in Complex Organisms, p. 12: The Rules of Physics.
43. Graham Scarr, *Biotensegrity: The Structural Basis of Life*, Handspring Publishing Ltd., Pencaitland, 2018, 2nd Edition:
44. Graham Scarr (2012) A consideration of the elbow as a tensegrity structure. *International Journal of Osteopathic Medicine* 15:53–65
45. G. Scarr, H. Harrison (2017) Examining the temporo-mandibular joint from a biotensegrity perspective: a change in thinking. *Journal of Applied Biomedicine* 15:55–62.
46. Robert Beverly Hale and Terence Coyle, *Albinus on Anatomy*, Dover Publications Inc, New York, 1979.

The Fascial Architexture

"Fascia is the connective tissue of the skin. It's the computer system of the body. It links all the body together in one big computer-like system. The largest organ in the body is the skin. The fascia connects with the muscles, and with the underlying nerve, tissue and bone structure of the body, in a way that we can have an instantaneous report throughout our body to our sense mechanism. Through the fascia the tissue moves, and with it signals surface in the mind - pictures of the past, traumas, holding patterns, the tension we hold, because it's releasing. It's as if we're hitting a computer button that says, 'Here comes this information you need'."

John Roger,[1] DSS, May 26, 1984.

The skin wraps the outside of us in a continuous, seamless structure, in the round. Unlike a neoprene wetsuit, that can be removed (somewhat like a skin), ours cannot be separated from what holds it up (us) as a volume; attached everywhere (by skin ligaments), in complete continuity with all that is organised inside it. It contains us and threads together the whole environment of our outside world and our internal world. From the outer skin and superficial fascia (effectively the back of the skin) to the innermost networks of the bones and the depths within them. We are formed as one toroidal "donut" with a long, squiggly, juicing-tube down the middle. It's a genius design and we each self-assembled to a similar, remarkable, blueprint.

That blueprint includes and facilitates apparently solid, liquid or gaseous exchanges and organisations within the forms (within the forms, within the forms). Everything structurally begins and ends in the fascial wrappings of the fascial pockets. All pockets and fluids within them are bound by the fascial architecture, as one continuous piece of biological organic origami. The bound fluids themselves constitute the fascial matrix, self-assembled during our embryological development and grown by us ever since (see Chs 4 & 5; nothing happens in a dry atmosphere of mechanical isolation). What varies endlessly (but not randomly) are the densities, thickness, stiffness and softness of the ways the fascial components' respective architectural shapes and textures are *organised*, while they remain in an intimately bound collective *organisation* – you.

All these *contents* are in a multidimensional, multidirectional and multi-sensory orchestra[2]; flowing and fluxing (at different *stages* and *states* at different times), translated *through* these internal architectural fabrics. Whatever names we give the different structures (defined somewhat *by their texture*), whatever functions we assign to them, our experience of them takes their behaviours so completely for granted, that it is as if fascia has been hidden in the obvious, by the ordinary, for centuries (see Ch. 2). Like cellulose to a plant, its various expressions allow our various expressions – of form, of gesture, of posture and of self. In our search for what I'm calling *biomotional integrity* we are dealing with one fabric, albeit expressed in as many textures and patterns as nature can usefully include. Your texture depends, to some extent, on who and how you are – *it is a responsive biological material.*

We could consider ourselves as a work in progress that lives as an organised collective, bound by fascia on every scale. The roots of a tree have a pattern that allows them to hold together the earth in the ground they bind, reciprocally related to maintain each other in a flow of nutrients and structural integration (Fig. 7.1). Every branch (similar pattern, reflecting the roots), every leaf and every seed have different textures of the same basic building materials. Their respective textures reflect the rates and rationale by which they photosynthesise and self-assemble to do so. They are bodies of biological fabric, distributing and managing water, light and nutrients, through the medium that holds them together in all its variety of textures.

Similar patterns of nature exist within our bodies, the way the lungs and the circulatory system mimic the patterns of trees – *even though we "humans being" bind our "ground substance[3]" on the inside.* The relationships between the forms, however, share similar properties and morphologies. Do we share similar patterns and textures that integrate the flow of water (Fig. 7.2) and interact with light (even if we don't call it photosynthesis as such), distributing our subtle energies?

How does fresh air get so beautifully organised between the trees and us,[4] then transformed into our blood stream (or their sap stream)? How does blood get made in our deep bone marrow (inside the crystalline texture of the bone), filtered through that and the periosteum, back into the right vessels, so that it *can be* oxygenated? Without taking detailed lessons in physiology, is there a foundation principle that can make some sense of all these fascinating, myriad exchanges that we ignore as the resilient daily miracle of a healthy body – while we seek to enhance it with our yoga practice? Could the fascial matrix hold the key?

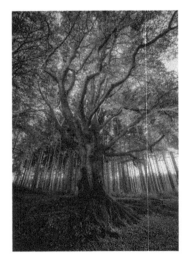

Figure 7.1

The roots and branches of a tree resemble the patterns of matter in the body.

"It is easy to forget that the concentration quotients of salts (NaCl, KCl, CaCl2) in interstitial fluid [in the body] and in water of an ocean are nearly identical. Our cells are, in a manner of speaking, swimming gel-like structures in an ocean of interstitial fluids, and we are carrying that ocean around with us."

Guido F. Meert[5]

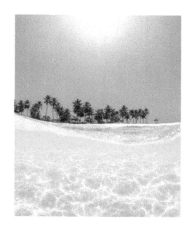

Figure 7.2

Notice the way water reflects fractal patterns of light that echo polyhedral morphologies in the interior architecture of the body (see Ch. 2, Jean-Claude Guimberteau).

Does this mean that salt water is a major component of that "everything" inside us? Why doesn't it slosh around as we walk, if the percentage of it in our bodies is so high (approximately 70% in adults and upward of 80% in babies)?

The term "embryonic mesenchyme" describing our earliest stages, refers to a kind of "embryonic soup" that van der Wal calls the meso ("middleness" or "innerness"), where fascia is produced to hold it(self) together, from the inside out. It doesn't originally stop at our skin border in embryological development. We also generate the placenta and actively engage in a spectrum of fluid, dynamic, self-assemblage, including all that we need to become. That is, to form and shape ourselves into the beings we develop into (Ch. 4). Van der Wal describes, in his "Embryosophy lectures", our "structural fabric".[6] We might think of it as a responsive "materia biologica", a growing and ever-changing version of the embryonic soup we were introduced to in chapter four, shaped by our gestures and shaping us in response to them. None of the skin (or skins within) are separate; nor is the stuff of the in between of the skins, wrappings and fabrics of this network of networks we call fascia. We are still that wonderful, origami-like work in progress – how *does* it work?

"Fascia is the fabric of the body; not the vestments covering the corpus, but the warp and weft of the material"

Stephen M. Levin, 2012[7]

According to Deane Juhan (referring to collagen):

"In the tendons and ligaments its tensile strength is superior to steel wire; in the cornea of the eye it is as transparent as glass; it accounts for the toughness of leather, the tenacity of glue, the viscosity of gelatin. Invest it to various degrees with hyaline, a nylon-like substance exuded by chondro-blasts and it becomes the various grades of cartilage; invest it with mineral salts and it becomes bone."[8]

One difficulty here is the expression "water of an ocean", and the implication that the cells are "gel-like" within it. It implies two things that we might trip up on: (1) the *type* of liquid we might expect in a large body of water, such as the sea. Apart from urine, none of the water in the body resembles that kind of fluidity, as we will explore. Moreover, (2) the idea that cells are somehow separate (gels) from the milieu in which they reside gives rise to the idea that water, cells, fascia and

The basic ingredients filling the majority of this internal fascial matrix as a volume are variations on the theme of water (which might be more than it seems), protein (*collagen* and *elastin*[10] and *reticulin*), and the various minerals and molecules that form the building blocks of our matrix (see Ch. 6). It is not so much a separate fibrous scaffolding, as it is a different texture of the same basic weave of the "materia biologica". Thus the term "architexture" to overlap the meaning of how the architecture is made of different versions of the same stuff that *is the wrapping fabric*. The pockets that wrap everything are all made of it, like various textures of containers on every scale.

Fascia – see Box 7.1 – (as a binding, bandage, active, animated, sensory, conscious skin within the skin) takes on shapes and properties (textures)

skin are all somehow separate *items* or ingredients of the body (not to mention the muscles, bones, viscera, vessels and so on). It implies they are all *separable* within the matrix *before* the anatomist or pathologist cuts them out of their natural environs. That is part of the issue; they are not separate, other than when they are separated to be studied. *They are made of the material that distributes the fluids* through *them*, holds the cells of each in the appropriate location and communicates all these myriad exchanges in balance, so that they can function as "items". **They are distinct, but they are never separate.** They are distinguished by their shape, their texture, their location, their organisation; their structure

The Question of Blood and Bone

and their innate properties and specialisations. However, nothing is separate – it is a miraculous interrelated collective. (See special piece at the end of this chapter by Mae-Wan Ho.)

Levin (and other protagonists in fascia research) would agree with Juhan that the bone is indeed a type of fascia, expressed in a particular (and more crystalline) form. It arises in the embryonic tissues as a "cartilaginous placeholder" that responds to forces; hardening as a function of growth, motion and development.[9]

Consider the idea of "sand" as a material in the building of a house. Depending entirely upon how it is treated, what it is mixed with (at what temperatures) and where it is placed, it can be a component of solid brick, sticky cement and transparent glass, among other things. These all have clear quantitative formulae and properties that result in their respective forms and textures. However, from a qualitative perspective, few architects would describe the texture of a

according to organisation, hydration and location. That includes, but is not limited to, the nature of fluid in living organisms, although fluid dynamics may play a bigger role than generally assumed. First, however, we have to accept that this high percentage of water within us (upon which we and all living forms on earth depend for life) has more to it than the three phases we are familiar with – i.e. solid (ice), liquid (water) and gas (vapour) as in Fig. 7.8.

It is difficult to imagine that the nature of the body, made up as it is of three fundamental things (according to Jaap van der Wal: "cells, connective tissue and the in-between"[11]), all belonging somehow to the definitions of fascia. Even the in-between, or the intercellular "space" isn't empty as such; it is all filled. According to Neil Theise[12] and colleagues, this "in-between" may also be considered another expression of fascia ("the Interstitium"; see Fig. 7.12). It includes the spaces within the in-between, which he and his colleagues further define as fascia, on the microcosmic scale (see Appendix A). That changes a lot – even the questions we ask!

Blood, which is defined as a form of connective tissue but is not considered fascia,[13] is produced in the bone marrow, deep within the bones. Imagining bones as separate, rigid components in the middle of the limbs (or around the torso), made of a different material to that which surrounds them and that which they contain, makes little sense. (Even though we are all taught to consider them as such, from classroom skeletons.)

We asked at the beginning of this chapter, how does blood get from inside bones to outside them, so it can circulate around the body and be oxygenated? It is one of those "may I ask the stupid question?" kind of questions, that I happily drive my mentors mad with. Fortunately, on the occasion I asked this "stupid question", it was directed at John Sharkey, who spontaneously came up with my favourite alchemical metaphor (see margin note) to clarify the answer.

To light-heartedly (but seriously) paraphrase John Sharkey, answering my question: "*Let me give you a metaphor: imagine you are making tea, from a tea-bag. You need just the right size holes in the bag, so that the tea filters through at the appropriate timing, temperature and filtration. If the bag was too thick and dense–it couldn't get through. If it was too loosely woven, you would have tea leaves in your cup. Everything in the body is made of membranous pockets; each with specific densities, filtration capacity and we could say "the right size of mesh" (or semi-permeable membrane), for the chemical and fluid exchanges. The blood cells produced in your bones (Reticulocytes) are immature; when it has to filter through that matrix to the rest of your body, to be circulated and oxygenated and so on. It is part of a cycle, through which it grows, matures, dies and is replenished by new, immature blood, constantly. (It's the same principle – in a sense – as giving birth; it has to be to an immature infant, not a two year old, while it is still small enough to move through the birth canal). It is the same principle here – different sizes of container/molecule to traverse and filter (via* brick-wall and a window as the same basic material. Fascia (in this realm of soft-matter living architecture) has many variations on the theme and one thing it tends **not** to be in vivo is a fibrous, fluffy material, somewhat like fibre-glass or kapok (industrial fibre for stuffing cushions). That "fuzz" is much more often a function of formalin preservation in cadaveric specimens. Other forms of preservation

The Skins Within

reveal a fluidic texture and interface which impacts the basis upon which classical theories distinguish function, as we will explore.

Regarding the term **alchemy**, there is a very simple practical explanation for the use of it here. According to Tom Kenyon (in his book *The Magdalene Manuscript*), he describes the daily brewing of his tea as such: "*The art of alchemy is simply changing one form into another. Most people think of alchemy as a medieval obsession for changing lead into gold. [Think Isaac Newton, Ch. 2] And while this is one form of alchemy, anything that causes a change in form is alchemy as well. Turning water into steam is alchemy. Changing a dry tea bag into tea is also alchemy… All successful alchemies must*

On the Large Scale

have three elements: 1) a substance to be transformed; 2) a container to hold the alchemical reaction; and 3) energy. Had I, for instance, stumbled into the kitchen this morning and poured water onto the burner instead of into a kettle, I would not have created alchemy. I would have created a mess."

Where Does the Fascia Begin?

tension and compression force transmission) through the bone matrix into the matrix on the outside of it. It's always the same principle; expansion (tensioning the tissues) and reducing them (in compression), as we breathe. The same forces animate the motion of blood; each part of us accomplishes these tasks at different speeds, flows and rates. The uterus can change rapidly; the bladder even faster; the bones, much more slowly. These are all time-dependent (i.e. temporal) functions of the same principle in action". I so love that explanation. Just saying. It makes perfect sense of why fascia would be everywhere in the body: on every scale!

The skin on the outside of us is more obviously "skin" perhaps, than the "skins" of everything inside of us: from the wrapping of muscles, fibres, organs and bones, to the tubular tunics and dura of vessels and the walls of cells and even the containing micromembranes of organelles within them. Fascia has time-dependent behaviours and characteristics, uniquely expressed on every scale; with the ability to modify and create variations in shape (morphology) depending on where it is and what it does (and what we do). That is, various *textures* according to the particular type of binding and what loads (i.e. types of gestures) that part of our architecture is used for (and used to). If part of its role has to include the filtration of fluids, then have we really begun to appreciate the scope and subtlety of what fascia can do and the significance of its texture?

Are we taking as much care of the fascia's sensitive subtle internal movement (that we don't see) *as the shape changes we do see*? It invites a huge paradigm shift, once we honestly ask about fluid dynamics – and what kind of fluid we really mean in this profoundly complex and detailed matrix? The subtle qualities of internal filtrations are not separate from the elastic recoil the more obvious fascial structures facilitate, that we see on the macro scale of whole body motion! (See Ch. 10.)

In yoga practice, we have to be fascinated by the ubiquity and continuity of this matrix, given that it unites all the muscles and suggests that their attachments are in totally interwoven continuity. Let's also ask, what of the more subtle aspects of yoga? Fascia, it turns out, is by no means limited to that macrocosmic aspect of our function; the larger movements of the postures and the shapes we are in, to make more shapes on our mats. Let's consider how the basic tenet of pockets enfolding pockets makes sense of far more subtle practices than simply describing the poses. How do the micromolecules of us move around on the microcosmic level? Does it matter to the more subtle aspects of us and our yoga practice?

To re-iterate, we learned in Chapter 4 that the fascial tissue arises from the so-called *embryonic mesoderm* that van der Wal calls the "meso" – because it is the "innerness" of the embryonic form – not a layer, as such (like a cream filling, placed between two halves of sponge cake, is a layer – or the plastering

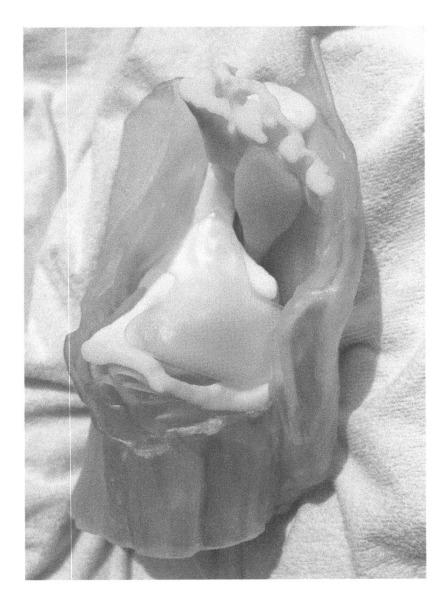

Figure 7.3

John Sharkey (in 2018) researched, designed and authorised this ground-breaking study to create this 3D printed render, taken from an fMRI scan of the right leg of a living human (female) body (in her 50s). It is the first in the world and it depicts a breakthrough in confirming the intimately containing role of the fascial matrix in the musculo-skeletal organisation/architecture. Sharkey points out that while it provides a fascinating view of the fascial matrix of the human thigh, at a certain depth/detail, in isolation (i.e. separated from the myofascia it would hold in place) it is just as false (in a way) as thinking only muscles and bones move us around. There is, indeed, a synergistic triumvirate of these three completely interconnected types and textures of tissues – and the fascia is but one essential component of this whole trinity. The muscle fibre is in a continuum with what we see in this image. In vivo, that fascia would continue through the muscles as well as between them. There is a size limit to the level of detail currently attainable in terms of reproduction of a 3D render. (In the left-hand image is the cross-section of the pubic symphysis (lower) and sacrum (upper), in front of which is the containing matrix of the psoas major muscle.)

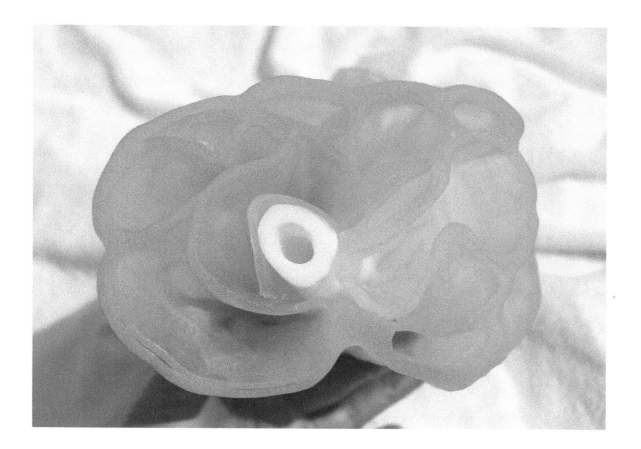

of a wall is a layer on top of the plaster board). It is the whole "middle world" filling the volume (between the inside of the outermost skin of the ectoderm and the outside of the innermost skin of the endoderm) in the embryo. Many tissues organise from the meso; however, this occurs in concert with a multitude of different expressions and forms on various scales, within that middle world of embryonic soup. These include various cells that produce fibres (*fibroblasts*) and connective tissues, such as cartilage cells (*chondroblasts*), bone (*osteoblasts*), marrow, muscle, blood, lymph, ligament, tendon, nerve, the lining of the body walls and wrappings of the cavities, the outermost coverings of the bones (*periosteum*), the joint capsules, and many of the folded tubes, pockets and pouches that form the organs, the urogenital system and ducts; not to mention what joins them all together (on every scale), including the milieu from/in which they arise. We have already noted how this ubiquitous fascial fabric binds everything to everything else, weaving all the internal structures into place, something like an "organ of organisation". Can we even begin to imagine the scale and detail at which it does (we do) that?

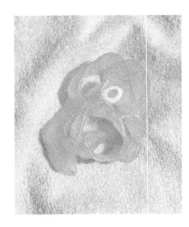

Figure 7.4

This smaller image of the sample render shows the fascial wrappings of this smaller cross-section of the thigh, with a small portion representing the femur bone in the middle. The hollow spaces represent where the myofascia (muscle protein) would be. Needless to say, in vivo, that would be invested throughout with finer fascia.

Deane Juhan and Mae-Wan Ho describe collagen (see Box 7.1) as the "most abundant protein in the animal kingdom".[14] Think back to the orange we examined in Chapter 3. Although the pith between the skin and the fruit is different from the membrane around segments, or that thinnest texture of the wrapping of the juice droplets, it is the same principle at work. That is, the architecture and *architexture* of forming structure: pockets within pouches and tubes, containing fluid (of varying consistencies) on every scale, in finer and finer folds and membranes of connective tissues and *textures thereof*. We saw this principle of formation in Chapter 4, describing the development of the human embryo and in soft-fix dissection of human or animal form, it is nevertheless a very finely organised fabric that permeates the whole system, relying ubiquitously on its essentially fluid matrix. It manages to hold our 75 trillion (see page 171) adult cells together and keep them where they belong *as we move, muddle and make our way through* our lives.

At each scale, a "skin" contains and wraps, in continuity with both its surroundings and the skin we see on the outside (known as the *integumentary system*). This is part of the difficulty and the quantum leap we have to make into **volumes at various scales** and more than two dimensions – even while we ask the questions, *volumes made of what?*

Box 7.1

The Web We Weave

The collagen molecule is one that we could say specifically exists to make netting and cabling in the body, as it originally forms in long tubular-like strands, within the extracellular matrix, or ECM. It also exists for weaving, flat fabrics and to form volumes (tubes for example, such as the tunicae of the blood vessels or the material of the gut tube; even bones are tubes, with variations in texture to define them).

This is where the distinctions of how function integrates with structure are finding new definitions, since the understanding of fascia and (what we are affectionately calling) "fasciategrity" began to emerge. Donald Ingber[15] presented on this topic (at the cellular level) at the First International Fascia Research Congress, held in Boston in 2007, at Harvard Medical School, Boston, MA. Here are two quotes from the summary of this talk.[16]

"Anyone who is skilled in the art of physical therapy knows that the mechanical properties, behavior and movement of our bodies are as important for human health as chemicals and genes. However, only recently have scientists and physicians begun to appreciate the key role which mechanical forces play in biological control at the molecular and cellular levels. ...."

Ingber continues, in his summary, to describe the results of what has been learned over three decades, from research that focused on the following:

"...Our research focused on the molecular mechanisms by which cells sense mechanical forces and convert them into changes in intracellular biochemistry and gene expression—a process called "mechanotransduction". This work has revealed that molecules, cells, tissues, organs, and our entire bodies use "tensegrity" architecture to mechanically stabilize their shape, and to seamlessly integrate structure and function at all size scales. Through the use of this tension-dependent building system, mechanical forces applied at the macroscale produce changes in biochemistry and gene expression within individual living cells. This structure-based system provides a mechanistic basis to explain how application of physical therapies might influence cell and tissue physiology."[17]

The Collagen Molecule

In the fibroblast, the collagen molecule begins its formation as a long chain of free amino acids in the cell's protoplasm. These amino acids link in an order, so the chain is made of repeated similar units. The attraction/repulsion nature of these complexes (they are electro-magnetically charged) results in the chain forming a left-handed spiral, as a helical chain. It is fragile and floats randomly. As they come into contact with each other these helical chains begin to spiral together in threes, twisting to form into a strand with a right-handed spiral. Thus they become like a three-stranded rope. The rope is electro-magnetically charged and responds to the forces being transmitted through the form. It is a relentless and intimate integration of bound forms responding to forces, to express each other as a whole *performance*.

Hydrogen Bonds

This chain (the three-stranded rope-like helix) is a single collagen molecule, eventually attaching to other similar molecules by hydrogen bonds. Once formed, they are exuded into the ground substance as discreet units, with no specific structure.

We note here the innate properties of polarity, paired to form a triune whole. This is not just the three-strandedness of the collagen chains. It is the left chirality of the individual strands, uniting in a right chirality arrangement when they twist together. Their combination forms one collagen fibre, as a lattice-like tube. In ancient yoga, this is "triune harmony". (It is a harmony innate to our geometry and fundamental to the metaphysical aspects of yoga.)

"Specific local qualities of the ground substance and the surrounding tissues then dictate the specific manner in which these molecules join together to create the collagen structure with the qualities needed for that specific area."[18]

The same sequence of location-specific events recurs. Just as the chains formed fibres, so the fibres then bind with further hydrogen bonds, overlapping in an alternating pattern (like bricks, but not stacked, spiral-bound) and forming strong tensile cables called collagen fibrils (Fig. 7.5). (These can be stronger than steel wire, which requires a load 10,000 times its own weight to stretch it.) We also have very compliant fibres called elastin. They are considered part of the suite of tissues the body calls upon in wound healing.[19] We rely on the very high resistance to deformation (stiffness) in the collagen for our true elasticity (see Ch. 10, The Elastic Body).

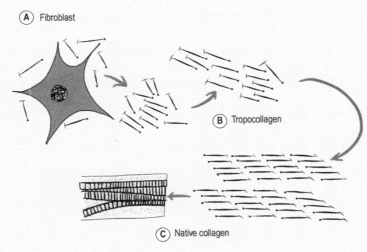

Figure 7.5

A fibroblast exuding tropocollagen (free collagen molecules). This will then
assemble into fibrils which will organise themselves into structures.

(Image after Deane Juhan, 1987, Fig. 3.17; see note 8.)

Connective tissue is also one of our most reliable repairing mechanisms, acting as a barrier to unwanted chemicals as well as healing wounds to restore integrity after injury. Fascia is everywhere in the body. It constitutes the immediate environment of every cell, "wrapping and uniting all structures with its moist, fibrous, cohering sheets and strands".[20] Modern schematic diagrams tend to show muscle tissues in preference to the fascia. Strictly speaking, a muscle cannot be, or function as, a muscle without connective tissue. What we have to realise is that the contractive power of muscle is completely useless without the tensioning cables of the connective tissues in which the muscle resides. It contracts to tension a tensional network that connects the body to itself and contains everything. It has to pull on something. The body is referred to as a pre-tensioned or a pre-stressed structure; the whole body is in a tensional network of these tissues. Everything moves everything and yoga can teach us how to moderate that (effectively to "tune it" with sensitivity and awareness.

Under the Skin

Immediately under the skin, as we can see in Guimberteau's films[21] of the soft "shearing zone" (see Ch. 3) of the so-called "superficial fascia", fascia appears open and fluid-like, something like the texture of egg white (in similar patterns to the water in Figure 7.2). Its variability (see Box 7.1) means it can appear as sheets (*aponeuroses*), and between muscles and around them (variously described as *perimysium* and/or *intermuscular septae*) as wrappings, slightly differently as muscle fibre (within the muscle itself, *epimysium*; and microscopically within the fibres, *endomysium*) and distinctly named for the wrapping of certain organs or cavities, e.g. as lung (*pleural*), abdominal organ (*peritoneal*) and heart (*pericardial*) sacs (all of which are better described as pockets, perhaps, since they are in complete continuity with the rest of the wrappings). Around the bones it is tightly wrapped, *periosteum,* the fibres (*Sharpey's fibres*) of which are deeply invested into the bony matrix; similar in principle to the way the skin ligaments attach to the deep fascia, keeping it woven through the superficial fascia to the deeper *fascia profundus* that wraps the whole body (see Fig. 7.11 for formal nomenclature). Between all these named features of our living form (that are cut out of the body separately by anatomists) lies the in-between; different textures of this fascial fabric and its fluid-like organisations (see later), in configurations that allow them all to glide and move without friction, *with every move we make.* How can it all be so various and all still be fascia? (We usually only notice when this gliding *doesn't* work and tissues become adhered, or inflamed, so we *can't* move them as easily and ordinarily as we expect to.)

The Textures of the Fluid Matrix

"Water is essential for life. Yet this simple, ubiquitous chemical compound has remained completely mysterious for centuries until quite recently. New evidence indicates that liquid water may be quantum coherent even at ordinary temperatures and pressure. It associates with macromolecules and membranes in a **liquid crystalline configuration** *that enables enzymes and nucleic acids to function as quantum molecular machines that transform and transfer energy at close to 100% efficiency.* **Liquid crystalline water at interfaces** *also provides the excitation energy that enables it to split into hydrogen and oxygen in photosynthesis, simultaneously generating electricity for intercommunication and for redox chemistry that ultimately powers the entire biosphere. Water is the means, medium and message of life – "the rainbow within that mirrors the one in the sky"."*

Mae-Wan Ho[22]

Interestingly, timber merchants are very familiar with the treatment of wood to account for what they call "bound water" and "free water". Since we live in a reciprocal relationship with trees to breathe, perhaps they can teach us more about our organisation. They live at the opposite end of the scale from stiffness to suppleness to us, but there are many more structural and systemic correlates between our natural forms. Different types of water are no surprise in this discipline! Indeed, in his chapter called Tree School, in The Hidden Life of Trees, Peter

Let us consider this watery behaviour as an essential motif in the story of fascial architexture, to all living biologic forms. All living things rely on the healthy *distribution* of hydration throughout their structure. A dry and fibrous tree or plant will be more brittle and less compliant (see Ch. 10) compared to the resilience of a young sapling, or a well hydrated tree. We asked earlier why the human body (70% water for adults or upward of 80% for the child's body) doesn't slosh around as we move, if such a high percentage of it is fluid. What do we mean exactly and why is it so fundamental to understanding the variety of forms of the fascia?

*"Up to 70% of the proteins in the connective tissues consist of collagens that exhibit constant patterns of alignment, as characteristic of **liquid crystals**. Collagens have distinctive mechanical and dielectric properties that render them very sensitive to mechanical pressures, changes in pH, inorganic ions and electromagnetic fields."*[24]

Mae-Wan Ho

Wohlleben[23] elaborates how trees have to learn to manage and preserve water over long periods of time, trained relentlessly by nature in self-preservation and as part of a collective in any given forest. As the basis of their ability to photosynthesise, they have to literally learn how to behave according to their location and community!

This beautiful excerpt from the book Mae-Wan Ho refers to (see note 26) was written by Harold Saxton Burr, Professor Emeritus, Anatomy at Yale University School of Medicine, in his book *Blueprint for Immortality, the Electric Patterns of Life*, Chapter 1: An Adventure in Science. It is useful to see why the bound nature of water and its behaviour at every membrane is essential to our understanding of fascia and its intimate relationship to fluid dynamics, of our most basic, life-sustaining ingredient – water!

In her work, Mae-Wan Ho integrates the subtle and various forces that we negotiate, with a philosophy that makes exquisite sense of our complexity while perfectly describing how the fascia behaves. Mae-Wan Ho offers explanations as to how essentially fascia binds and interacts with water, as a profoundly important aspect of our health and vitality. It was new and different at the end of the last century, however there is now a growing body of work that Mae-Wan Ho endorsed and, reciprocally, validates the many connections she made to support her methodical scientific research. What we are looking at here is the suggestion that the water at every *boundary* in the body (membranes of cells, organs, vessels, deep to muscle fibre and the fascial matrix interface that we have pointed to above) behaves with what Mae-Wan Ho calls "quantum coherence". In other words, it acts in certain ways, like the silicon chip in your computer (see opening quotation). Not only is it part of the structure, but **it is the communication network**; the soft-tissue hardware of your body's software; the anima/animus that programmes the applications. We are all wet, breathing volumetric architectures; close-packed in space over time; transmitting the most subtle chemical, electrical, electro-magnetic, quantum fields of information. Isn't that somewhat (metaphorically at least) like the crystal chip[25] in your computer?

"New evidence suggests that the L-field[26] is generated by, and embodied in, the quantum-coherent liquid crystalline water that makes up to 70–90% of organisms and cells, and is essential for life.

Water forms quantum coherent domains at ordinary temperatures and pressures. Within organisms, coherent domains become stabilized as liquid crystalline water on the vast amount of membrane and macromolecular surfaces, effectively aligning the entire body electrically to form a single uniaxial crystal."[27]

EXCERPT: *"Electro-dynamic fields are invisible and intangible; and it is hard to visualize them. But a crude analogy may help to show what the fields of life – L-fields for short – do and why they are so important:*

Most people who have taken high-school science will remember that if iron-filings are scattered on a card held over a magnet, they will arrange themselves in the pattern of the 'lines of force' of the magnet's field. And if the filings are thrown away and fresh ones scattered on the card, the new filings will assume the same pattern as the old.

Something like this – though infinitely more complicated – happens in the human body. Its molecules and cells are constantly being torn apart and rebuilt with fresh material from the food we eat. But, thanks to the controlling L-field, the new molecules and cells are rebuilt as before and arrange themselves in the same pattern as the old one.

Modern research with 'tagged' elements has revealed that the materials of our bodies and brains are renewed much more often than was previously realized. All the protein in the body, for example, is 'turned over' every six months and, in some organs such as the liver, the protein is renewed more frequently. When we meet a friend we have not seen for six months there is not one molecule in his face which was there when we last saw him. But, thanks to his controlling L-field, the new molecules have fallen into the old, familiar pattern and we can recognize his face.

Until modern instruments revealed the existence of the controlling L-fields, biologists were at a loss to explain how our bodies 'keep in shape' through ceaseless metabolism and changes of material. Now the mystery has been solved, the electro-dynamic field of the body serves as a matrix or mould, which preserves the 'shape' or arrangement of any material poured into it, however often the material may be changed."

New Paradigms

In his book *Cells, Gels and the Engines of Life* (to which Mae-Wan Ho refers), Gerald Pollack[28] discusses some of the basic features of cell dynamics:

"Thus, the gel-like character of the cytoplasm accounts for the basic features of cell biophysics.

Think of jelly or jello. It is 98% water, yet when you pour it as a liquid, with the 2% protein stirred through it, it sets into a shape that holds itself up in space. You can cut it into a million pieces, however not one of them will leak water. There is no pure, running water in the body; it is invariably bound with (or by) other elements. However we will consider the research that suggests that water can indeed bind, to varying extents, with or without additional protein. Perhaps this is part of the deeper mystery of the paradoxical fascia; that stuff that connects and disconnects our parts, while simultaneously holding them all together as one cohesive (quantum coherent) whole?

The focus then shifts from statics to dynamics. Here again the question is whether adequate explanations can emerge from the cell's gel-like character. Contrary to the common perception, gels are not inert. With modest prompting, polymer gels undergo structural transitions that can be as profound as the change from ice to water, which is why they are classified as phase-transitions. Polymer-gel phase-transitions are commonly exploited in everyday products ranging from time-release pills, to disposable diapers. They have immense functional potential."[29]

Pollack is among the scientists showing that water has a fourth phase (see later) which is that of a *liquid crystal state*; neither liquid nor solid, it has properties of both, but cannot strictly be defined as either. It fundamentally changes how we view not only the cell, but the Extra Cellular Matrix in which the cells reside, as we will see. Pollack suggests that phase-transition is the single unifying (simplifying) explanation of all cellular function. This level of paradigm shifting feels similar to the way in which fascia is changing the traditional understanding of how the human body is structured and moves (and is moved) by the forces of life. They go hand in hand when you consider the percentage of water in the living body, held in place by the connective tissue matrix; the materia biologica – fascia!

The human body as a bound and rounded volume, made of soft matter, is organised by different principles than those of hard matter, where more traditional, linear theories of biomechanics remain. Every aspect of living organisms is non-linear, denoting them biologic forms – and they abide by the same rules as our organic planet in the cosmos and every other living thing it supports. Hard matter (such as buildings are made of) abides by different rules of physics (see previous chapter) that apply to architectural designs made of hard-matter materials (see Ch. 6). They are generally better designed to be static than in motion. They are basically different – and so are the explanations for understanding them.

Soft-matter, biologic forms live in (and by) different rules, although they share the same forces of the environment (e.g. gravity, ground reaction force and so on) but can express *transmission* of those forces in very different ways. The texture of their structures is hydrated and animated by respiration and consciousness – and essentially, it is in flux, all the time. They (we) are self-assembled, which is a feature of crystals in nature. The fundamental ability to respond is quite (and essentially) different to hard-matter, manufactured forms, yet classical biomechanics are still based largely upon hard-matter laws. Unlike hard-matter structures, we are pre-disposed to move around and, less so, for stillness; *it is something we practice* that yoga fosters. What if it is our *softness* that gives us clues to how we really move and hold ourselves together? Our general cultural inclination is towards acquiring physical strength and power; but what if the innate subtlety of our *soft tissues* is where the wisdom lies and the power to transform energy essentially resides? Surely it is a balance of all the extremes that we really seek. What if fascia unlocks the code to finding that innate balance, in more than just the realm of physical function and form?

What Is a Liquid Crystal and Why Does It Matter?

Why do soft-matter fluid dynamics matter so very much in understanding fascia as a liquid crystal matrix? Pollack invites us to understand that water is being reconsidered in the light of its ability to bind and release.[30] It is now possible to demonstrate it has four, rather than three, phases.

Considering the Fourth Phase of Water

This fourth phase refers to water as a "liquid crystal", where the molecular structure is more organised[31] and bound in the tissues (bound water) rather than freely flowing (bulk water).

Mae-Wan Ho's research endorses this shift in how we "think" water. Using light microscopy, Mae-Wan Ho was able to investigate living organisms and identify her reference to the "quantum coherence domain" (CD) of water's ability to bind and store energy as well as permit its flow and transference of signals[32] **at the interfaces of membranes.** Thus her work refers to "interfacial" water (pronounced inter-fay-shal – not *inter-fashell like fascia*), referring to the **interface** of membranes with their surroundings, rather than specifically the fascia, as such (even though the membranes are made of it). Mae-Wan Ho's research suggests compellingly that the interfaces of membranes behave quite distinctly and the water at these sites is specifically bound in a particular way (see Pollack, below). Everything in the body we have referred to as a "skin" could be considered a membrane of sorts, albeit at a different scale to the denser skin that seals us from the outside.

Gerald Pollack has spent recent decades researching the nature of water, presenting the story of his journey at the 3rd International Fascia Research Congress in 2012 in Vancouver, Canada. It turns out this work, beautifully tied in by Mae-Wan Ho, with Ingber (see Ch. 6) and Oschman (see Ch. 13) and other researchers, is crucial to understanding fascia and how we contain it and how it moves us *as containers of our "mothering sea"*, which is essentially salt water! Pollack[33] shows that not even plain water in a glass is all the same kind of "bulk liquid" from surface to base, in the sense we might expect it to be. In some ways this becomes obvious when we add gel to the story; or perhaps more accurately, understand that with protein, water *becomes* gel and binds in what might be considered **an even more stable way**. However, even without a binding "agent", it seems one of the innate properties of water *as a collective* **is to respond**. It responds in a particular way to any hydrophilic (water-loving) substance that is intimately related to how living human tissues conduct charges.

Pollack explains that all water is not the same. Referencing the work of Sir William Hardy (see Ch. 2), he distinguishes a "Fourth Phase of Water", which he refers to as "bound water". Simply put, according to Pollack's research, an ordinary glass of water is not all the same molecular structure. Nor is it "just a substance that is either solid ice, liquid H_2O or vapour". The "surface tension", we learn, goes much deeper than the surface; the water in the upper section of the container is in fact a different-shaped molecule. The research shows that in the presence of a hydrophilic (water-loving) interface (think boundary or gel), the surface water forms a negatively charged band (or exclusion zone) that extends **in the presence of light**, separating the boundary (surface) from the positively charged band of molecules on the other side of it.

"We took a gel, that's the solid, and we put it next to water. And we added some particles to the water because we had the sense that particles would show us something. And sure enough you can see what happened is that the particles began moving away from the interface between the gel and the water, and they just kept moving and moving and moving. And they wound up stopping at a distance that's roughly the size of one of your hairs. Now, that may seem small, but by molecular dimensions that's practically infinite. It's a huge dimension."[34]

Pollack suggests that not all the container contains precisely the same *shape of water molecules*. He refers to this upper section as the Exclusion Zone or EZ water; as it is more tightly bound than the bulk water (the type that pours out of the tap or faucet) in the remainder of the vessel. This has multiple implications. All the water in our bodies contains particles of our mothering sea (see Meert, above); so the suggestion is that *within* the nature of the water is a coherent dance, within the skins of the forms, between the membranes of the molecules. It means that the water responds, specifically and especially (according to Mae-Wan Ho) *at the interfaces*.

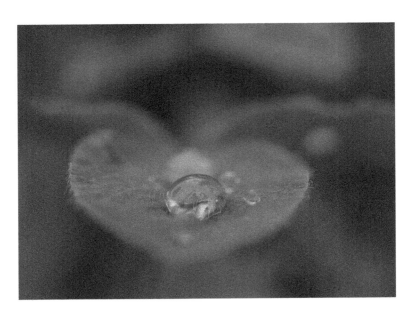

Figure 7.6

Water is bound fluid and demonstrates far more detailed properties than are assumed by its classifications as having only three states: solid, liquid and vapour.

(With grateful thanks to Aaron Burden on Unsplash.)

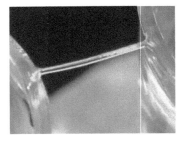

Figure 7.7

With electrodes in the water, a drop can be extended from one jug to the next to form a tubular structure of bound water. Then they can be moved up to 4 cm apart and the water forms a bridge that holds up without support, which "bulk" water could not do. This bound water behaves differently, yet it is clearly not a solid, such as ice.

Pollack explains that every particle creates a negatively charged band, beyond which a positively charged region accumulates. The negatively charged zone (EZ) is structured, in an hexagonal organisation which is really H_3O_2, because it has formed one extra hydrogen and oxygen bond. Its presence is evident at a *phase-transition interface*, within any given container of water. Because it is charged, it acts like a battery and can be set up, with electrodes, to form a bridge between two containers (a tube of water) that, even when the two containers are 4 cm apart, can hold itself up as a bridge of "stiffer" water than the H_2O (Fig. 7.7).

That is a simplification, however it is important as we are invited to expand the ways in which water can be considered and the idea that it is bound at all, let alone the pattern of its bound organisation. Furthermore, this research shows that sunlight (and infrared rays) are what powers this "battery effect" that the nature of contained water manifests in the presence of light.

"So, we began looking, of course, more into these extremely interesting properties. And what we found is, if we stuck electrodes into the EZ water [exclusion zone], because we thought there might be some electrical potential, it turned out that there's lots of negative charge in that zone. And we used some dyes to seek positive charge, and we found that in the bulk water zone [around it] there was an equal amount of positivity."[35]

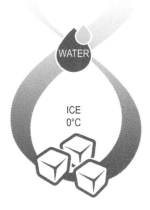

STEAM
100°C

WATER

ICE
0°C

Figure 7.8

We might suggest that anything such as the standard graph of stable states of water is an insufficient view. Given that the Fourth Phase of Water includes a range of subtle "inter-states" expressing bound water as a gel of varying thixotropic densities; the colour gradients in this graphic suggest a range of liquid crystal states along a spectrum of possibilities.

(Graphic Design by Bex Hawkins. Reproduced with kind permission from Art of Contemporary Yoga Ltd.)

When you cut meat or put it through a mincer, you don't get water and fibre in a bowl; you just get smaller bits of meat – no water. Nor do you get much juice cutting an orange or an onion in half (Fig. 7.9). You have to put fruit or vegetables through a pretty intense process to extract liquid juice from the

It turns out that this band of negatively charged water is not just a "layer" in a glass. It also acts something like a shield around even a single droplet of water; which you might expect to simply disappear into more water and coalesce (see Fig 7.6). However, it has this negatively charged "exclusion zone" around it, like an aura around a globe. It doesn't instantly dissolve into its surroundings. It behaves, within a glass of water, in a variety of close-packing arrangements and reveals the behaviour in tissues expected of tensegrity-based organisations, i.e. phase transitioning according to multiple variables.

If all the droplets are exhibiting these charged properties, then between them (think of the tetrahedral patterns of round things close-packed in Chapter 6) there is a subtle "interface" of positive charges, accumulating just beyond the band of negative ones. Far from "like poles of a magnet resisting each other" (as the researchers expected), the **interface** *between the water molecules, wrapped in a negatively charged EZ,* carries the accumulated positively charged particles just beyond the EZ water: opposites attract. This effectively *binds* the water into a close-packed hexagonal organisation resembling that of bee honeycomb (in 2D). Hexagons in three-dimensions remind us of the same pattern in endomysial fibres at the microscopic level of muscle fibres within muscle (see Ch. 3) and many other *liquid crystal-type structures*. They all rely on the only one of the five platonic volumes, with a geodesic shape that can phase change rapidly – that of the Tensegrity Icosahedron (see Ch. 6, Fig. 6.13). The geometry goes deep and Pollack's research would suggest that water abides by similar quantum rules.

Pollack explains how this provides a new dimension to the standard, linear spectrum classically assumed to distinguish only between ice, liquid and vapour. The difficulty in showing it on paper is that it can't be represented as a linear graph of a temperature gradient, of the easy-to-understand type that works in a flat, straight line and assigns water to just three stable states (Fig. 7.8).

If, as Pollack suggests, between ice and vapour there is a liquid-crystal *phase*, then it requires a more three- (or multi-)dimensional approach that allows for gradations and gradual differences in phase transition. Water would include a spectrum *within the linear spectrum generally assumed*, of variations on the amount of *binding* that the body shows. It would depend on a particular location/action/moment in space and time/availability of energy (e.g. light) and suitable interfaces. The presence of protein, salts and other chemistries would play a role in this multidimensional aspect we are invited to consider, to understand fascia. It takes the idea of "quantum coherence" to unimaginable detail – especially if we consider we are (already and naturally) doing it anyway!

The fourth phase of water (the Liquid Crystal phase) is less of a "set" division and more of a spectrum of (subtle) changes, if we can even consider it in a generalised and somewhat simplified way (see Fig 7.8). It is, however, important in the scheme of things, to understand fascia more fully and the fluid dynamics of variability that we experience in movement.

A liquid crystal phase is something that can respond rapidly to changes in various conditions and harden and stiffen (or soften and become more flowing), gradually. That is according to a number of nuanced emergent properties fibrous structural matrix. Essentially, you have to vigorously destroy and separate plant fibrous structure; tearing it apart and/or compressing it; to get liquid juice out of it (notably, often with a spiral extraction mechanism). Even in a grape or a berry, a seed or a nut – the *water is bound*. (Cut a

within the milieu, all of which are time-dependent. It allows for "phase change" or shifts in consistency of a fluid medium, calling into play precisely the kind of soft-tissue behaviours that the fascia can express under various forces and organisations. (It also allows for transition because the formation is in response to force changes.) While Pollack suggests "phase transition" is a function of cells, it may make sense of the function of us, on the macro scale.

*"In particular, **a cylinder of bound water** surrounds the triple-helical molecule, giving rise to an ordered array of **bound water** on the surface of the collagen network that supports rapid "jump conduction" of protons. Proteins in liquid crystals have coherent residual motions, and will readily transmit weak signals by proton conduction, or as coherent waves."* [36,37]

Mae-Wan Ho [10]

grape in half – it won't leak its high water content without compression or tension; you have to either pull it or squeeze it to break the bindings. It will stand a surprising amount of weight, naturally resistant to counter-force as part of its geometrical structure – which is the basis of biotensegrity, see previous chapter.)

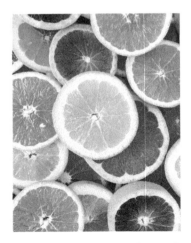

Figure 7.9

Cutting fruit doesn't mean its juice pours out. The cellulose in a plant is like the fascia to a living animal body; the high water content is bound.

(With grateful thanks to Rayia Sodeberg on Unsplash.)

This research suggests that the behaviour of water, at interfaces, plays a vital role in how collagen and our fluids interact. It is known that the fascial matrix conducts light through the body [38] – is it part of the puzzle of how energy interacts with this exquisitely sensitive and complex matrix?

One of the difficulties in describing fascia is accounting for its variability and the sheer range of expressions and properties it incorporates. Once we understand the nature of liquid crystalline substances, however, those "emergent properties" begin to make some sense – even at the scale of the movement classroom. That is a place where we expect change and harness change to express ourselves and explore our movement practice. Understanding how liquid crystals behave sheds some light on how widely the fascia supports our biomotional individuality. **Is there a correlate with how light (literally) and *lightness* of step (symbolically) and lightness of spirit (metaphysically) integrate with fascia?**

The idea of a liquid crystal matrix sounds complex in abstract theory, however we are all actually very familiar with liquid crystal behaviours, if we consider for a moment a popular organic substance: most people's favourite – chocolate (see Box 7.2).

The fascial matrix exists in the body as a *bound fluid medium*. It displays so many similar characteristics to chocolate that I can only imagine the general affinity to this confection somehow resonates with us, beyond the story of its origins. It can be a seriously inspiring and emotional subject and it has taught me much. Not least of which is the ESSENTIAL understanding of the phrase "emergent properties" and the impact upon *our* form of the "five T's" – fundamental to working with cacao and its derivatives, but providing an interesting metaphor for teaching yoga!

Box 7.2

Chocolate – the story of a liquid crystal matrix[39]

Chocolate, as a substance, can be solid, brittle, squishy, gooey, elastic, plastic, powdery, flaky, fluid (of varying viscosities), crystalline or dust. It is essentially made up of fat (cocoa butter), cocoa mass and various added ingredients when turned into variations on the cacao theme. It is basically hydrophobic (water can devastate its condition if you don't know what you're doing with it), but it is organic and, as such, displays many of the liquid crystal properties that Mae-Wan Ho, Pollack and others suggest in the cells and gels that form the "engines of life". It's much easier to describe these properties if you imagine enjoying eating your favourite kind while we discuss them, metaphorically but with a keen eye on how similarly our bodies respond to detail and subtle change.

Emergent Properties

Definition of Emergent Properties: An **emergent property** is a **property** which a collection or complex system has, but which the individual members do not have. In other words, **emergent properties** are **properties** of a group of items, whether insects, atoms or buildings, that you would not find in any of the individual items. Understanding what the term "emergent properties" means is an essential part of appreciating the nature of the fascia. Let us simplify and storify this to some extent, to paint a picture that leads us into the importance of fluid dynamics and begins to bridge some of the harder-to-understand and multiple aspects of the fascia and its behaviour in the living body.

The Five T's in the World of Chocolate

The five T's are:

Type. Temperature. Temporality. Tempo. Temper. (All of which are relevant in the study of the human body, given that the fascia is its main constituent material – and we might beg poetic license and bend the word "temper" to "temperament".)

There are other elements to making chocolate (and chocolates), however all these features affect each other. Once they combine in a particular way, the properties emerge that give us our favourite confections. We will consider each property, in the context of working with chocolate, to clarify why understanding *emergent properties* and understanding fascia are synonymous. Appreciating the liquid crystal nature of a form unlocks its code. Without it, you will be limited to understanding fascia as if it fits in the 2D world of linear forms, which it never does. (Please forgive the brevity of these explanations if you are a chocolatier – I'm making a metaphorical point here, illustrating fascial architecture and architexture – not describing how to make chocolates!!)

1. **Type.** There are many different types of chocolate, depending on their proportions and ratios of cocoa mass to cocoa butter. To make them palatable (as confectionery), the blends include different

kinds of cocoa beans, to create subtle flavours. Then other commodities are added, such as sugar and milk (and sometimes colour – although mainly it is natural) to change the appearances (which changes the behaviours!). Within the actual range of beans, however, (much like grapes to wine, and coffee beans to your favourite espresso blend) cocoa beans from different countries, climates and cultivations have distinct flavours. Each flavour will have its own optimum variables/properties of the other four "T's".

2. **Temperature.** Chocolate, whatever its type, must be at the right or optimum temperature *for its type* and for the *environment in which it is being made*, throughout the process, at each stage. That optimum changes *during the process* and if it is not appropriate to the point in the process, the result will be sub-optimal. (Basically, it won't work!) You will still have a chocolate mass, but far from a delicious palatable confection that is compliant to shape-change, you may literally have a chocolate-coloured porridge that isn't fit for purpose, because it cannot express the properties for the particular purpose you intended.

3. **Temporality.** The timing of all the above, over multiple heating and cooling procedures, is crucial. That is in terms of dosage, degree and the *length of time* (periodicity) at each temperature depending on the specific point in the procedure and purpose for which the chocolate (and its type) is being created.

4. **Tempo**. This refers to the motion and rhythm and *rate of change* in working with this material. To turn the cocoa beans into chocolate, they have to go through certain processing (roasting, grinding, "melanging", conching, etc) to release the mass from the liquor. Conching is blending (evenly distributing) the assorted particle sizes achieved in the grinding or "melanging" process and at the same time releasing the unwanted volatiles that would otherwise adversely affect the flavour profile you are trying to achieve. This gets the particle size to an appropriate texture and distribution (a suitable balance of structural integration). Once melted and treated in the various possible ways it can be used, stirring continues (it must be moved) or it just solidifies, if it is in an environment cooler than its melting point. (If you are in a working temperature higher than its melting point, it will just soften into a soggy mass of undifferentiated goo.) The movement is essential and it has to have a suitable rhythm if you want the chocolate (at each stage) to behave in a manageable way. Each process and each form (or morphology) has its own viscosity, crucial to the success of the shape to be created. Stillness is used as a means to cool it, so that it sets and becomes brittle. The time it takes to harden is the window of manipulation to achieve the desired outcome. There is a rhythm to each stage and if it is honoured, it contributes to the excellence of the results – depending on what you intended to create (you being the artisan chocolatier – the one assembling the results!).

5. **Temper.** Chocolate, like steel, has to be tempered to form the appropriate architecture and textures at later stages. This is technically referred to as the "pre-crystallising phase".[40] This means it is heated, cooled and re-heated (subjected to specific temperature variations over specific periods for each type) so that its crystalline properties can adopt and hold different morphologies when it sets. Once it has been produced, this final stage – tempering – produces a homogenous mixture of stable and unstable crystals with the object of the stable crystals "overwhelming" the unstable crystals in order to eventually set. (Therein lie the timing skills!) The reason you still want unstable crystals present is so that the chocolate will remain workable

for whatever purpose you have in mind, for long enough to achieve it. In order to maintain the equilibrium you have to keep stirring (moving it) and at a temperature that keeps the chocolate workable. (It is *temperamental* material!!)

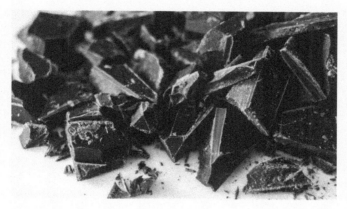

Figure 7.10A

Chocolate, when tempered, is hard and crystallised. It is still soft-matter, however.

(Photo by Charisse Kenion on Unsplash.)

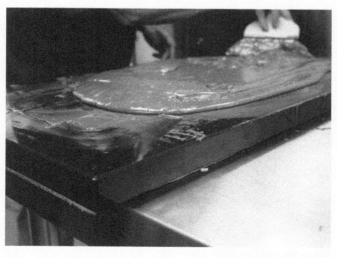

Figure 7.10B

Once its temperature is raised it enters a new liquid-crystal structural phase.

(Photograph by Bex Hawkins at Vantage House; Chocolate Development Kitchen, Henfield, East Sussex.)

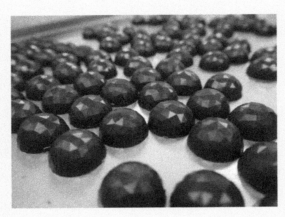

Figure 7.10C

When all the variabilities of phase-change have been harnessed, the chocolatier can create a variety of different shapes that demonstrate how this liquid-crystal material can be crafted into forms.

(Photograph by Bex Hawkins at Vantage House; Chocolate Development Kitchen, Henfield, East Sussex.)

Understanding these Properties

I was a chocolatier for 20 years in my earlier life and as such the notions of emergent properties lived deep to my daily experience in the artisan craft of making Belgian chocolates; not that I described it as such, at the time. Recognising the significance of emergent properties makes perfect sense to an exploration based on living fascia, be it movement or manual (or even meditative) practice. If nothing else, it leads to a certain expansion into the idea of how an organic material can phase-change, flow, vary and become soft or solid, to the extent that the body can; and that is on the basic physical level, before its quantum nature can be considered.

Essentially chocolate crystallises into forms and responds to forces moved/moving through it and the timing of that. We are considerably more specialised, sophisticated and various than the cocoa bean, not to mention alive and conscious! However, the *behaviour* of a "liquid crystalline" substance need not be so astonishing, when we realise that its *natural patterns and forming principles* have something in common with any other liquid crystal medium.

Type, temporality, temperatures, temper(ament) and tempo and their crucial interdependent co-creative properties bring about the right *texture* – if you know how to initiate and balance them!! It is a dance of emergent properties, responding to forces transmitted through the material in particular ways.

Fascia, in the living body of all animals, is (in a way) the mistress (matrix comes from "mater") of all emergent properties. Essentially the role is to adapt and operate within certain parameters, adopting the morphology that optimises the conditions (and vice versa; seeking the optimal conditions to adapt a suitable morphology – it is a co-creative, collective matrix).

We talk about "being in shape" or "getting into shape", which is precisely what this is about. The body of any being adapts to its genetics, kinetics, environment and situation *over time* and *at the time*. We are far more akin to the functional variations in the story of chocolate than the mechanical lever-based systems of a Pinocchio, in our natural motion patterns, needs and variability.

We are more than "non-linear biologic forms". Our architecture and shape reflect many similar properties, but we are self-assembled, self-regulating, self-motivated and essentially self-*animated conscious beings*. Perhaps what we are reaching into here is the recognition that we have, as Mae-Wan Ho terms it: "body-consciousness" as well as "brain-consciousness".[41] Mae-Wan Ho refers to the molecular behaviour of the internal fluid matrix as the "quantum jazz of life". Her extensive research and books (see special end piece and notes) endorse the deeper aspects of Pollack's research and invite consideration from other scientists that explain the essential role of collagen in binding biological water into a "liquid crystalline matrix".

Seed Crystals and Bound Water

Chocolate that is tempered (ready to crystallise in a particular, stable organisation; see Box 7.2) can be added to melted chocolate (that is not ready to crystallise, unstable) and it will "seed crystal" the surrounding molecules. The structures seem to have a kind of "architectural language" that changes them, according to how the five elements described above (see Box 7.2) mix and manage the forces through the material. The substance shifts to appropriate structuralisation *in response* to change. I call this the *architextures* of the matrix. They change according to the pressure, speed, temperature and treatment of the material – and its natural temperament.

We also respond variously to temperature, temporality, temper(ament) and tempo and treatment, according to type. Our tissues display these at different *stages* of our development – different *ages* and different situations. (That is not limited to purely physical function any more than the practice of yoga!).

We emerge and merge the elements of our various crystallisation processes. In the embryo, we saw the cartilage (think thick fascia, with hyaline added to it) form the precursor to the limbs, providing a placeholder for the bones. It mapped the cartilage architexture, within which the tissues were able to respond (through forces of genetic, kinetic and morphological organisations) *as denser crystallisations of the bound fluid* within the same matrix. They "seeded" the growing morphology within the potential architectural constraints, of the bone (think crystallised fascia, with calcium salts [hydroxyapatite] added to it). These are *responses to tension–compression forces* moving a particular type of liquid crystal matrix, surrounding it and maintaining more variables than we can easily imagine (see end page of this section). In living bodies, we call this process *mechanotransduction* (see Ingber, note 15) and it makes more sense if we understand how liquid crystals can behave.

Fascia is a mostly liquid gel that forms strands, fibrils and tubular networks at a variety of densifications, to live in (and as) the "wet tropical jungle" Schleip refers to in Chapter 5. The body is a wet, breathing, changing milieu, formed under tension and compression forces to hold the various fluids it contains in their distinct pockets and tubular pathways, bound together within and between them. Some of the various fluids act as binding agents, such as the effect of protein on water (see margin note). *Is it possible that the water itself is bound by the same patterns?* It seems that the water at the interface of membranes (between cells, organs or tubes) is more bound than that

Architextures is a word I made up to explain something that has a qualitative nature, emerging from (and responsive to) the structural conditions and response as a material integrating with its environment. A material that varies in its essential role as the basis of our physical, organic architecture.

within the membrane; and architecturally (or haptically?) it knows where it is. According to Mae-Wan Ho, it can "phase change" rapidly or slowly and ignite surrounding molecules to communal behaviours. This matches how chocolate behaves in response to seed-crystallisation.

The chocolate metaphor simply helps us to understand that *emergent properties* influence shape, or morphology. Fascia, being a living organic material, can express *itself* as a multitude of tissue types, depending upon (and presenting) the emergent properties of the material over time and the fluid matrix of that particular location.

Formal Fascia Distinctions

Re: Figure 7.11. Note that in this terminology, bone, cartilage and blood are excluded.[42] They are considered to be connective tissue rather than fascia. In the case of bone, for example, this is due to the fact that bones are considered *discontinuous* whereas fascia is technically considered to be continuously tensioned throughout the matrix. There is controversy over this fact. Jaap van der Wal, for example, suggests the periost precedes and mediates the bone and Levin, Sharkey and Scarr all concur, endorsing Deane Juhan's proposal (see previous chapter). (Levin describes bone as "starched fascia".) In tensegrity models, the compression members *are discontinuous by texture, not separate by design*. However, in the human body they are all made of different textures of the same fabric, co-existing in a mutual synergistic relationship with all the fascial forms; which powerfully challenges the grounds upon which they might be excluded as fascia.

The nomenclature in Figure 7.11 is offered by a selected committee, within the Fascia Research Society. It suggests clarification of the general terminology that the term *fascia* encompasses. The reason why so many clinicians are keen to use one term is exactly why yoga benefits from understanding fascial anatomy. Its **unifying** nature throughout our form is relentlessly present and connected. By naming each aspect of it separately, the invitation is to break it down into parts and risk misunderstanding its wholeness.[43]

It is the very continuity of the fascia that shifts certain perspectives and allows us to see it as a communication system, a force transmission system, an organising matrix, a means of sensory refinement and proprioceptive self-awareness. That it is ubiquitous (everywhere) cannot be emphasised enough. In the end, it is the unity of these characteristics that makes it so compatible a basis for the understanding of yoga in all its variety of forms.

In the more advanced practices of yoga, the subtle qualitative aspects of the energy system, or field, are noted. Perhaps this is the direction in which the process of languaging the fascia is going.

Essentially there is one fascia, from the original embryonic forming process. It is one piece of tissue, self-organised into a toroidal pattern, made from two spheres touching, joined by respective membranes, to form with a tube down the middle of the ensuing toroid, as we have described. A toroid is a donut. If you imagine a donut joined by respective membranes, to form with a long hole down the middle – a very, very long, wiggly, twisting, turning, folding tubular tube – you have the soft-tissue architecture between the mouth and the anus of a very sophisticated juicing machine, with a mind of its own. It seems it has a body-mind of its own too, perhaps! (Its metabolic role as a "juicer" is beyond the scope of this work, however the integration of fluid dynamics *and the quality of those fluids* might have more to do with fascia as a filter than has yet been researched.)

Everything else is a variation on the theme of tension–compression geodesics – close-packed cells forming tubes and pockets of various architextures that are all attached everywhere under their liquid crystal, fasciategrity-based, architectural design. This gives rise to the peristaltic motion we rely upon for fluid exchange and opens us into a huge field of microbiology and links the pathology of the interstitium (see later) described by Theise. When the various architextures pack super close and short, under pressure from the bones, they tend to form themselves into ligament-like dense interfaces (between bones).

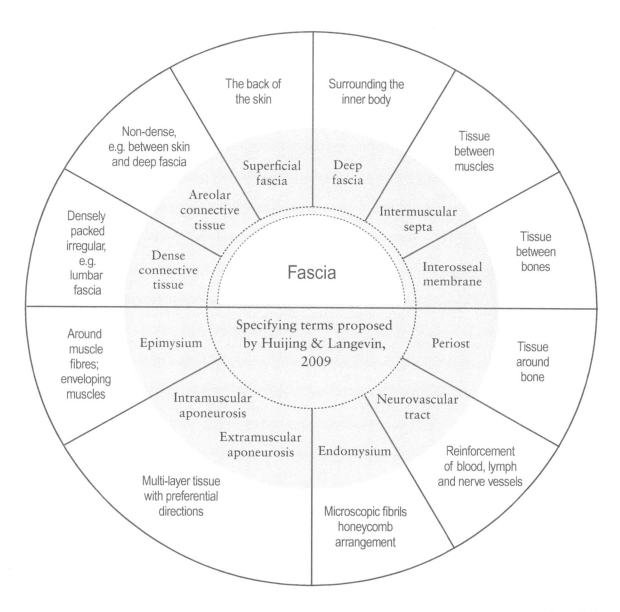

Figure 7.11

These are the twelve main classified distinctions of the fascia within the body. Besides each one is a note of the particular area or quality it refers to. Note that in this terminology, bone, cartilage and blood are excluded. They are considered to be connective tissue, rather than fascia. In the case of bone, for example, this is due to the fact that they are discontinuous whereas fascia is technically considered to be continuously tensioned throughout the matrix.

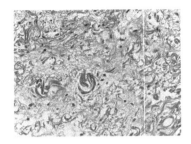

Figure 7.12

This is the tissue of the interstitium; the "in-between" that the research of Neil Theise and Rebecca Wells and their colleagues are able to demonstrate is part of the living fascial matrix.

(From Dr Neil Theise and Dr Rebecca Wells.[48])

When they crystallise with calcium deposits they become outer bone and within that, porridge-like bone on a spectrum within a spectrum of the harder *architextures* of this type of fascia.[44] The story goes on and on, effectively describing every architecture of the soft-tissue body as a different type/location/timing field of the one "materia biologica"; always uniquely expressed and invariably *translated* by our unique movements, diet, environment and variables.

Bones are really tubes, like muscle fibres or intestines, with different "harder soft-matter" architextures. They have more compressed emergent properties due to the location, chemistry, genetics and kinetics (which influence the tension–compression forces they are exposed to), force transmission and structural integration.

The principle we have to upgrade to, to fully appreciate the fascia, is that its architexture (its quality, according to where, how and who it formed) changes from birth to death, from day to day, from location to location, in time and space. Its morphology occupies space and changes constantly over time. Once we understand its spatial behaviours we begin to recognise how essential it is that we appreciate influencing factors such as type, temperature and temporality as keystone elements in how the matrix moves and behaves over time. It is temporal and temperamental! *As is the business of being human!*

"Mechanical physics has banished organic space-time from our collective public consciousness, though it never ceases to flourish in the subterranean orphic universe of our collective unconscious and our subjective aesthetic experience. In a way, all developments in Western science since Descartes and Newton may be seen as a struggle to reclaim our intuitive, indigenous notions of organic space-time, which deep within our soul, we feel to be more consonant with authentic experience."

Mae-Wan Ho[45]

If we consider yoga as what Mae-Wan Ho describes as an "authentic experience", then the inclusion of visual resonance (light currents) through the Yantras (see Ch. 13) and the audial resonance (sound currents) through the Mantras (see Ch. 13) is perhaps congruent with our multi-dimensional physical architexture in all its mysterious detail. Perhaps these are actually very sophisticated ways to self-regulate and "tune our system" – along with the physical yogasana.

Fascia is known to conduct light through the body.[46] It is suggested that the pre-stiffened, tensegrity organisation (which is the basic nature of the fibrils and fibres throughout the cells and the entire system) resonates with tissue-specific frequencies.[47] That suggests fascia is highly sensitive to sound currents – as might be expected from a tension–compression structure. (Most instruments are based on such a design – see below and in Ch. 10). In many ways, the science is returning us to the deeper philosophic basis of yoga.

This theme of seeking balance is so deep to the nature of us and the most microscopic aspects of our form that it may be valuable to amplify it in practice. Perhaps we can allow our attention to find that wonderful combination of awareness, of awe and alchemy taking place within us, whether we recognise it or not!! Whatever the song we sing or the rhythm each of us dances to; perhaps, underneath the mind-chat (*chitta-vritti*) Mother Nature is playing it through us, anyway. Perhaps all we need to do is listen in and wonder?

Excerpt from Mae-Wan Ho, *Meaning of Life and Universe: Transforming* – Chapter 3:
Organism and Psyche in a Participatory Universe.

A Theory of the Organism

There are about 75 trillion cells in our body, made up of astronomical numbers of molecules of many different kinds. How can this huge conglomerate of disparate cells and molecules function so perfectly as a coherent whole? How can we summon energy at will to do whatever we want? And most of all how is it possible for there to be a singular "I" that we all feel ourselves to be amid this diverse multiplicity?

To give an idea of the coordination of activities involved, imagine an immensely huge super-orchestra playing with instruments spinning an incredible spectrum of sizes from a piccolo of 10^{-9} meter up to a bassoon or a bass viol of a meter or more, and a musical range of perhaps 70 octaves. The amazing thing about this super-orchestra is that it never ceases to play out our individual song lines, with a certain recurring rhythm and beat, but in endless variations that never repeat exactly. Always, there is something new, something made up as it goes along. It can change key, change tempo, change tune perfectly, as it feels like it, or as the situation demands, spontaneously and without hesitation. Furthermore, each and every player, however small, can enjoy maximum freedom of expression, improvising from moment to moment, while maintaining in step and in tune with the whole. I have just described a theory of the quantum coherence that underlies the radical wholeness of the organism, which involves total participation, maximizing both local freedom and global cohesion. It involves the mutual implication of global and local, of part and whole, from moment to moment. It is on that basis that we can have a sense of ourselves as a singular being, despite the diverse multiplicity of parts. That is also how we can perceive the unity of the here and now, in an act of "prehensive unification" according to Whitehead.[1] Artists, like scientists, depend on the same exquisite sense of 'prehensive unification', to see patterns that connect apparently disparate phenomena. To add corroborative details to the theory of the organism, I shall give a more scientific narrative beginning with energy relationships.

[1]Whitehead, A.N. *Science and the Modern World*, Penguin Books, Harmondsworth, 1925.

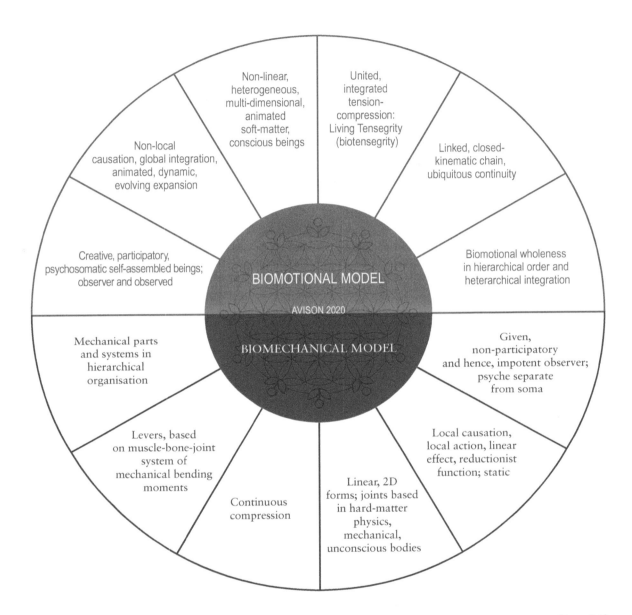

Figure 7.13

Proposed integration of new consideration for ideas based upon the distinction between classical biomechanical properties and contemporary biomotional properties.

(Adapted from Mae-Wan Ho research.)

Notes

1. John Roger, Doctor of Spiritual Science, May 26, 1984. Peace & Theological Seminary and College of Philosophy, LA, California
2. See "A Theory of the Organism" by Mae-Wan Ho on page 171.
3. If you look up 'Ground substance' on Wikipedia (https://en.wikipedia.org/wiki/Ground_substance), the definition you will see is something like: Ground substance is an amorphous gel-like substance in the extracellular space that contains all components of the extracellular matrix except for fibrous materials such as collagen and elastin. Ground substance is active in the development, movement, and proliferation of tissues, as well as their metabolism.
4. Trees inhale our waste gas (carbon dioxide) as we inhale theirs (oxygen) in a reciprocal relationship.
5. Guido F. Meert, "Fluid dynamics in fascial tissues", Ch. 4.5 in Robert Schleip, Thomas W. Findley, Leon Chaitow and Peter A. Huijing, *Fascia: The Tensional Network of the Human Body*, Churchill Livingstone/Elsevier, Edinburgh, 2012.
6. Jaap van der Wal, lectures in Embryosophy, https://www.embryo.nl/english-1?sitelang=EN
7. S.M. Levin, D.-C. Martin D-C. "Biotensegrity – The Mechanics of Fascia". Chapter 3.5 in: R. Schleip et al (eds) *Fascia – The tensional network of the human body*, pp. 137–142. Edinburgh: Churchill Livingstone, 2012.
8. "Connective Tissue", Ch. 3 in Deane Juhan, *Job's Body: A Handbook for Bodywork*, Station Hill Press, Barrytown, NY, 1987.
9. Levin's article on Bone is Fascia – published on ResearchGate and as a special contribution within the Introduction of Susan C. Lowell de Solórzano's *Everything Moves: How Biotensegrity Informs Human Movement*. Handspring Publishing Ltd, Pencaitland, 2020.
10. Adjo Zorn and Kai Hodeck; Erik Dalton, *The Dynamic Body*, Freedom from Pain Institute, Oklahoma, 2010; http://erikdalton.com/products/dynamic-body/
11. Jaap van der Wal, Dundee University Life Sciences Department, 2018, Presentation on the Nature of Fascia in Soft-fix Theil dissection.
12. P.C. Benias, R.G. Wells, B. Sackey-Aboagye, et al (2018) Structure and distribution of an unrecognized interstitium in human tissues. *Sci Rep* 8, 4947.
13. See note 44.
14. Ibid
15. Ingber; presented at the first International Fascia Research Congress, October 2007, held at Harvard Medical School, Boston, MA.
16. Donald E. Ingber (2008) Tensegrity and mechanotransduction. *Journal of Bodywork and Movement Therapies* (2008) 12:198–200.
17. Ibid.
18. Deane Juhan, JobsBody.com.
19. Adjo Zorn and Kai Hodeck; Erik Dalton, *The Dynamic Body*, Freedom from Pain Institute, Oklahoma, 2010; http://erikdalton.com/products/dynamic-body/).
20. Ch. 3, "Connective Tissue", in Deane Juhan, *Job's Body: A Handbook for Bodywork*, Station Hill Press, Barrytown, NY, 1987.
21. Jean-Claude Guimberteau, See Dr Guimberteau's work (www.endovivo.com/en/dvds.php). His DVD: Interior Architectures, is available on the same site. See also *The Architecture of Living Fascia: The Extracellular Matrix and Cells Revealed Through Endoscopy*, Handspring Publishing Ltd., Pencaitland, 2014.
22. Mae-Wan Ho, *Meaning of Life and the Universe: Transforming*, World Scientific Publishing Co. Pte. Ltd, London, 2017. From: Ch 15, Water the Means, Medium and Message of Life, opening quotation. p. 349.
23. Peter Wohlleben, *The Hidden Life of Trees*, Greystone Books, Vancouver, Berkley, Chapter 8, pp. 43–49.
24. M.W. Ho and D. Kinight (1998) Liquid crystalline meridians. *Am J Chin Med* 26:251–263.
25. https://www.extremetech.com/extreme/208501-what-is-silicon-and-why-are-computer-chips-made-from-it
    Silicon chips in computers that hold memory are crystals. Silicon isn't the only semiconducting substance on Earth — it's not even the best semiconductor on Earth. What it is, is by far the most abundant semiconductor on Earth. Silicon is readily available, all over the world; you don't need to import it from special African mines, or do months of expensive and polluting treatment just to get some. It's easy to work with and, most importantly, scientists have come up with reliable ways of growing it into perfectly ordered crystals. These crystals are to silicon as diamond is to carbon. Growing enormous, near-perfect silicon crystals is one of the primary skills in modern computer chip manufacturing. These crystals are then sliced into thin wafers, then engraved, processed, and treated in sometimes hundreds of different ways before being diced into the individual die and packaged into commercial processors. It's possible to make superior transistors out of things like carbon, and even more exotic materials like germanium, but none of them allow the sort of bulk manufacturing silicon allows through large crystal growth — at least, not yet.
26. L-field means fields of life, according to Harold Saxton Burr, Professor Emeritus, Anatomy at Yale University School of Medicine. in his book *Blueprint for Immortality, the Electric Patterns of Life*, Neville Spearman Ltd, London, 1972.
27. Mae-Wan Ho (2015) Life is water electric. *Bioelectromagnetic and Subtle Energy Medicine*, 2nd Edition 93–104.
28. Gerald Pollack, *Cells, Gels and the Engines of Life*; Ebner and Sons Publishers, Seattle, 2001.
29. Ibid. Preface.
30. Gerald Pollack. *The Fourth Phase of Water: Beyond Solid, Liquid, and Vapor*, Ebner and Sons, Seattle, 2013.
31. Mae-Wan Ho, *Living Rainbow H2O*, World Scientific Publishing, Singapore, 2012.
32. Mae-Wan Ho (2015) Life is water electric. *Bioelectromagnetic and Subtle Energy Medicine*, 2nd Edition 93–104.
33. Gerald Pollack. *The Fourth Phase of Water: Beyond Solid, Liquid, and Vapor*, Ebner and Sons, Seattle, 2013.
34. Excerpt from the full transcript of Dr. Gerald Pollack's TEDx Talk titled *The 4th Phase of Water* at TEDxGuelphU conference.
35. Ibid.
36. A.S. Mikhailov and G. Ertl (1996) Nonequilibrium structures in condensed systems. *Science* 272:1596–1597.
37. Mae-Wan Ho, *Meaning of Life and the Universe: Transforming*, World Scientific Publishing Co. Pte. Ltd, London, 2017. From: Quantum Coherence and Conscious Experience, pp. 272–273.
38. M. Cifra, P. Pospíšil (2014) Ultra-weak photon emission from biological samples: definition, mechanisms, properties, detection and applications. *J Photochem Photobiol B*. 139:2–10.

39. Vantage House; Chocolate Development Kitchen, Henfield, East Sussex

40. Fine Chocolate, Great Experience; CallebautUitgeverij Lannoo nv. Tielt, 2004.

41. Mae-Wan Ho, *Meaning of Life and the Universe: Transforming*, World Scientific Publishing Co. Pte. Ltd, London, 2017. From: Ch 3, Organism and Psyche in a participatory universe. pp. 80–103.

42. Definition from Note 41: "The fascial system consists of the three-dimensional continuum of soft, collagen containing, loose and dense fibrous connective tissues that permeate the body. It incorporates elements such as adipose tissue, adventitiae and neurovascular sheaths, aponeuroses, deep and superficial fasciae, epineurium, joint capsules, ligaments, membranes, meninges, myofascial expansions, periostea, retinacula, septa, tendons, visceral fasciae, and all the intramuscular and intermuscular connective tissues including endo-/peri-/epimysium. The fascial system *surrounds, interweaves between, and interpenetrates* all organs, muscles, bones and nerve fibers, endowing the body with a functional structure, and providing an environment that enables all body systems to operate in an integrated manner." (Changed wording in *italic font*.)

43. John Sharkey (2018) Biotensegrity – Anatomy for the 21st century informing yoga and physiotherapy concerning new findings in fascia research. *J Yoga & Physio* 6(1):555680.

44. John Sharkey (2019) Letter to the Editor. *Journal of Bodywork & Movement Therapies* 23:6–8.
    Article by Stephen M. Levin - 2018/08/21, SP , Bone is Fascia - published on ResearchGate and as a special contribution within the Introduction of Susan C. Lowell de Solórzano's *Everything Moves: How Biotensegrity Informs Human Movement*. Handspring Publishing Ltd, Pencaitland, 2020.

45. Mae-Wan Ho, *Meaning of Life and the Universe: Transforming*, World Scientific Publishing Co. Pte. Ltd, London, 2017. From: Ch 3, Organism and Psyche in a participatory universe. p.87

46. M. Cifra, P. Pospíšil (2014) Ultra-weak photon emission from biological samples: definition, mechanisms, properties, detection and applications. *Journal of Photochemistry and Photobiology B: Biology* 139:2–10.

47. D. Curtis, et al (2010) The efficacy of frequency specific microcurrent therapy on delayed onset muscle soreness, *Journal of Bodywork & Movement Therapies* 14(3):272–9. Joseph M. Mercola, Daniel L. Kirsch (1995) The basis for microcurrent electrical therapy in conventional medicine. *Journal of Advancement in Medicine* 8(2).

48. See Appendix A for more information and detail.

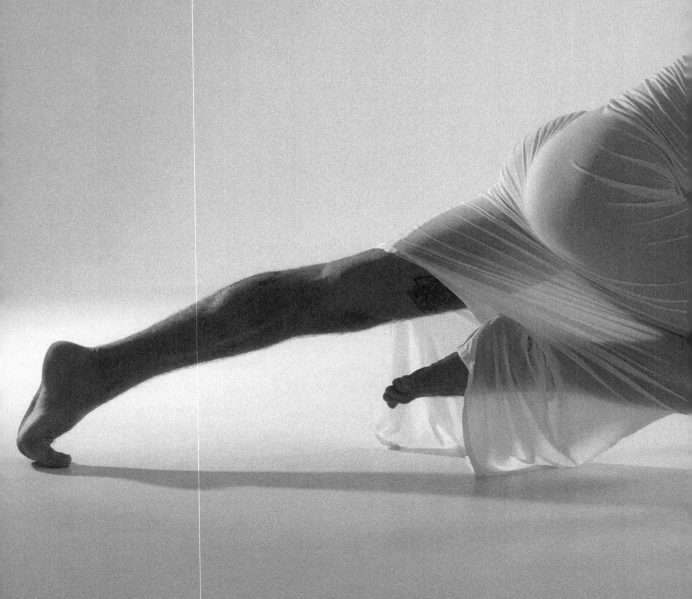

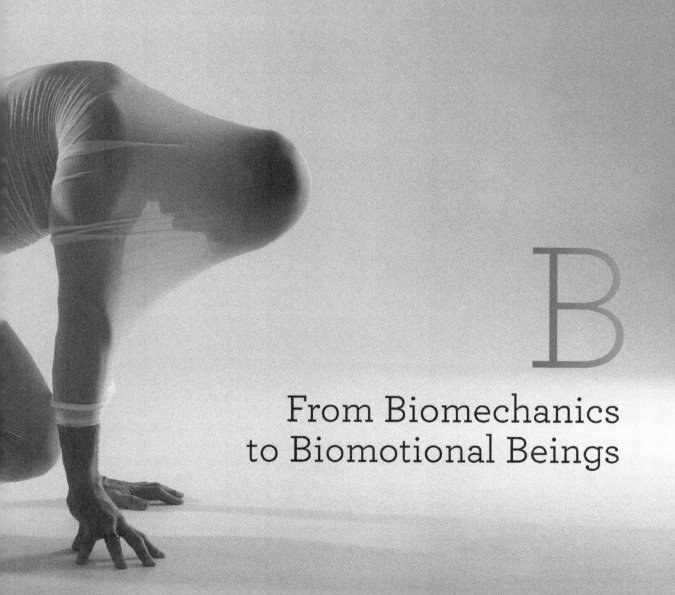

B

From Biomechanics
to Biomotional Beings

8

From Biomechanics to Biomotional Beings

In considering the anatomy and architecture of our living form, if we are truly hard matter structures it makes sense to describe our motion via levers, pin joints, unidirectional forces and layers. If, however, our true architecture is soft matter arrived by self-generated, self-emerging, self-organised, self-orchestrated and self-aware tissue, then we must use the principles and laws of soft matter physics. Soft matter physics is associated with shaving cream, gels, polymer solutions, surfactants, liquid crystals, and colloidal crystals."[1]

John Sharkey, Clinical Anatomist

We have begun to reconsider some of the traditional views of the anatomy system to include the fascial matrix as its connecting "transanatomical architecture".[2] Does that connectivity and continuity influence our classical definitions of the individual muscles and how they are considered to move us, or breathe us, now that we are learning we originally *feel our way* into form? Does it change how we teach movement and yoga? Does it account differently for the motions of breath, bones and skin as the sensory architecture feeds back how the adjoining segments of the body move and manage motion? (See Part A.)

The new distinctions of the fascia[3] shift how we see what I like to call the "whole biomotional body architecture" and invite new questions about how actions are allocated to individual muscles, or even if they really are. Research presented at the worldwide International Fascia Research Congresses[4] suggests the accepted lists of muscles and the specific movements traditionally assigned to them via the nervous system are simply not a reflection of how we, as animated beings, really move and organise our bodies. According to Robert Schleip:

"when discussing any changes in motor organisation, it is important to realise that the central nervous system does not operate 'in muscles', i.e. a muscle is never activated as a whole."

"To give an example: in real bodies, muscles hardly ever transmit their full force directly via tendons into the skeleton, as is usually suggested by our textbook drawings. They rather distribute a large

portion of their contractile or tensional forces onto fascial sheets. These sheets transmit these forces to synergistic as well as antagonistic muscles. Thereby they stiffen not only the respective joint but may even affect regions several joints further away."[5]

Let us dive into what this means by taking, as an example, one particular popular muscle in dissection. If some of the traditional actions that classical anatomy assigns to the movements of individual muscles are not necessarily how we move, then what happens to muscle groups such as the "hip flexors", for example? Does it change the way we describe the designated "breathing" muscles? We will consider the breath in a chapter of its own, from this point of view, in Chapter 11. Let us ask here, what happens in the yoga classroom, *biomechanically* to the hip flexors (as one example of many) – and what is meant by *biomotional integrity* as a distinction?

Whole Movements

In classical biomechanics, we learn that the body moves via first-, second- and third-class levers, organising functions so that we can place ourselves in positions. However, when we do Eagle Pose (*Garudasana*) we do not activate one arm, lever by lever, or muscle by muscle. Whatever linear description we might use in technical, biomechanical terminology, we can intertwine the arms around the torso in a fluid, integrated gesture. Then we entwine the legs and stand upright, balanced and counterbalanced in global organisation, on one foot (Fig. 8.1) on the mat. In practising this pose to each side, we ask our body (as a whole) a kinaesthetic question *in its own language*. We physically pose the question of mediating easy respiration, balance and equilibrium through-out the entire organism, while gently breathing and centering ourselves. We ask (perform), "How can I express this pose? And can I find stillness here?", or "Can I transition to the next pose gracefully?", or "Am I moving consciously?" in a kinaesthetic conversation, *in action*. We do not deduce the technical plan first (as a list of intellectual commands) and then move as a result.

Reducing the movement to an explanation of how we do this biomechanically, by rules of levers and muscle–bone–joint anatomy, can make it appear to be a very complex process. Technically, it cannot make sense in body language, since there are no levers in non-linear biologic forms and while they may appear *like* levers (if you were to project them in silhouette against a white wall, like a shadow-puppet show), every limb is a volume and *never* contains (or moves) itself via levers. It is simply the wrong definition for a rounded, soft-matter form. By rules of tension–compression, however, we are experimenting with balancing and counterbalancing forces through the whole body in response to the ground, *constantly*. We are balancing the inside with the outside, the front to the back, the spiral to a counter-spiral as a whole dynamic architecture. That includes all the various soft tissues *to varying degrees* – all at once in a gravitational field, bound as we are to abide by its cosmic laws, locally and globally.

Through physically experiencing the posture we are effectively asking the body "How is this now?", over and over again, moment by moment, through

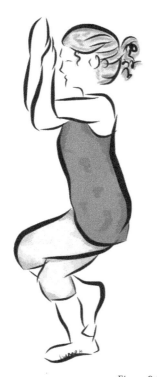

Figure 8.1

Like all the poses, Eagle Pose (Garudasana) is a whole-body posture.

practising how we make this particular gesture or morphology as an *anti-gravity force transmission*. In other words, we are the radial counter-force (as a volume) countering the forces of gravity in the round, surrounding us (aka your ability to sit or stand up, in a gravitational field). By imitating, repeating and mimicking (the teacher, or what we did before), the body learns the poses, eventually remodeling the shapes instinctively (i.e. without having to think about them at all). Even with the choreography down, each occasion is new and the pose is experienced uniquely every time. We can also explore and accumulate our own sense of balance and variation in different positions and transitions and variations. The body "speaks" or rehearses these movements, in the *language of balance and variation* – as an orchestration of different properties. It amounts to *sensing a feeling* of poise, a kind of biomotional feedback loop. This felt sense might be a significant factor of structural integrity, in terms of somatic value (Ch. 5). Like the embryo (Ch. 4) we are sensing our way into form, as a whole, as we go – every moment, every day with every new gesture. That's essentially how we learn to move as a child and *move better* as an adult. We practise!

Tissue Glide

Physiologically, at a global and regional level, we are also inviting tissue glide, flexibility and various internal fluid exchanges by centripetal and centrifugal expansions and in-drawing (breathing: by drawing in and out – see Ch. 11 for definitions), folding and unfolding, tightening and holding different parts of the limbs at variable angles, or vectors, according to their morphologies and the geometry of the posture *in relation to the ground*. We ARE the *ground reaction force* expressed as a biomotionally intelligent, whole form (which can be said of every one of our cells, too).

By practising the different poses (*asanas*) we are training the ability to focus and organise our awareness and our attention, expressed in a co-ordinated manner. As we might practise a language in different situations to expand our vocabulary and eloquence, so we expand physical literacy in body language by inviting different positions, with curiosity. We explore balance and containment by varying the shapes and listening to the different parts of the body doing the weight-bearing or providing the anchor for load and distribution in space, as a volume. At the gross, or macro level of movements, however, we do not do separate things and wait for them to behave as if they are joined together. We work as a whole; **we come from our original connectedness and continuity**. We animate this body-wide signalling system[6] that communicates at different amplitudes throughout the inner matrix, to explore the outward *appearance* of the outer shape (the asana, or postural form). Such sensory listening might be the key to understanding these tissues (Ch. 5), particularly in motion and dynamic stillness.

Doing the different asanas varies the angles and forces through the joints. We can consciously foster the benefits of mobilising and hydrating the joint fluids and tissues so that they express the pose (asana) and our balance in a congruent, healthy way. Numerous subtle things are taking place that make sense if we seek to define them in terms of the whole matrix. They become

360 degrees of experience, as felt on the occasion. It gets quite tricky in a movement classroom to work on still frames in an analytical, two-dimensional format. It leaves the movement centre disengaged. This is the body language seeking to be heard. It speaks for itself in a sense. It

cumbersome if they are reduced to merely anatomical descriptions or classical biomechanical functioning/processes.

Yoga teachers are not required to be surgeons or scientists in the classroom, nor are we managing machine parts. The muscle-by-muscle description of a movement can take longer than the movement itself. ***Ours is a participatory medium.*** We want to **be in motion** between speed and stillness, rather than describing it. How do we use biomechanical terms if the basis of describing muscles as units is lost to the fact that they *do not operate* that way?

Keeping Both the Baby and the Bath Water

Tempting as it is to run with the new and abandon the old, fascia alone is not necessarily the answer to everything either. Is it possible to unite classical wisdom with contemporary research and come up with something that makes more sense of both? Where can we look to make more meaningful

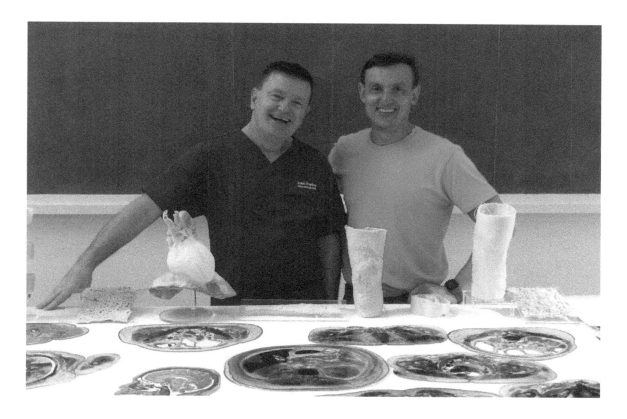

Figure 8.2

John Sharkey and Dr Vladimir Chereminskiy[24] in 2019 in the Anatomy Laboratory at the Centre for Anatomy and Human Identification, School of Life Sciences, University of Dundee, Scotland. These are the plastinates of the human heart and diaphragm; a very complex dissection process, designed by John Sharkey at the earliest stages of the FNPP project (more detail in Chapter 3).

certainly does not speak English. It also fails miserably at naturally speaking Biomechanics, as their classical language does not translate easily, even into 21ˢᵗ century anatomy. This is something like the difference between *seeing* the Mona Lisa and describing it afterwards; they are distinct areas of our experience that don't match – they have different operating systems.

You can try describing Eagle Pose anatomically and/or biomechanically and making sense of the experience of doing it in your practice. It is fun to attempt this exercise because

The Rift

it highlights the rift between the intellectual description of the pose and what your body experiences while doing it, instinctively, throughout the matrix. The details of the postural mechanics somehow bypass the feeling of accomplishment and sense of balance you experience when you find the pose in your own way, on both sides! Balance is a kinesthetic and aesthetic experience of quality, rather than an anaesthetic, quantifiable assessment. It is a distinct domain of experience and on the yoga mat we foster the former.

If the purpose of a given movement and the individual yogic postures are divided into categories of purely biomechanical function and positional references, it is possible to lose the somatic point. Reducing the body to anatomical fragments at best creates

The Power of Distinction: An Example

distinctions in this triumvirate of locomoting tissues, in biomechanical terms, for the whole body, based on what actually happens? Bones, muscles and connective tissues *only* work together, within the fluid sensory wholeness of the entire matrix. That is what self-regulation relies upon – accurate and intimate biofeedback, beyond our ability to analyse it.

The research into the fascial network of tissues raises new questions but it does not answer them by itself, on its own, by definition. How do these *united* tissues function in a united form?

In Chapter 7 (Figs 7.3 and 7.4), we showed the 3D printed model render of the human thigh. Sharkey points out that this provides us with a new orientation, a new view or perspective on the living matrix. However, while it demonstrates that the fascial connective tissue provides a whole and complete architecture, forming pockets in which bony calcification and proteinous (muscles) arise, it is still only part of the wholeness. Taken in isolation, it is just as false a picture as considering only muscles and bones as key players in the locomotor system. "They all work together in life."

We feel through the skin and feedback from the ground, in the round, whichever way up we are. Our sense of the pose we are in and our relative location in space and the duration of the gesture all matter and accumulate. We guide (or we are self-guided) to optimise the ease and grace with which we can flow or spring or hold or deepen a position for a given time. How do we do those "in-betweens", moving into and out of the asanas? Which biomechanical laws make sense of all of them, *in real time*?

Is there a biomechanical explanation for that whole experience? Are there physical laws of movement expressed by the range of postures that honour the variable ways we can do them? Are there theories that account for what happens, including standing on one leg and balancing on hands or shoulders? Or functional principles that include the **stillness**?

The body does not stop or wait to think about it, once we have become physically familiar with the choreography by practising on the mat, or resting on it. Arguably this is the point of yoga: to create a kind of moving meditation where the mental commentary can actually quiet down. Then we can begin to occupy our physical body from the point of view of the witness, the attentive observer, seeing itself as the observed. Listening to *itself* as the guiding matrix.

Somewhere in all this complexity, semantics begin to dominate somatics if we hunt for a linear explanation in classical biomechanical terms. For people who live happily in (and teach from) their kinaesthetic centre, this would be putting things back to front. It creates a huge rift between the so-called function and the actual experience: movement is not an intellectual process.

Given that movement is not an intellectual process (it bears repeating), there are many instances in biomechanical explanations for movement, when semantics *govern* somatics, reducing experience to something that becomes an inaccurate reflection of it. One such case arises in considering the psoas muscles as a powerful example. This is important because we are searching, incongruency in terms of speed and translation into actual movements in the classroom. It tends to leave us in the rift between, on the one hand, the charts in the anatomy book and, on the other, the people on their mats waiting for instruction. Furthermore, the named actions of given muscles and muscle groups cannot always account for the subtleties of motion, awareness or micro-movements we (and all our students) are capable of exploring. That is not only in the held postures, when we are seeking stillness and balance, but also in the joined-up kinetic writing of the sequences in fast or flowing yoga practices, such as Vinyasa. We do not "fall off" the asanas in transition or pump ourselves up with enough breath to make a dash for it before the oxygen runs out. We find ways of organising the breathing movements fluidly, moderating the breath accordingly and sensing where we are from moment to moment through reflecting exactly those possibilities in action, at biomotional speed (appropriate to the style of class).

I have since spent many hundreds of hours in the anatomical laboratory at Dundee University, Centre for Anatomy and Human Identification, with the privilege of seeing this myofascial organisation in Soft-Fix Theil dissection, where it appears in a more natural state, than that of fixed dissection (where the muscles remain in rigor contraction). It has deepened my passion for this work and dedication to transforming our notions of biomechanics deduced from dissections in which the fascia is stratified and discarded. Worse still are the effects of over-arching extrapolations of biomechanical theory, based upon muscles in rigor contraction. It is not what physical *architecture* suggests *before* the surrounding, investing and ubiquitous fascia and connective tissues are anatomically cut and removed.

essentially, for a new language in the new paradigm, to describe clearly what is happening, such that we can encourage better movement. How does this intriguing muscle (commonly known as a "hip flexor"), for example, appear in the body before it gets into the anatomy books?

I recall teaching a class after I had spent a long week in the Laboratory for Anatomical Enlightenment in Boulder, Colorado[7], with Tom Myers and Todd Garcia[8] (2003), being trained in human dissection. It was the first human dissection programme focused solely on the individual Anatomy Trains™[9] described in the book of the same name, by Thomas W. Myers.

We were each invited to choose a favourite muscle and ask to see it on every cadaver.[10] I requested the psoas muscle, intrigued as to why it is often referred to as one thing: the "iliopsoas complex" (Fig. 8.3). (Table 8.1 shows the muscles of the posterior abdominal wall, including the psoas major, in the classical presentation. This table separates all aspects of the anatomy and physiology of the psoas and refers it to iliacus for its actions, assigning them a joint role as one muscle.)

Nothing could have prepared me for the detail I saw in the dissection programme, or for the clear discrepancy between the classical definition and the architecture of this muscle-in-tissue, deeply embedded in its original, although not living, context.

A number of things about the psoas became apparent from careful observation:

- It is intimately connected, myofascially, with the legs (crura) of the diaphragm (fascially it is continuous). I have since seen that it is in fact completely continuous with (not just "connected to") the diaphragm itself.

- It is woven into the fabric of the spinal soft tissues, deep to the discs and "spaces" between the lumbar vertebrae and the spinal fasciae. (These are strong, tough fibres; the spine does not appear as a clean bony surface as it is shown in anatomy books.)

- Its connection to the spine seems much more elaborate than that of iliacus. It appears as a kind of guardian of the lumbar curve from the inside, joining the lumbar vertebrae to the legs, over the pelvis. Thus, it would seem able to contribute to pelvic tilt, especially if you *include* the fascial continuity. Iliacus appears to have a distinct role despite their close affiliation; it lines the iliac bone (lying in the iliac fossa) rather than having direct connection to the spine, although it shares continuity. Iliacus and psoas have very different shapes and geometries.

- If psoas plays "best friend" to iliacus, then it is "close cousin" to quadratus lumborum myofascia (lying immediately in front of it). This intimate relative is clearly a muscle of breathing. (It anchors a *floating* rib to the back of the pelvis (iliac crest) and spinal tissues.) While psoas might play a role in responding to movements with the diaphragm, its cousin might ensure a reciprocal balance behind it for the rib basket. (In some cadavers the quadratus lumborum can appear very small, so a strong structural role seems unlikely. It appears as an anchor, securing a floating rib.)

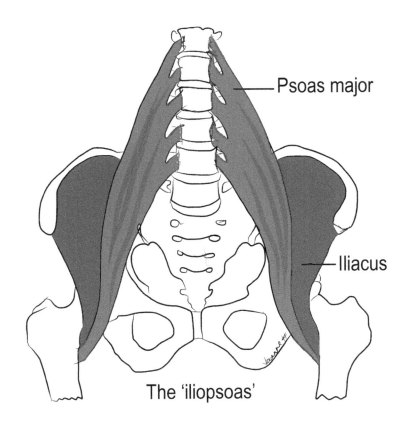

Figure 8.3

These muscles are commonly taught as the "iliopsoas complex". I was curious as to why they are combined and called "hip flexors" (what we call things makes us think they "are" their names and, therefore, function as such).

- Psoas at the front and piriformis at the back of the sacrum are most definitely BFFs (best friends forever) in terms of going nowhere without each other's cooperation[11] or "kinaesthetic comment". It is in the architectural co-ordinates when you see them together, managing as they must the *geometry* of forces moving through the pelvis.

- The relationship between psoas and iliacus and all the other neighbouring continuities is far more integrated than any segregated sections of an anatomy book could imply or reveal from the cartoon-style images we mostly see and their segregations.

- Paradoxically, however, putting psoas and iliacus together appears to be a somewhat arbitrary affiliation, in that several other muscles could be contenders for the role and be put together as a "complex" or "composite" such as this (if all they have to do to qualify is be neighbouring structures). They may share certain attachment but so do the psoas muscles and the

Table 8.1					
Muscles of the Posterior Abdominal Wall					
Muscle	**Origin**	**Insertion**	**Nerve supply**	**Action**	**Blood supply**
Diaphragm	Xiphoid process, lower six costal cartilages, lateral and medial arcuate ligaments, crura (LI and LIII), median arcuate ligament	Central tendon	Phrenic (C3 to C5)	Chief muscles of respiration	Percardiacophrenic, musculophrenic, superior and inferior phrenic arteries
Quadratus lumborum	Iliolumbar ligament, iliac crest, lower lumbar transverse processes	Rib XII and upper lumbar transverse processes	T12 to L3	Fixes rib XII, flexes trunk, flexes vertebral column laterally	Iliolumbar artery
Psoas major	Lumbar vertebrae	Lesser trochanter	L2 to L4	See iliacus muscle	Lumbar arteries
Iliacus*	Floor of iliac fossa	Tendon of the psoas major muscle and lesser trochanter	Femoral nerve	Flexes and rotates thigh medially, then rotates the thigh laterally, flexes vertebral column	Iliolumbar artery
Psoas minor**	Vertebrae TXII to LI and intervertebral disc	Pectineal ligament and iliac fascia	L1	Helps flex vertebral column	Lumbar arteries
*Joins psoas major to form iliopsoas muscle. **Frequently absent.					
(After Table 32.1 in K.P. Moses, J.C. Banks, P.B. Nava, D. Petersen, Atlas of Clinical Gross Anatomy, Elsevier Mosby: 2005.)					

diaphragm if they are cut out anatomically from the fascia differently. It is easier to dissect the psoas from the iliacus than it is to cut it off the spine and its intimate continuity with the diaphragmatic crura (which become the diaphragm). You have to cut that out, as if it is discontinuous in the body – which it blatantly is not.

- All these "close-to-the-spine" (paraspinal) muscles live together in association, intimately forming a composition of myofascial organisation, deeply woven into the soft tissues around the spine. The anatomy seems to tell a very different story when looking for connectivity, rather than components or *contiguity*. Together they manage and contain a cavity and if fascia is a force transmission and communication system, then our range and detail of **integrated motion and breath** in the yoga class relies upon it. It calls, however, for new distinctions to make sense of the parts as unified organisations within our wholeness, rather than separate bits, described as affiliations.

In Anatomy Trains, the muscles are referred to as "myofascial units" within their designated "myofascial continuities". We learned this in Chapter 3 – the fibrils, fibres, fibre bundles forming muscles and groups of muscles are often considered to be wrapped in the "cotton wool-like" weave of the fascial network. This is not altogether accurate, as in the living body there is less fibrous tissue (often an artefact of formalin dissections that preserve the muscles in rigor mortis) and much more gel-like integrated fabrics that are hydrated and interwoven like the gels and soft-tissue structures referred to in Chapters 6 and 7. This liquid-crystal matrix appears everywhere inside and around the muscle tissues. (They reside within it. The deeper within a so-called "muscle" the fascia is, the finer it is, being invisible to the naked eye at the innermost microscopic depths [called endomysium].) As such, we will often refer to myofascia where the word "muscle" might usually be used, since muscle tissue is entirely invested with fascia and, in our bodies (that we bring to class), much more hydrated in healthy living motion than appears in general dissection. That fact matters. It changes the matter materially – it's a whole other thing.

"Same but Different"

John Stirk[11] planted a seed of curiosity about the psoas and its links to breathing and walking, in one of my earliest yoga classes (in the early 90s). He asked: *"What if we consider the psoas as a breathing muscle and the diaphragm as a postural muscle. What happens to the yoga postures or walking or sitting?"*

We might think we know from the semantic label what the somatic effect of this muscle will be. However, seen as part of the fascial matrix (even deceased), its intricacy and detail is overwhelming. Once invited to look for it, the fascia clearly contains and

Besides the different views of the psoas myofascia, it was also arresting to note the anatomical differences between individual donor bodies. Without realising it, one can assume that what is in the anatomy books is what will be in the body. While we all expect to look different on the outside, it is a surprise to discover that we are equally different on the inside too. (The anatomy of variation is "what is so" from the point of view of a continuous matrix: we might dare to say that the exquisite weave between these components is more reminiscent of Indra's Net[12] than as shown in our Table 8.1.)

Needless to say, from this fascinating encounter, and many since, a similar "story" could be written about many (indeed all) "muscles" (myofascia) of the human anatomical form. None appear as segregated or able to exist or function in isolation. As we saw in Chapter 3, they are all attached throughout their forms; they all arise within the fascia and they are all deeply invested with the fabric of the body.

Classifying the psoas as a "hip flexor" or calling it an "iliopsoas complex" does not make sense after one has seen it so intimately organised with the spine.

A Psoasic Matrix?

connects and encloses everywhere in the three-dimensional form. It is exceptionally difficult to come from such an experience and return to the same dry conclusions, based on schematic diagrams of parts, labelled for their mechanical actions. In fact, it is impossible, especially if that includes levers, since there are none in the living body, *by definition*.

The myofascial role of the psoas is closely situated with the legs (crura) of the diaphragm (diaphragmatic crura) and appears to "anchor" the breathing diaphragm to and along the lumbar spine. What could be its role in mediating exactly the moving relationships between the breath, the spine and the legs that we explore in so many different ways through yoga? Given its position relative to the spine (Fig. 8.4), it must surely be considered to play an intimate role in the shape of the spinal curve and its position in relation to the legs and the breath. When we fold our legs at the groin (hip flexion), does that action make sense of this muscle's classification as a hip flexor, as if it can be treated exactly the same as iliacus? Or looking at it the other way does calling it a hip flexor explain its movement, or risk reducing its scope and assets?

Many of these questions are addressed in Tom Myers' Anatomy Trains®, assigned to the Deep Front Line. Whether or not the train lines are considered anatomically correct or universal, the point here is that these so-called myofascial meridians pose new questions when seen as global contributors to movement. My experience of the dissection programme had no small impact on my work in manual and movement therapy and training; it transformed my thinking and led me to a different quest. The new question became "How do we move as a whole? How do we organise in the round? When do we self-regulate in bits, or bands for that matter?" Truth is – we don't, EVER.

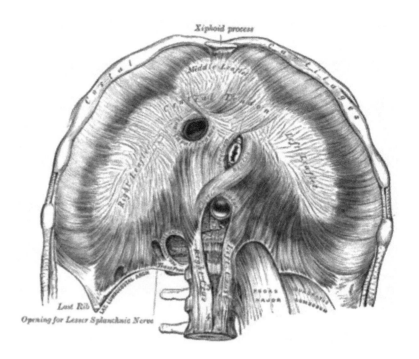

Figure 8.4

This image from an old edition of *Gray's Anatomy* shows how close the psoas is to the diaphragmatic crura. The visceral organs and vessels have all been removed and the visceral and neurovascular fascia, as well as the ligamentous fibrous covering of the spine, have been meticulously excised to reveal these deep structures. The outer connective tissues are necessarily discarded to enable the illustration to be drawn as a very "clean" image of the diaphragm, psoas and quadratus lumborum, so that they appear as quite separate units. In fact they would originally have been ensheathed with strong fascial coverings forming total continuities and relationships of varying densities that can no longer be observed.

I found myself privately wondering, if I referred to the psoas as the "psoasic matrix" in my mind, would it help to make sense of the dissection I was seeing and the fascial tissues weaving it in to the context of the rest of the body, particularly the spine tissue? Clearly, folding the leg at the hip is a movement involving the psoas. However, one could readily see it plays a part when the leg would be extended, or rotated, or many other positions. Seeing it in the laboratory, before it is extricated from its natural environs, evokes questions and possibilities of something much more refined than hip flexion. Something that makes more sense of what I see in classroom and clinic.

In the classroom, in poses such as Eagle (Garudasana), Half Moon (Ada Chandrasana) and Triangle (Trikonasana), for example, how would this so-called hip flexor be authorising or assisting the integrated leg movements (not to mention animating the breath, balance and poise)? How would it express what happens differently from one side to the other? Graceful transitions are something life (with or without yoga) demands. It seems evident that there is a difference between the detailed sculpture of the tissues in situ, the movements assigned to them and the classification of "iliopsoas as hip flexor". The semantic label reduces what happens on the mat, making it less than the actual architecture might imply and, it seems, be able to animate in finding biomotional integrity.

New Distinctions

During a later dissection opportunity, Robert Schleip responded to my endless questions around this intriguing myofascial complex by saying, "rather than considering it as a hip flexor, think of it as a spine stabiliser and it will make much more sense to you". Considering iliacus (with rectus femoris) as a hip flexor, while designating the psoas as a spine stabiliser also makes more sense of their roles in yoga, especially in the more complex poses.

I liked the idea of multiplying up to a range of functions that moves towards our experience of subtle corrections and balances. When an asana calls for the breath to be integrated with balance and folding quite differently from one side to the other, the ability to find and respond to the position, breathing steadily, is far better explained this way (Fig. 8.5). A close relationship between the psoas and the spine, *seamlessly including the diaphragm*, has to be available in the living body, anchoring and structuralising the roundness of the breathing torso. It is evident in the architecture and the experience. In many postures, the pair of psoas muscles (the psoae – *plural of psoa*[14]) have to negotiate differently from left to right, obviously, in concert with many aspects of the surrounding architecture and the breath. This is what yoga explores and I began to see why the question posed by John Stirk was so valuable.

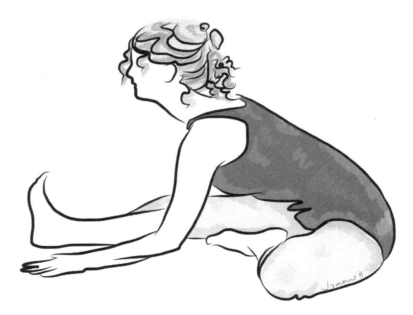

Figure 8.5

En route to full Head to Knee Pose
(Janu Sirsasana).

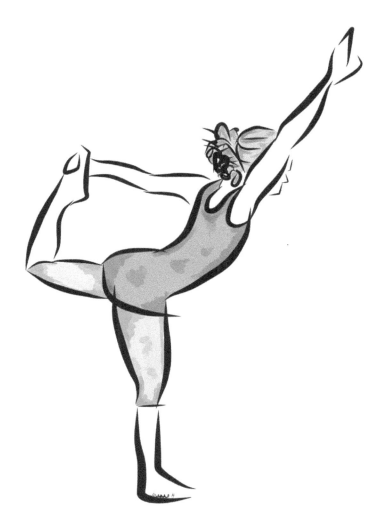

Figure 8.6

Lord of the Dance Pose (Natarajasana).

In postures where the left psoas has to do something different from the right psoas (Fig. 8.6), the common denominator is the spine, not hip flexion. Doing the pose to both sides is an enquiry into instinctive balance. It is the variation and possibility of loading patterns whilst maintaining integrity of breath and poise that is the purpose of our enquiry. Do we bring variability and range by practising this ancient art, so that these deep structural myofasciae can get on with the integrated task they know anyway, in spite of our opinions or what we call them?

I have grown to appreciate and respect the psoae as mistresses of integration in breathing, walking and spinal stabilisation; that is, in rotation, counter-rotation, side bending (lateral flexion) and forward and back bending (flexion and extension) postures. They are in close partnership with far more than their adjacent iliaci. However, before further discussion about any one particular member of our body-wide myofascial family, let us bear in mind that such a story can be told about many individual muscles, before they are cleaned up for presentation as isolated units in classical styles of dissection. The role of the psoas here is as a symbol of a new challenge. How can we meaningfully expand and evolve our thinking to a more global context that makes sense of the whole spine within the collagen matrix? How can we name the hundreds of myofascial units operating in this whole tensional architecture called "human being doing" or "you in action" in an appropriate way without reducing them to "actions" that they are not limited to?

Maps and Territories

The London Underground (subway) map provides a useful schematic, a topographical diagram that indicates only the approximate location of the system's stations relative to the others on the line. It is very useful, as long as there is no expectation that it shows the correct distance between stations, or that the stations will look the same in the real-life experience of arriving at one of them.

Prior to the first dissection I experienced, it was apparent that I had lived with similar topographical notions of human anatomy as if they were the territory. I had collapsed the distinctions of anatomy and natural or so-called "functional movement". One is clearly not derived from the other, unless you restrict the definition to a very limited version of what can actually happen in the classroom.

Even my work learning and eventually teaching with Tom Myers, in Structural Integration and Anatomy Trains™, had not prepared me for seeing muscles so intimately interwoven and continuous in longitudinal, lateral and lattice-like, woven relationships with all our parts and forms in the round. They are anything but discrete units, even in cadavers. They are completely connected to each other and surrounded. Not even a suite of muscles can operate without affecting the rest of the matrix; it becomes obvious once whole body cadaveric dissection begins. Once again, Indra's Net[15] seems a more appropriate model than Table 8.1.

The problem lies in the assumption that the "map" (and the action assigned to an isolated schematic of a muscle) explains functional movement and the *form* (or structure) of the territory. Maps are two-dimensional, topographical guides and thus distinct from the experience of the of the *topological* territory. They are an entirely different quest to understanding yoga in the living body, which is unique to each of us. This is the shift to a bigger explanation for global movement of the whole body. It brings into distinction the communicating network of tissues within our whole form, interrelating. It absorbs the classical annotations into a bigger context. The psoas does indeed play a part in hip flexion; however, while that may be its occasional job, its vocation is evidently to a higher, more sophisticated calling.[16]

Anatomy may provide a kind of grammar, but it does not necessarily tell the different stories these architectural components can present depending on how each of us uses them. Any yoga practice, dance modality or physical performance is like a tale told by a kinaesthetic author: the person in action. The point is we speak that somatic language pretty fluently in as many and various dialects as we have bodies to express. Yoga can serve to support the range and subtleties we have access to, as can many movement modalities; they don't reduce easily to classical biomechanics. Somatically, they are too "big for the [semantic] box".

What Then?

Seeing the "psoasic matrix" in vivo ignites curiosity on four key things that stand out: (1) the unified whole-body cavities; (2) the lateral diaphragms;

(3) the *one-and-the-all* on every scale; (4) the proportion and primary role of the spine in the body.

(1) Unified (whole-body) cavities

Experiencing how completely unified all the tissue weave and cavities of the torso are, begins to bridge the gap between the *books about* motion and the *experience of* movement. With the organs removed, the abdominal cavity appears as a whole container. The depths of transverse abdominis, internal and external obliques, rectus abdominis, pelvic floor and the diaphragm overlap and wrap to form roundness of the whole container, backed and supported by the lumbar spine curve, whatever its shape. They enclose the abdominal (peritoneal) cavity in all its volume. Rather than considering them as if they are separate (a front, a back, a side, a top, a base), if we look at them together, they multiply up to a complete and relatively thinly clad chamber. They are pierced above and below by the continuity of the gut, the neural and circulatory vessels and the urogenital openings, but are otherwise entirely unified by the connecting tissues of these variously soft walls. They do not experience themselves as separately organised units in isolation, whatever exercises we think we are imposing on them, one at a time (like abdominal crunches, for example). We saw in Chapter 4 how the embryo forms these cavities by enfolding them, in the original "bio-organic origami" process of embryogenesis. We are self-assembling forms, kinaesthetic architects of our own developing design – at all times; a whole work in progress.

(2) Lateral diaphragms

In a more recent dissection, I was working on the diaphragm and the peritoneal sac – and it was continuous with the viscera at the lower depths, also. While I knew "technically, intellectually in my head" from working with John Sharkey and being trained by him and Jaap van der Wal in tissue sparing dissection, nothing prepared me for actually experiencing the continuity of the diaphragm and the mesentery and the entire soft tissue architecture of the viscera. They are literally continuous: as in the same piece of tissue. Not just "connected" as if by some fibrous net, but *of the same continuity*. John laughed at my astonishment: "you knew it was all one piece, you've written a book about it" – yet there I was, stunned, that the embryological forming of one single piece of biological origami *really is one piece*. Come and sit down with that thought for a moment. Imagine your heart actually beats ALL of you at once because it is continuous with all

The second aspect is experiencing the diaphragm as an arched, lateral myofascial sandwich that is tensioned across the whole torso, between the abdominal (peritoneal) cavity below and the thoracic cavity above (Fig. 8.7). It is deeply integrated with the heart and forms the base of the heart (pericardial) and lung (pleural) cavities: all are attached to the soft tissues of the thoracic spine and supported by its curves. (This is no surprise to us after learning the basics of embryogenesis, but somehow, they are more intimately interrelated than we might generally imagine from separate maps of them.)

The heart and lungs are all enclosed by the ribs, which are like wrapping, curved, specifically angled bones of a corset, tightly bound stiffeners issuing from between the vertebrae, deeply wrapped in the fascial bandages containing them (and the spine and these organs). They encompass the upper torso but remain profoundly integrated with the body walls and distinguished by their respective cavities, all held open under tension; like a marquee or a parachute – albeit anchored to (or by) the spine. In a soft, living, breathing body they can act like stiffeners in the breathing, pulsing upper-body wall *so that it can hold its volume*. Always, in the round!

In a later dissection in the programme,[17] the myofascia of the pericardial tissues surrounding and forming the heart cavity demonstrate continuous connections with the throat and tongue. This makes perfect sense in embryological terms, because of their forming sequence (Ch. 4); it is part of our most original developmental pattern. We speak from the heart both physically and metaphorically, if the interconnecting continuity of the fascial web is included and acknowledged.

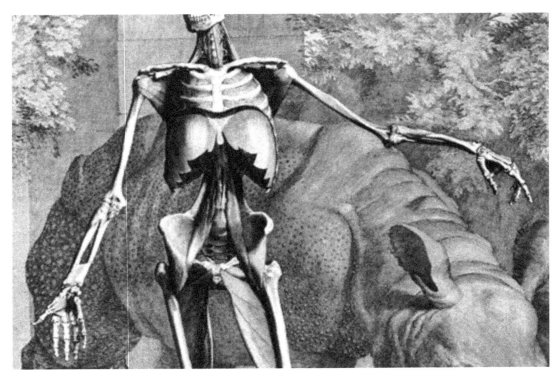

Figure 8.7

Image from *Albinus on Anatomy*. The diaphragm forms a double dome across the entire cavity, attached in 360 degrees to the inner body wall. We "know" this. However, seeing in dissection that the pericardial and pleural sacs are distinct but nevertheless exquisitely shaped by each other's neighbouring forms (including the uppermost aspect of the diaphragm) emphasises their intimate and original forming relationships (see Ch. 5). Seeing how their respective cavities are shaped by the neighbouring tissues shifts the perspective irrevocably, inviting us to appreciate the intimate relationships between the cavities of the torso in any movement.

of you at once. At one. All the time. In total and relentless continuity. It changes something exquisitely gracious about the complex simplicity of every **one of us**.

Technically, there are no "spaces" as such in the human body; everything is contained and filled with something. They are considered "virtual spaces" when we refer to "joint space" or "joint play", however this is a language of convenience, as the body doesn't contain empty spaces, as such. The spaces between cells, for example, form the extra cellular matrix and there is always something there (see Chapter 3 and reference to the work of Neil Thiese et al, see Appendix A).

The breath and bones and body wall of the torso are not separate anywhere. Mediated by the soft tissues and septae, their relationships and ability to glide, expand and impand and release are the foundation of our functional movements, that is, the moves we make to do the poses and the internal organisation that follows naturally, as we breathe (Ch. 12). Indeed, function and form appear to be intimately co-creative elements of our living bodies. I no longer see the logic in naming specific muscles as "breathing muscles" or "accessory breathing muscles". Part of our ability to breathe is in response to gravity, so can we wisely segregate the intimately related muscles of breathing and walking? Is there a way to describe the whole roundness of it all?

There is a pattern of organs contained by cavities, cavities contained by the body walls – adult versions of the embryonic tubes and folds. As John Sharkey points out, strictly speaking they are pockets, because they are all connected to each other in (and as) one tissue. We appear, from the outside, to move these

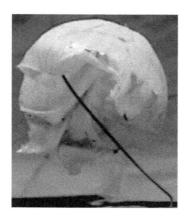

Figure 8.8

Some of the fabric of the fascia inside the skull and around the brain, dissected intact by Todd Garcia (see note 21) and photographed by Shane McDermott (reproduced with his kind permission). This enclosing tissue does not stop where it has been cut here; it is continuously expressed as a continuity throughout the form.

as a whole, pre-stiffened or tensioned by our tension–compression organisation (see Ch. 9).

Books describing the lateral myofascial bands and diaphragms[18] begin to make sense of the body, divided across or sectioned by the more subtle descriptions of the yogic bandhas described in yoga practice.[19] There are whole cylinders within cylinders, tubes within tubes, as Stanley Keleman and others have pointed out.[20] The brain sits in the highest position overall, enclosed within the toughest walls of the cranial vault and its own continuous container of connecting tissue (Fig. 8.8).[21] There is continuity between these cavities, not just from the spine. The wrapping and interwoven nature of the tissues connects them all to each other, yet distinguishes them *from* each other at the same time. There is a paradoxical aspect to it. In a sense, the fascia connects and disconnects simultaneously.

How did we come to consider the parts of the body as anything other than entirely continuous? They are united by the fabric and forms of the axial (except girdles and limbs) and appendicular (girdles and limbs) skeleton, wrapping them in the continuous matrix of tissues and continuously wrapped in periost: *the fascia around all the bones*. In the embryo, everything grows from the original conceptus. In the adult, the connectivity of the whole form is still in place. Nothing is separate; everything can be traced back to everything else, via these tissues. They span the apparent spaces as well as the organs and bones, forming the extracellular matrix. Is there anywhere connections and continuity cannot be found?

(3) The one and the all

It becomes hard to separate any one (anything) from the all (of everything). Yoga is about the whole body, honouring all of its detail. This invites me as a yoga teacher into the rift, or chasm, between general, academic, classical anatomy/biomechanics and living, moving, breathing people, in all shapes and sizes, who do poses. Do we limit someone's ability by designating a muscle as responsible for a single action? More to the point, whether the psoas is a spinal stabiliser, or a hip flexor, do we need to know that in order to do yoga well? Yoga has been practised beautifully for centuries, without necessarily knowing much about the psoas, or that possibly the least of its roles is as a hip flexor. Yet the practice of yoga can and does free many a stuck pelvis or disorganised lumbar spine, when used appropriately, through the sensory refinement of the individual practising it (and the guidance of their practitioner). It can facilitate the body to sort itself out and relieve pain (see Ch. 5). Does intelligent movement become more kinaesthetically conscious if we name the parts involved? Can we make a bigger difference by appreciating the relationships between those parts as having more than a subordinate role? While it is clearly so useful to know the topographical map, how do we usefully guard against making it mean something it doesn't? We are actually expressing the body as a *topological transformation* by moving it – they are not the same! In short, we collapse the distinction between the map and the territory.

(4) The proportion and primary role of the spine and axial skeleton

The fourth point is about the scale and strength of the spine, the spinal joints and the tissues that hold them together. It is about knowing that, in places, the collagen formation holding our bodies together has the equivalent tensile strength of steel wire (Ch. 10).[22]

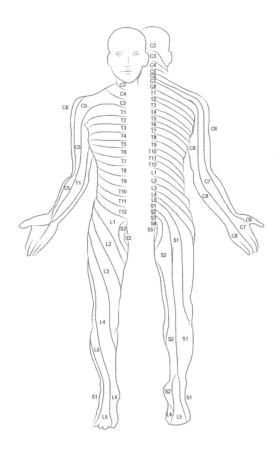

Figure 8.9

The dermatomes are illustrated on the body, sketched as rings with the related vertebral level, to show approximately where the skin is considered to be innervated segmentally.

"Each of the yoga poses is accompanied by breathing and it is during the process of exhalation that the spine can stretch and elongate without effort. We learn to elongate and extend rather than pull and push. Elongation and extension can only occur when the pulling and pushing have come to an end."[28] (n.b. Scaravelli is not referring in this context to the biomechanical term "extension", i.e. back-bending. Her work was devoted to a "feeling of extending" a natural sense of "elongation" of the spine that had nothing to do with stretching or forcing it by pulling on it. She sought to reveal the innate, effortless elasticity of our form. See Ch. 9.)

The spinal segments are the dominant feature of the "axial body". The larger part of the depth (front to back) of the torso is taken up with the spinal vertebrae, from the front of the vertebral bodies to the ends of the spinous and transverse processes. Their arrangement and the spaces (discs, foramen, etc.) between them authorise the shape of the body wall and deeply connect the myofascia, viscera and vessels, guarding the neural tenderness of the soft tissues. They invite us to recall the somites (and their echo in the dermatomes) from Chapter 4 (Fig. 8.9).

The body wall reflects the segmental rings first prescribed by the embryonic somites (they are organs of the body wall in our earliest stages of formation). They played an original part in creating these lateral rings – presented in the skin as dermatomes (see Fig. 8.9). (See Ch. 4, Fig. 4.16, for an illustration of the somites.) Their role in "spacialisation" of the spine designated the spaces between each of the vertebrae, where nerves exit from the spinal cord, discs organise and ribs and psoas (and all paraspinal myofascia) integrate. We are more familiar with these segments grouped as sections of the spine, i.e. tail (sacral), lower back (lumbar), upper back (thoracic or dorsal) and neck (cervical).

The spine does not make sense if it is described only in sections, as if the sections are separate or as if any section functions on its own, as it appears in the typical classroom skeleton. It forms one continuous structure, the larger proportion of the entire torso. Our sense of its wholeness in yoga, in postures and in meditation, seems to be exceptionally valuable once it has been seen so entirely connected in dissection.

How can we separate breathing from sensing and moving our innermost bones and outermost skin, communicating from the ground in any movement class, especially once we know that we are moving *one tissue* – one matrix, as a whole? Perhaps yoga luminary Vanda Scaravelli was right about how important our focus is on the strong, graceful wave of the "awakened, resilient, thinking spine" (my paraphrase). In practice, it shapes the breath and is shaped by it, continuously, *as a continuum – in relentless continuity.*

Now What?

Naming a muscle and classifying it is one thing. Finding out that muscles do not work as functional units is another. Understanding how a myofascial suite of tissues plays a role within a body-wide web (possibly uniquely for each participant) is yet another thing to consider. How is it possible to understand something whole and connected, something more fundamental than the naming of functions and labelling of parts, especially if that makes each part (i.e. muscle) restricted to specific actions, when they are not? I was left wondering what could actually make a difference to my classes and give the teachers and students I work with something that makes sense for them. (It has since become a course!)

A Fascialogical Context

With the fascial tissues in place, different questions arise. As we learn more about them, the need to shift how we see movement in an animated body is obvious.

Anatomists portray what they see, but they see it through the lens of a historical viewfinder that traditionally removes the fascia in order to see the parts "cleanly". Once removed it can't be put back. Removing the ubiquitous fascial matrix (and presenting the parts as if they work in function without it) misrepresents wholeness, however you look at it. Despite the common acceptance of its legitimacy as a dissection method, (i.e. clean dissection that ignores the fascia) in the face of whole function of the moving human architecture, it is simply inaccurate. Anatomy as traditionally presented may be an exquisite view of clean dissection; what is left behind after fascia is meticulously removed and placed in the cadaveric bins, but it is claimed to be something more. It is presented as being the best way to learn about how our parts work, biomechanically. It can even suggest functional efficiency in certain exercise techniques, as if we can isolate muscles in movement practice and improve ourselves by only moving or training individual parts. **There is no such thing in terms of function.** We organise different parts in different ways, but they all have a role – even if it is (dynamic) stillness. Biotensegrity, as the explanation for structure, applies in movement and stillness. The amplitude of a movement changes, but the ability to affect the whole body (be it inhibited from moving, poised in a particular position or kinaesthetically ignored) remains the only rule of body language; one singular tissue speaks it fluently, throughout the form. Our innate skill is to move *only* what we choose to. The rest is in dynamic, neuromuscular stillness. If everything is connected, then that is a very nuanced skillset that remains hidden in the ordinary unless we lose it.

Paradigm shifts can be uncomfortable, however enlightening they are. If we stay tuned to the yoga experience while we traverse the landscape in the rest of this book, though, we can expand to include new possibilities that account for what actually happens in class as we learn to move better. We recognise that we experience the body as whole and complete by virtue of moving it, *anyway*. These are new distinctions, but they make sense of our senses; our proprioceptive sense of where we are in space – and how we "know" that.

It may sound simplistic or even obvious, but in some ways seeing the united parts as one coherent whole clarifies everything. It takes us from the numerous different parts shown in the books towards the unified whole being that walks into the classroom. We breathe, move our own soft-tissue skeleton, embedded in and containing the fascial matrix. We sense where we are segmentally and globally as we do so, cavity by cavity, segmental wave by wave, microfilament to microfilament, all with breath, bones and dermatomes intact. That whole organisation, is our daily miracle; the one we learn with, transmit forces through, animate the language of and express uniquely through our own *biomotional intelligence* that we self-organise and animate. This is less about learning to find biomotional integrity, as it is about *revealing it as it is* and enhancing it as we can, on the moment-to-moment basis upon which we live in it; the architecture that we, as the architect, sustain biomotionally, to express ourselves *as the architect!*

Notes

1. John Sharkey, Centre for Anatomy and Human Identification, School of Life Sciences, University of Dundee, Scotland. Keynote at the Massage & Myotherapy Australia National Conference at the Gold Coast in June 2018. *Myotherapy Magazine* article: Summer 2017. '*Massage & Myotherapy Australia*' is a brand of the Australian Association of Massage Therapists Ltd. pp. 12–17

2. Wal JC van der (2009) The architecture of the connective tissue in the musculoskeletal system – an often overlooked functional parameter as to proprioception in the locomotor apparatus. *Int J Ther Massage Bodywork (IJTMB)* 2(4): 9–23.

3. John Sharkey (2019) Can medical education be enhanced by the world's first 3d printed fascia models and plastinated specimens of fascia superficialis and profundus? *Biomed J Sci & Tech Res* 15(4).

4. International Fascia Research Congresses 2007, 2009, 2012 and since can be found here: www.fasciacongress.org and Fascia Research Society: www. fasciaresearchsociety.org.

5. Robert Schleip, "Foreword", in Luigi Stecco and Carla Stecco, *Fascial Manipulation: Practical Part*, English edition by Julie Ann Day, foreword by Robert Schleip, Piccin, Padua, 2009.

6. H.M. Langevin (2006) Connective tissue: a body-wide signalling network? *Medical Hypotheses* 66(6):1074–1077.

7. Laboratory for Anatomical Enlightenment, Inc: https://lofae.com/about-us/

8. Ibid.

9. Thomas W. Myers, *Anatomy Trains: Myofascial Meridians for Manual and Movement Therapists*, 2nd edition, Churchill Livingstone, Edinburgh, 2009. Also note the DVD with this second edition as a resource.

10. The author would like to express her reverent gratitude to all donors and their families for the value of their donation.

11. Thomas W. Myers (1998) Myofascial meridians for manual and movement therapists. *Massage Magazine* 75:38–43. Or in Body³, published privately and available at www.anatomytrains.com.

12. Indra's Net Wikipedia (https://en.wikipedia.org/wiki/Indra%27s_net). Indra's net is a metaphor for the non-dual nature of all.

13. John Stirk, Osteopath and Yoga Teacher, comment during a training session, 2000. Author: *The Original Body*: https://www.handspringpublishing.com/product/original-body/

14. Etymology of the word: Originally Greek: **psoas (n.)** dates back to 1680s, from Greek *psoa* (plural *psoai*) meaning "muscles of the loins." - A feminine noun [*psoa*], was mistaken by the French anatomist Jean Riolan (1577–1657) for the "correct" form of a (nonexistent) masculine noun. It was he who introduced this erroneous form into anatomy. [Klein]

15. Indra's Net Wikipedia (https://en.wikipedia.org/wiki/Indra%27s_net). Indra's net is a metaphor for the non-dual nature of all.

16. Liz Koch, *Stalking Wild Psoas: Embodying Your Core Intelligence*, North Atlantic Books, Berkeley California, 2019.

17. See www.anatomytrains.com for DVD of this dissection programme.

18. For example, R. Louis Shultz and Rosemary Feitis, *The Endless Web: Fascial Anatomy and Physical Reality*, North Atlantic Books, Berkeley, CA, 1996.

19. The Bihar School of Yoga. The teachings of Swami Satanyanda.

20. Stanley Keleman, *Emotional Anatomy*, published in 1985 by Center Press. Stanley Keleman, director of Berkeley's Center for Energetic Studies.

21. Todd Garcia, Laboratory of Anatomical Enlightenment, Inc. (https://lofae.com/about-us/).

22. Dean Juhan, *Job's Body: Handbook for Bodywork*, 3rd edition, Station Hill Press, Barrytown, NY, 2003.

23. Vanda Scaravelli, *Awakening the Spine*, 2nd edition, Pinter and Martin, London, 2012.

24. Dr Chereminskiy is head of the Anatomy Department at the Gunther von Hagens Institute in Gueben, Germany. He also participated in the first presentation on Fascia at the IFAA in London, August 2019. (See Ch. 3.)

9

Curved is the New Straight

"The commonly accepted 'tower of blocks' model for vertebrate spine mechanics is only useful when modeling a perfectly balanced, upright, immobile spine. Using that model, in any other position than perfectly upright, the forces generated will tear muscle, crush bone and exhaust energy. A new model of the spine uses a tensegrity-truss system that will model the spine right side up, upside-down or in any position, static or dynamic. In a tensegrity-truss model, the loads distribute through the system only in tension or compression. As in all truss systems, there are no levers and no moments at the joints. The model behaves non-linearly and is energy efficient. Unlike a tower of blocks, it is independent of gravity and functions equally well on land, at sea, in the air or in space and models the spines of fish and fowl, bird and beast."[1]

Stephen Levin

As movement teachers we have to hit the ground running. People who sign up for a yoga class want you to join the dots at the speed they can move and understand the ways they can do it. They want those ways optimised, so what aspects of biomechanics do we need to learn in order to enhance and ensure this optimal practice? In the last chapter we considered that muscles do not, in fact, function as units, which changes how we might explain their role in any actions. There is still a difficult gap between classical biomechanical explanations of movement of our parts and the natural experience in the yoga classroom of how participants animate, in stillness or in sequences. Finding accurate distinctions is especially challenging when considering the fascial matrix as a tension–compression network under the biomotionally intelligent model of living tensegrity architectures. How can we bridge the difference between anatomy and architecture, classical and connected forms and "Cross the Rubicon",[2] from biomechanical to biomotional?

Moving Architecture

In standard biomechanics, the first thing a new student is invited to do is work from an imaginary axis, a central vertical line down the middle of the body that acts as a reference point for the planes: sagittal (lateral, median – *divides* the body into left and right sides), coronal (frontal – *divides the body into front and back*, or dorsal/ventral or anterior/posterior) and transverse (axial, horizontal – *divides the body into upper and lower* – superior/inferior, cranial/caudal). These planes separate movement into right/left and front/back and upper/lower (rotational motion) aspects, in order to describe human actions by reference to these planes and dimensions (Fig. 9.1).

However, we do not in reality have a straight line down the middle of us, and we do not move in straight lines or flat planes, nor does our body divide easily into symmetrical halves, in any dimension. We do not naturally stand in the anatomical position and our spines do not behave as vertical columns that have to be upright to function; let's agree with da Vinci that the spine is curved. It is a useful method to describe planes of motion. However, it becomes painfully difficult to make sense of yoga in these terms, even on paper, let alone at the speed of a classroom full of self-contained whole bodies in asymmetrical volumes, moving in *any* and all directions.

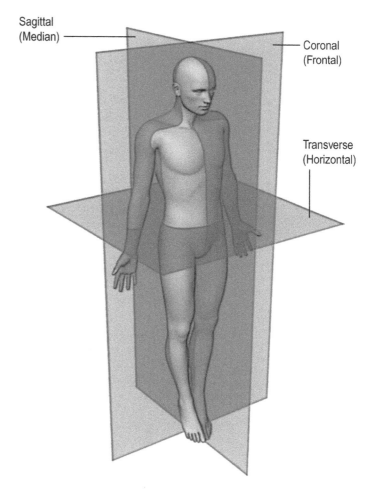

Figure 9.1

Body planes.

Image by Bex Hawkins. Reproduced with kind permission from Art of Contemporary Yoga Ltd.

It keeps us under the spell of the "straight spine". Does nature's propensity for working with roundnesses in volumes invite us to search for a more useful starting premise than this imaginary straight pole, divided into perfect quadrants on x, y and z axes? Ontogenetically (since conception), we challenge this from the relentlessly curved performances of the embryo. From an evolutionary viewpoint, there are more clues to suggest that curves are fundamental to healthy motion. According to Serge Gracovetsky, Stephen Levin, John Sharkey, Jaap van der Wal and others (see the notes and suggestions for further reading at the end of this chapter) it shapes our shape and fundamental movement patterns profoundly, which calls for explanations that make more sense of them. It is accepted as a language of convenience, if we remember that is *all it is*.

Contemporary Questions for Classical Assumptions

The Spine as an Engine; the Story Behind a New View

Into this inquisitive gap between the classical theories and contemporary interpretations walked Serge Gracovetsky PhD, to present at the first Fascia Research Congress in 2007, at Harvard Medical School, Boston, Massachusetts.[3,4]

Gracovetsky emphasises that the human form is entirely designed for agility, not for rigidity (as if the spine was stacked, as denoted by the term "column"). His spinal engine theory (see also notes and further reading) is like water in the overheated arguments of a dry biomechanical desert. It is complex; however, it breaks many spells by showing logically how the whole spine moves in all its various segments and natural curvatures. It is dependent upon the intimate relationships between muscles and the collagen matrix in which they reside, to transmit forces (between the head and the earth, via the rotation of the shoulder girdle and the counter-rotation of the pelvic girdle and through the feet), to and from the ground. That is, via the gears (locking facets) of the *essentially curved* and *essentially rotational capacity* of the human spine and its *appropriate* motions. He points at the complexity in the detail that is reduced to an axis, if we underestimate the spine's authority in motion.

According to Gracovetsky, when we bend forward or lift an object, for example, the spine naturally switches back and forth within fractions of a second between tension and inhibition (see Appendix B). That is the tensional strength of the collagen and the active contraction/inhibition of appropriate neuro-muscular responses. That is at specific frequencies for the load/interaction at the time. This is, effectively, a fast reaction between tension and compression forces, *through the motion* and *architecture* and *morphology* of the *curved* spine. Rotation and counter-rotation drive the spinal engine, based upon its *curved structural* design and "neuro-myo-osseo-fascial" (my phrase) organisation. It responds rapidly to tension/compression signals of motion through its myofascial–collagen network. Standard biomechanical suggestion that the torso is carried along by the legs as a sort of passenger, stacked upon the pelvis, is properly challenged (see further reading). Gracovetsky suggests that the spine comes first; the limbs come after as an *advantage* to energy management and conservation, *refining* our basic spinal movement signature rather than dominating or dissecting it. (Which is compelling, since it recapitulates our embryonic sequence of self-assembly – see Ch. 4.)

It is not a common event to see a standing ovation at a scientific research congress. Nevertheless, Gracovetsky made so much sense of what we experience in the real living spine, founded in fundamental laws of motion and the geometry of the collagen matrix, that the audience celebrated his candid and highly researched reasoning with cheers. He pointed out that because there was an assumption that movement was based upon the musculoskeletal system, measuring devices were developed over the centuries that based calculations almost exclusively on examining muscular action. This reinforced the musculoskeletal bias of classical anatomy and subsequent theories of function that largely ignore the integrated nature of the fascia. Thus, any living (in vivo) testing perpetuated the assumptions and allowed science to bypass the crucial role of the collagen matrix in movement; *it wasn't considered, let alone measured.* Traditionally, the fascia was overlooked both anatomically and biomechanically, at least in terms of its ubiquitous continuity – certainly in terms of its sensory signaling and force transmission roles. It was simply left out of most of the equations. That is turning out to be a crucial omission.

Recently, advances in equipment and methods of investigation, particularly more sensitive ultrasound and MRI devices,[5] have allowed the reading of fascial structures in vivo to endorse the essential role of collagen everywhere in the body, including the spine. Science has also begun to ask different questions, hence this paradigm shift and the advent of a whole new level of curiosity and enquiry. Biotensegrity features heavily in many of the emerging models, since it fundamentally explains volumes, round things and curvatures that are self-assembled into whole adaptable, shape-changing creatures.

"The wide range of human physical activities obscures the relative simplicity of the physics behind movement. From the moment the legendary fish emerged from the water and landed on solid ground, the development of anatomy was shaped by the need to conserve energy. In this context, the Earth's gravitational field became another natural resource that our species learned to exploit."[6]

In the gravitational field on earth creatures move around as a constant management system (or physical interpretation) of ground reaction force.

"GRF simply means that the ground is pushing back to whatever is pushing down on it. (Newton's 3rd law, for every action there is an equal and opposite reaction; if you push on a wall the wall is pushing back equally.) If someone is walking or running, F=ma (Force = mass x acceleration; Newton's 2nd law), so the GRF would be greater."[7]

Serge Gracovetsky explains it another useful way, to emphasise further how completely we rely on this force in all interactions on the earth: using the legs to translate the energy we store temporarily with every step. We take it so completely for granted, we are not even aware of it as a distinct balance of forces that account for our homeostasis; the self-containment of being here – standing or sitting on a mat – is already an achievement!!

"To understand the concept, first note that you are not in a free fall, even if your body is subjected to the earth's gravitational field. This happens because the ground under your feet opposes a force equal to the weight of your body and hence your feet are in equilibrium. If something happened to the ground (a sink hole that would open up) then your body would fall towards the center of the earth."

Serge Gracovetsky

The hummingbird, we learned, cannot maintain its ability to beat its wings at a rate of approximately 100 beats per second based on classical theories of muscular energy production. The mathematics (upon which biomechanics are generally calculated) of the energy required means the hummingbird would generate so much heat it would burst into flames. On a similar basis, Olympic weightlifters raising anything over 50 kg would routinely explode if they really were relying on "intra-abdominal pressure" as the basis of their power to lift, due to the forces involved, were they *really* to be relying on this functionally. Gracovetsky debunks what he calls the "myths and fairy tales of musculoskeletal anatomy". *He challenges the standard theories of biomechanical force transmission, based on levers moved by muscles at joints that* don't necessarily stand up to mathematical scrutiny, however long they have been believed.

Since the first edition of this book, I understand from Dr Stephen Levin that Gracovetsky espouses biotensegrity as a founding explanation for his theory.

Collagen, he explains, plays a "fundamental role" in spinning (elastic recoil – see Ch. 10) a hummingbird's wings, shaping and moving the spine, whether or not it has been understood or accurately accounted for. Importantly he emphasises natural spinal curvature, in upright posture as an asset of *"biomotional integration"* (my phrase). Gracovetsky walks us scientifically towards a fuller appreciation of *curved* motion mechanics (if they can be called that), challenging some basic, long-held classical assumptions.

The ground reaction forces are nothing more than the "equaliser forces" to gravity, keeping you in balance (*allostasis*) during your everyday life.

"When you walk, the ground must oppose a force to your foot (precisely and exactly equal to your mass) and that is what is called the 'heel strike pulse'."

Serge Gracovetsky

At the conference, the idea that "intra-abdominal pressure" sufficient to weight-lift 50 kg would cause the weightlifter to explode, was hilarious – and Gracovetsky has done the math! He wryly recommended that personal trainers make sure they get paid before their clients lift anything, just in case such classical myths are accurate!

When you sleep, your body shape is imprinted into the mattress because the mattress is soft and crumpled when the ground reaction forces push UP into your body.

In real terms, we animate different ways of expressing this relentless dependence on the mutual relationship between gravity and its counterforce (ground reaction force; GRF[8]). We can dance "lightly" or stamp "heavily" depending upon how we animate our tissues, moment to moment, so the experience of it can change – due to the *internal forces*. The GRF remains the same, but we can actively modify how the forces move *through* our connected tissues. We can tension and compress their connections elastically; using the ground (constantly), as a temporary energy store. We can move over it, as if it was a trampoline or a treadmill, using our own bodies as the elastic recoil mechanism (see Ch. 10, The Elastic Body).

If the ground is covered in snow or sand, as distinct from being a dense, hard, flat road for example, then the way in which our tissues respond changes accordingly. We then have to react and organise *internal forces* to account for that difference in "heel strike pulse" (i.e. energy return). Our experience then, might be less of a "bounce back" and we need to adapt and generate more (*myofascial effort* and *metabolic*) energy to move over that softer terrain, when its particles are not so dense or close packed: which means they don't *return* the energy of the heel strike pulse as rapidly or directly. *There is less resistance to deformation* (see Ch. 10). We naturally navigate this all the time, consciously or not. Your body *already* knows how to do this instinctively. It lives in a mutual balance between gravity's radial pull towards the centre of the earth and (any creature's) ability to occupy space in response *from* it, i.e. in direct response or reaction from the ground (thus the term *ground reaction force*).

Our bones (which Levin refers to as "starched fascia"[9,10]) are originally formed *as a result of* the day-to-day management of forces, of our reaction to the ground (and the balanced, mutual pull, or pressure, of gravity towards it). We exist as three-dimensional form in relationship to this force-and-counter-force balance. We are not crushed; we are able to stand up and move around, away from the ground. We don't float off it, either; we can spring off, however we are literally and symbolically *bound to return*.

We could say this innate ability is a unifying of triune forces. In a tension–compression system we have three elements: (1) tension, (2) compression and (3) combined tension–compression, which is a *whole* volumetric material, expressed in a certain pattern, as a certain organisation of tension and compression forces. (The way they are combined, i.e. the pattern, matters.) We also have three elements of gravity and ground reaction force: (1) gravity, (2) GRF, and (3) their combination, which shows up **as our structural integrity** – the result of their combined forces as our physical *expression* of wholeness. Your ability to move around as a living volume, is an expression of how you interpret gravity and ground reaction force through your physical structure at any one moment in time; in your body's own language at the time. Essentially, your ability to stand still, given that muscles only contract,[11,12] is an asset of a healthy nervous system that can *inhibit that contraction appropriately* at a given point in time and any given point in your myofascial home (aka your body architecture). Homeostasis, or allostasis, is not just about movement; it is the ability to stabilise at will, given our innate mobility and motility and the environment we move it around in (and the muscles' innate predisposition to contraction). It is dynamic balance, rather than default prejudice.

The ground interrupts the relentless pull towards the centre of the earth all the time. Our human ability to resist this pull affects and expresses the health of our whole system, so much so that we do not even have to think about it. We are already its consequences in space and time. We rely on these mutual forces for our structural integrity. We do this instinctively, whether or not we understand them intellectually.

From an evolutionary point of view, we have acquired the ability to manage ground reaction force (perhaps what Scaravelli[13] refers to, in yoga, as our "anti-gravity reflex") in ever more refined ways. Newton is credited with discovering the distinction of gravity but, according to Levin, there are different interpretations for the way that biologic soft architectures move, independently of that gravitational pull. It may be also a question of how literally we translate Newton's laws. An equal and opposite force is at work in living tensegrity structures (tension and compression) at all times. However, they resist deformation naturally in omnidirectional ways (in yet another equal and opposite system of force transmission, expressed as gravity and ground reaction force). Studies of how our tissues *really* respond to stress and strain suggest they do so in non-Hookean (i.e. non-linear) ways.

"This [tensegrity structural behaviour, measured in a stress-strain graph] is radically different from the Hookean, linear behavior of most non-biologic materials and structures. In Hookean structures for each increment of stress, there is a proportional strain until the point of elastic deformation, just before it breaks. Hookean structures weaken under load. In the tensegrity structures, there is rapid deformation with the initial load but then the structure [responds and] stiffens and becomes more rigid and stronger."[14] *[n.b. it is self-regulating]*

Levin details how tensegrity structures explain our omnidirectional strength and ability to resist deformation. This challenges the "spring and dashpot" model as somewhat contrived and suggests something actually more direct for the way we explain structure, given how we naturally move and respond *as living tensegrity volumes*.

Evolutionary
Movement
Requirements

According to Gracovetsky, our spines originated (evolutionarily) in creatures that had to be able to move over slippery mud when they emerged from the sea and had to adapt accordingly, to evolve. The side-to-side (lateral) motion of fish was not so efficient over land (Figs 9.2A and 9.3B).

The forward and back motion (flexion and extension) had to develop from an evolutionary point of view, if the animal body was to move over rocky terrain and eventually find upright motion.

To do this, these two planes of motion gave rise to the helical motion potential (see Fig. 9.2B) that could exploit the gravitational field, rather than be defeated by it. This was rotation and counter-rotation between the shoulder and pelvic girdles (the key drivers of the spinal engine[15]). This occurred in concert with the developing appropriate curvature of the spine and the

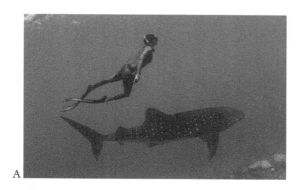
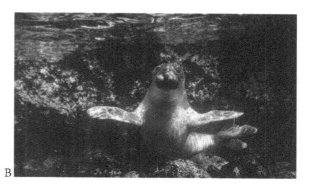

Figure 9.2AB

(A) Human motion. This freediver (Michèle Monico) naturally moves in a human motion pattern (flexion extension based) compared to a shark, which relies on a lateral motion pattern. (B) Here the elephant seal shows exactly how the "Law of Coupled Motion" works: extension and lateral flexion, giving rise to rotation.

Photographs by William Winram © Freediver Michèle Monico *blessed with the company of a beautiful Whale shark (Rhincodon typus)* Reproduced with kind permission from William Winram©

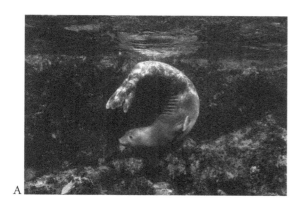
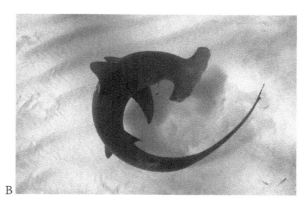

Figure 9.3AB

This elephant seal (A) can arch its back in a mammalian full extension pattern, whereas the hammerhead shark (B) relies upon only lateral flexion for its movement range, to propel itself forward.

Reproduced with kind permission from William Winram ©.

evolutionary development of the limbs and extremities on land. The evolving gait patterns produced an integrated whole-body movement capacity greater than a contrived lever-based mechanism that fits the sum of the parts together (as in building Pinocchio).

Spine First

"Locomotion was first achieved by the motion of the spine. The legs came after as an improvement, not as a substitute."[10]

Many theories of upright two-legged (bipedal) human movement suggest the legs authorise or initiate gait and the torso, or axial body, "travels along as a passenger" (to quote Gracovetsky). As he points out, from an evolutionary point of view (that recapitulates the embryonic forming sequence), the legs developed as an asset for living on land. Lower limbs are among the later structures to grow, some embryological time after the spinal structures are in place and after the arms (upper limbs).

Gracovetsky debunks the theory that the lower limbs drive gait by asking what happens if there are none. Would that mean the spine does not work (or "walk")? He filmed and monitored (with sensors along the spine) a man without *any* limbs, who could nevertheless move along the ground in a natural walking gait-pattern. Gracovetsky analysed the torso movements, which match those of a person with legs to walk on and arms to swing. Any theory of walking that presumes initiation in the legs is challenged by this research. (In close-up video footage of the spine it was impossible to detect that the person walking had no arms or legs and in fact walked directly on their sitting bones (ischial tuberosities), rotating and counter-rotating the torso to move over the ground.)

Gracovetsky shows that in human walking, the lumbar curve of the spine is paramount in the translation of forces to and from the ground, via the legs. Rather than a passive passenger, carried along by them, it is the *author* of gait. According to Gracovetsky, the spine drives the limbs from above, which allows the legs to translate the *amplitude* and *quality*, or *resonance* of the movement forces to and from the ground using it step by step as a temporary energy store (via the heel strike pulse). As yoga teachers, we are well served by understanding this organisation and Gracovetsky provides cogent reasons why it is an advantage to keep the body supple and mobile, to naturally translate energy as efficiently as possible (his work is referenced throughout the notes and in the further reading suggestions at the end of this chapter).[16]

The spinal engine theory is in fact congruent with Levin's tensegrity-truss model and Flemons' tensegrity models (see Ch. 10, Fig. 10.6); if you remember, they are modeling force transmission, not body parts. As closed kinematic chain[17] models, they naturally evoke the law of coupled motion (see later in this chapter). It begins to make sense of our ability in the yoga classroom to balance on hands and head, shoulders and elbows at various angles of poise in all but flat planes and the anatomical position. The spine becomes the common denominator: rotation and counter-rotation work both ways up. We could say that lying in Corpse Pose (Shivasana) resembles the anatomical position. However, even then, we can use that pose to experience and sense our natural curvature on the ground, using it for feedback directly (see Ch. 11 for a specific exercise). We do not experience ourselves as flat to the mat; nor would we want to.

This exercise makes sense of Gracovetsky's view suggesting that the spine acts, albeit upright, in the same way as the spine in any sea mammal, with the limbs adding balance and ballast and further facility, rather than necessarily driving or originating the movement pattern (although they can orchestrate movements in a seamless integration). A bird's spine also has to navigate the different forces transmitted through flying and walking; once again, we discover that biotensegrity offers a model that binds on land or in the air or sea.

"Lordosis [lumbar curve] emerges as the single most important parameter in controlling the force transmission between the legs and the upper extremities."[18]

Gracovetsky shows that the limbs help to translate forces, driven by the spine, to and from the ground, refining them to the most appropriate amplitude, or shape, for the spine to receive and respond energetically, to the forces transmitted through it.

Exercise: Sitting in Staff Pose (Dandasana), it is possible to fold the arms, slightly bend and stiffen the legs and "walk" up and down the mat on the sitting bones, sliding the legs along the mat (bend the knees and lightly place the heels on the mat). It reveals the natural rotational reflex through the spine to make these motions. After "walking" up and down the mat on sitting bones, try it on the knees and then in standing with the additional "lift" of the legs. It seems to immediately facilitate a lightness of step and quality of elastic momentum. There is a change in amplitude but not in the fundamental ability to make the movements. It can be experienced as the same rotational pattern at different frequencies through the body, depending upon how close the spine is to the ground.

Primary and Secondary Curves

The curves of the spine (Fig. 9.4 and seen in Fig 9.2A) can be considered, as has been pointed out, from both an evolutionary (*phylogenetic*) and a developmental (*ontogenetic*) point of view. The reason the spinal curves are named primary and secondary is that the primary curves are formed before we are born (in utero) and the secondary curves develop over time, later (ex utero), through movement patterns and their force transmission, becoming a pattern in the soft tissues.[19]

One or Two Legs?

Levin goes further to suggest we are designed for *unipedal*, rather than *bipedal* posture. Once we learn to stand on two legs, we frequently use them one at a time. Indeed, in walking we spend up to 80% of our movement on one leg and in sprinting, the body travels through the air and is invariably on only one leg or the other. We even tend to favour standing on one leg rather than two. (Ask your students which is their favourite standing leg – most people prefer one as a default pattern.) We can certainly afford to explore this idea with some enthusiasm, given the most basic list of yogic asanas that develop exactly that aspect of balance and physical literacy, training us to do postures to each side and bring the same level of ability and agility and balance to both.

Animating our Curves in Three Dimensions

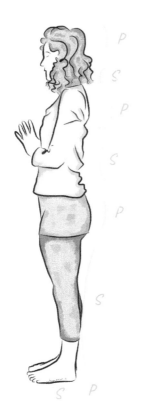

Figure 9.4

We can actually consider the back of the body as a sequence of curves; considered to be primary (formed in utero) and secondary (formed ex utero) that form as we develop. The front of the body is a continuum of this principle, if you consider we are formed in the round. (see Fig 9.2A)

Curved Poles

Gracovetsky shows that various laws of movement are animated by the fundamental design of a curved spine. His research makes sense of our yoga practice by acknowledging whole spinal performance. In walking, running, dancing and even sitting, we actually use the whole body, as we breathe. Gracovetsky emphasises the value of a curved/counter-curved central axis, rather than the primary curve structure such as our primate cousins embody. He embellishes the purpose of the primary and secondary curves. We have the natural ability to rotate, counter-rotate, side, forward and back bend. (We can do a lot more besides, incorporating subtle movements and spirals, in between these main classifications that are not so easy to label in classical biomechanical terminology; see Ch. 18.) The spinal engine theory clearly makes sense of the natural design of our structural relationships to the ground. We will explore this through practice in Part C (Chapters 14 & 15).

Very soon after birth, the forward-folded form of the curled ball (primary curve) of a healthy newborn (neonate) will attempt to lift its relatively large and heavy head (pressing down on mother's shoulder to push up, for example) and naturally begin to activate (through instinctive usage patterns) a curve at the neck (extension). This is the first of the two secondary curves of the spinal "S", crucial to our ability to spring and to the spine's ability to rotate and counter-rotate once we begin to fulfil our soft-tissue, architectural promise.

Lumbar lordosis, the secondary curve at the back of the waist, is formed after the secondary curve at the neck. It is prescribed as the baby learns to push and lift up from the ground and to twist.

Animated by natural curiosity, a baby uses rotational movements and side bends, as well as forward bending and back bending, to roll over, lift its head (and eventually chest) off the surface it is resting on. It mimics the evolutionary patterns describing our emergence from the sea, perhaps unsurprisingly! Ultimately it strengthens its back enough to raise head and torso, curving the spine back (secondary) as well as forward (primary). This takes months, sometimes years, to fully elaborate to the point of standing. To fulfil the potential of balance on two legs rather than four (commonly termed *upright bipedal posture*) and walk (refining *unipedal* balance) takes time, and the human pelvis develops gradually over the first six years of growth in response to these efforts and their cumulative loading patterns. The pelvis is a cartilaginous ring in the neonate and slowly but surely stiffens and hardens into bones as a direct result of force-transmission, animating the required minerals to be laid down as denser material, i.e. bone, as the baby becomes a toddler and eventually runs around as a child. The forming of the pelvic ring (as bone) is the result of forces transmitted through the form.

What if we start from an imaginary curved pole through the middle of the body instead of a straight one? *The laws of movement governing curved poles are very different from straight poles.* Furthermore, the biotensegrity model challenges entirely the notion of levers, which apply to linear structures. A standard lever, such as classically described for the movement at the elbow, for example, is represented as a "2-bar open chain mechanism" (Fig. 9.5). This

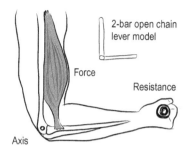

2-bar open chain
lever model

Force

Resistance

Axis

Figure 9.5

A lever is an open two-bar chain, shown here as a model for the arm (notably excluding other joints and structures), where the Triceps and Biceps muscles act over the upper limb bones to form a lever between them.

One of the not uncommon misunderstandings presented in movement research is the distinction of hopping. Some animals "hop" on two (hind) legs. Human beings hop on one leg. The same word means different things depending on the species it is applied to. When we walk, although the transition is seamless, the balance is unipedal. If we learn to sprint, we effectively animate a series of powerful (one-legged) hops, in joined up kinaesthetic writing, at increasing speed. Rabbits (and Kangaroos) hop using both their *hind legs* as one. In running, animals are also unipedal, even if they look

refers simply to the fact that there are two bars (the upper and lower arm) and one pin (the elbow) representing a (pinned) hinge joint. There are none in healthy bodies.

Living tensegrity architecture explains how forces move through the form of a living structure, joined together as one global architecture – like us. We are seeking explanations for *what we can actually do in a yoga classroom*, which far exceeds the limitations and range of lever mechanisms. We do not move in straight lines with levered joints, which don't exist anywhere in the body, however popular the term has been in the last four centuries of literature. In Jaap van der Wal's tissue-sparing dissection of the elbow, there was no angle at which the entire joint architecture was *not* under tension. This expands the context to a new explanation that can be found in "closed kinematic chains"[20,21] (see margin note and Fig. 9.6).

From the ground up, closed kinematic chain structures [**closed** (*because the body functions as a closed, enclosed system*) **kinematic** (*geometry of motion*) **chain** (*interlinked*) **structures** (variations on the connective tissue theme)] give rise to multidirectional and unpredictable motion patterns that describe what happens on a yoga mat, in more variety and detail than many classical theories can account for. In considering some of them, the reader is invited to explore from experience and read further (see suggestions for further reading at the end of this chapter). In Part C, we will consider these questions applied to adjustment in yoga specifically. They change the viewpoint considerably, from classical to connected biologic forms.

As human beings, we might organise from a "centrifugal sense", or a "centripetal" sense; however, there is no straight vertical axis for the body in its physical experience; we do not self-assemble as a compression-based architecture. The spine is curved. Our "null point" of embryonic development (see Ch. 4) forms ideally into a changing, continuous S-shape (just as Leonardo da Vinci first drew it (see Ch. 2). We can use it as an upright *reference* but that is a balancing act in itself. We can say we "straighten it"; however, its default design is a series of beautiful curves that allow us all the privileges of helical motion. (See Ch. 14, A Simple Practice, where we consider this in practice.)

"Developing a deeper appreciation and understanding of the helical nature of human anatomy through dissection is now further supported by modern day imaging techniques including ultrasound, MRI, and tensor magnetic resonance linking morphology and function to the true nature of our structure. New imaging techniques allow us to see what is not always possible to visualize immediately with the naked eye. We know bacteria exist however we cannot see them with the naked eyes. The same can be said for the most delicate of fascial laminas visible only (initially) by modern day imaging technology. Understanding fascial planes leads to less invasive medical and surgical clinical procedures. This results in faster recovery and retained functionality. With appropriate knowledge of fascia, the Yoga teacher can also play an important role in pre and post-operative care of patients ensuring a return to normal functionality and pain free movement"[22]

as if they are stamping from front to back legs. If you watch a cheetah (or a horse) running in slow-motion capture, you will see that each leg touches the ground in sequence, one-at-a-time. So, too, the rabbit's forepaws meet the ground one-at-a-time – does that mean they are really tri-pedal?

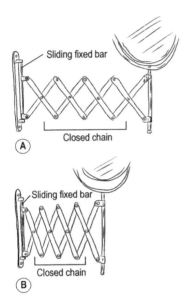

Figure 9.6

This is a four-bar linkage system with a fixed bar (where it is attached). It can squeeze together and open out (given its sliding hinge at the fixed bar) and remains in a closed kinematic chain. The "levers" are all joined up to form an enclosed linkage system that, in this symmetrical example, has the properties of a lattice. In a steam engine, the bars have different lengths, as they do in biologic systems.

Why Levers Give Way to Lattices

People are made up of three-dimensional shapes occupying space in roundish forms (tube-shaped volumes, essentially). We are tubes within tubes, folded to form various architectural origamis that are mostly able to change and modify, within a range, in a balance of motion, internal motility and poise. We are constantly interpreting (from "inter" meaning "between" and "translate" – *translate between*) internal and external forces in graceful balance, *all the time*. The geometries of living tensegrity architectures and the adaptable fabric of the fascia are the common denominators of all these forms. Notions of biomechanics dependent on flat planes, straight lines and exact symmetries (or spinal stacks) were originally deduced, at least in part, from dead bodies that were moved by the anatomist, rather than on observation of (or the technical ability to measure) living forms that animate themselves. The difference between the two conditions is vast, however established the linear, right-angle theories are of hard-matter forms. Recognising this changes completely the basis upon which we teach and read motion patterns. Once the spell is broken, we can wake up and cross the Rubicon towards new distinctions.

We have to actively *stabilise*, establish, release and *re-stabilise* ourselves from moment to moment (as anyone holding a yoga pose, for even seconds, experiences). It is an integral part of our movement skills; so how can we make sense of that architecturally? We become deeply interested in spiral balance and elastic recoil. In Chapter 10 we will look deeper into elasticity and make sense of this as our experience as a pre-stressed, non-linear, biologic system that changes itself (as a whole) from one moment to the next, just by breathing, just by being alive. It harnesses a new and valuable logic for the contemporary yoga teacher, to guide adjustment and honour natural, animated movement.[23]

From classical, quantitative theories of motion, levers were devised as an explanation for how we move, joint by joint. In the absence of connective tissue, a lever (a two-bar open chain linkage) answers the question of a muscle moving a bone at a joint, like a hinge, in one plane – in a very simple mechanism. This would give rise to the classical theory of antagonistic pairs of muscles to balance and counterbalance the lever. (It also *appears* to satisfy Newton's third law that to every action there is an equal and opposite reaction.) But we now know we do not (ever) move one muscle at a time (or even just two, one on either side of a joint) and we do not move one joint at a time either. This is a "local" reductionist view (of a mechanical lever-arm puppet-like construction) and it is a struggle to make sense of it in describing the natural context of global biomotion, in the living, soft tissue, human body.

In Figure 9.7B, for example, the model is doing a typical squat. What is actually happening here is a co-contraction of muscles (if you stop at the local forces) in which the following is taking place:

"When sitting, our rectus femoris, the largest of the quadriceps muscle group, is hypothetically in a shortened phase as the hip is in a flexion phase. Rectus femoris runs over the anterior aspect of the flexed knee enveloping the patella and associating with the tibial tuberosity by means of the patellar

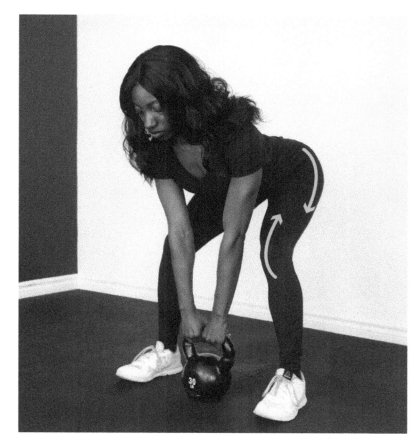

Figure 9.7A

This classic dead-lift involves a co-contraction of both Quadriceps and Hamstring muscles (see text) that challenges the lever theory; no muscles are relaxed in either leg.

Image adapted by Bex Hawkins, with grateful thanks to Unsplash/Sergio Pedemonte.

ligament. It is, therefore, hypothetically lengthened at the knee when sitting but shortened at the hip. Meanwhile the hamstrings are lengthened at the hip and shortened at the posterior knee. When we move from sitting to standing our hip must extend and our knee must also extend. Rectus femoris therefore hypothetically elongates at the hip and shortens at the knee. John Cleland MD was Professor of Anatomy and Physiology at Queen's College, Galway, in Ireland from 1863 until 1879. It is interesting to read Dr Cleland's amazing paper entitled 'On the actions of muscles passing over more than one joint', in which he wrote ' ....I have made the measurements of the distance from the superior to the inferior attachment of the gastrocnemius muscle, when both knee and ankle were completely flexed, and when they were both completely extended, and have found that the distance remains unchanged. If we sink upon bended knees, flexing the limbs completely and remaining balanced on the toes then to rise to our full height on tiptoe, the length of the gastrocnemius remains unchanged in the movement'. From the biotensegrity-anatomy of the 21st century viewpoint these are classical examples of how tissues neither lengthen nor shorten but rather shape change throughout range of motion similar to prismatic architected materials changing shape and reconfiguring their morphology without any individual part becoming shorter, longer, wider or narrower. This calls into question the idea of 'agonist' and 'antagonist' from the classical neurological description (i.e. when an agonist contracts its antagonist relaxes)."[24]

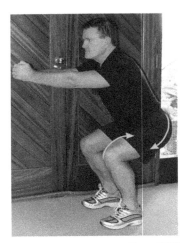

Figure 9.7B

The tensegrity model is not trying to "be" a body. It is a model. The issue the protagonists have with classical biomechanics is that we forget a classroom skeleton is a model of *how the bones would arrange, if the connective tissue was still in place.* Quite how we allow ourselves to pretend that the absence of that tissue can be ignored, should raise alarms at every level of anatomy training. Tensegrity models do not pretend to represent connective tissue or bones *per se* - rather the manner in which they self-organise, via optimum force transmission. It offers a model of resistance to elastic deformation (see Ch. 10).

In a Tensegrity model, the "lines" of both the compression struts and the tensional strings represent *lines of force transmission in the living structure*, not lines of form. It is possible to make extremely complex models that more closely re-iterate the forces moving via the paths of least resistance to *dissipate* through the form, than actually pretending to *be the form*. A typical tensegrity model (the T-icosa - see Figs 10.6 and 10.7) isn't a muscle and bone model. It is a model of tension and compression **forces** inside a closed-kinematic chain system, one that constantly changes in our bodies, depending upon which movements we are making, where the loads are and how they can be optimally distributed. It demonstrates how we bounce back, running across a field (or jumping on a trampoline, or hurdling) or doing a Vinyasa Flow sequence on a mat. We don't succumb to the laws of plastic deformation or deform, like a fluid substance that takes the shape of its container. We retain our natural elastic *reformation* by moving about with ease, adapting moment-to-moment. Just like the tensegrity model, that bounces back (see Ch. 10, The Elastic Body).

Perhaps one reason it is so complicated to learn about levers and human "bending moments" and classical biomechanical explanations of movements is because levers do not represent what actually happens in moving humans. After all, these theories were deduced when the omnipresent and ubiquitous fascia was routinely discarded by anatomists. Deduction was made in the absence of the connectivity and continuity of force transmission we rely upon *to move*. We incorporate more intelligent means of leverage; as we have noted repeatedly, **there are no levers in biologic forms**.[25]

The key thing is that in the living body, unified, the webs form various types of lattices, or weaves, or helical envelopes or fractal polygons between structures, *on every scale*. Their range of motion or scope and type depend on where they are in our form and how they are used. That is "in the round". However you describe them, "straight they ain't" in the body. We cut and straighten the fascia out into flat pieces to examine it or look for straight connections to make diagrams of them, but that does not lend them linear mechanical properties *as forms*. It may even mislead us, as the samples are no longer connected and continuously enclosed, such as they would be inside the body. How do we account for that coherence?

Closed-Chain Kinematics

Everything in the body is enclosed and linked together by that which encloses it (fascia). Thus the "chains" of moving parts, if we call them such, are also continuously connected. If the chain is "closed", then the bars cannot be levers, by definition. They become what is called a four-bar (or multi-bar) linkage system, which happens to be the minimum to represent our movement. (Three-bar mechanisms are fixed – see margin note.)

The structure becomes self-contained and the control mechanism changes completely (in that the lever explanation becomes redundant). In a closed system, the control at one end is reiterated throughout the structure. In his article "The Scapula is a Sesamoid Bone",[26] Dr Levin suggests that the control of the arm and hand comes from the spine, via the shoulder blade (scapula), to the fingers. Thus, it can authorise the integrated movement and subtle coordination we appreciate, based on a model such as the four-bar or multi-bar linkage[27] system. If the hand and fingers were in a line or sequence of levers, the *least* control would exist at the distal end. We enter a much more sophisticated realm of geometry, congruent with our biotensegrity architecture, the one we share with all other living biological forms. It suggests the possibility of the kind of dexterity and variety we can enjoy; we have the *most* dexterity in our fingers and toes. It is something that makes sense of the postures, the way we do them.

Something magical begins to happen to the geometry of a structure at four bars (or more) in a closed linkage system. They acquire a shift in stability and enter a state of potential mobility at different angles and position, at higher frequency (see margin note for a simple explanation). The slightest movement is communicated throughout and affects the whole connected structure *because it is linked* structurally, everywhere.

Theo Jansen's structures[28] are made out of multi-bar chain mechanisms that are driven to ambulate with no batteries or motors, just the wind or the shape of the landscape. They help to demonstrate that forms (albeit sculptures) suitably connected as one closed system (animated by *external* forces) move in multi-bar linkages of a closed kinematic chain sequence. That is but one of our many resources. Neither Jansen's sculptures, nor our bodies, rely upon levers for motion. They don't have the subtlety of motion we enjoy, through our sensory, soft tissue, fluidic architecture – however they do demonstrate the essence of CKC motion and why it is an essential upgrade in sophistication over levers. The levers are invariably *part of* multiple closed linkages – not open two-bar chains, as if they could exist separately-but-tied-together to move a limb – they are never open at both ends. That makes no sense at all, when you appreciate that the image of an elbow, for example, is cut out from the approximately seven "levers-in-continuity" of the upper limb, from breast-bone to finger tips. "Joined-up levers" don't work the way we do – you cannot simply cut one out from the continuity it exists as (i.e. an entire limb) and then describe it as something it isn't! (Even if that has been done for 400 years, it doesn't mean it is accurate.) All bars in the body are closed chain mechanisms.

There is integrity of form and movement: any change is communicated and transmitted kinematically (i.e. through the geometry of the structure). Even when it is squeezed, the structure "closes" but it does not reduce to a straight bar or a lever. *It multiplies up to a lattice*. At the very least number of

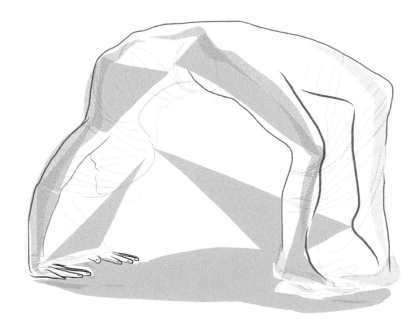

Figure 9.8

Through our yoga eyes, we see the whole movement, integrated via the fixed bar of the ground. It is seen in its entirety as a multi-bar linkage. The system is compliant and self-motivated – a closed kinematic chain.

What is a closed kinematic chain? Kinematic refers to the geometry of a structure, independent of the kinetic forces acting upon it. A closed chain means each link is attached at both ends. A lattice is an example of a closed kinematic chain, where every movement moves the parts, as a whole. The minimum number of bars in a closed kinematic chain is four. (Three bars give you a rigid triangle, that is

dimensions (two) it is a woven fabric. If, as Kenneth Snelson[29] suggests, weaving is the mother of tensegrity, then a pathway of enquiry from a woven lattice (the fascial matrix) to a four- to multi-bar system (of architectural design) seems worthy of some careful research. In other words, when the fabric is connected to itself, it forms a tube, in 3D. When the tube moves through itself, it forms a toroidal pattern, that is considered to be 4D (see Chapter 10, Figs 10.1–10.4). It models the spinal disc pattern and many other aspects of the human structure.

A multi-bar structure such as a Hoberman's Sphere (Fig. 9.8) can "expand" and "in-draw" without losing its structural integrity (see Fig. 9.6) or inter-relationships. Five-bar systems have one fixed bar, from which the rest of the closed chain can be animated in a coordinated, intercommunicating way. Whatever movement occurs, despite the different amplitudes, the whole structure is part of the organisation *at all times*. That is what is so, on a yoga mat! (Or any other movement!)

If the bars in a closed kinematic chain have different lengths, they can modify the available shapes, movements, range and overall organisation that is expressible by the structure, in response to forces around or through it (see Jansen's models on the beach – further reading). However, they still remain intimately interdependent and related. With ball and socket joints added to the variety of frictionless hinges (like our joints, which van der Wal refers to as "*disjoints in the continuum*"), the arcs and ellipses they can describe become three-dimensional under control of the organising motor. If the spine is the central "motor" or "engine", as Gracovetsky suggests, then control of the limbs a stable structure.) We are essentially unstable structures that actively self-stabilise. This too makes sense of our yoga. The work is not so much to be able to do a handstand, or one-legged posture, but to hold it there. A multi-bar closed-chain structure has one fixed bar, from which it moves the rest. (See the shaving mirror in Fig. 9.6, for example.) Consider the ground as our "fixed bar", changing every time we place ourselves upon it, depending on which part we place and where. Basically, we take the ground with us, wherever we move; *it is our fixed bar*.

can express the kind of patterns and shapes we *see when we move them the way we actually do* (which is never in a flat plane with a single pin at the joint, holding two bars together. It just isn't possible in a living organism – it is literally the wrong engineering terminology for round, living things that are invariably *volumes*).

When you consider the different shapes we make and balances we manage in a yoga class, the spine tells a much more mobile, multi-directional and intelligent story than a straight or stacked segmented pole can begin to account for. Our central "midline" is a "mid-wave" through a curved tube that allows us to do what we do on the mat, with all our helical movements and deep twisting and binding postures to account for; *as we breathe*.

We see three essential features of our movement patterns arising in a multi-bar closed-chain linkage:

- The structure is self-contained, enclosed and variable within the range of the one whole organisation.
- One "motor" can drive the whole shape economically. Nothing is redundant or separated from the whole form.
- Everything affects everything else in a self-regulating architecture, based on its innate shape and the coordinating angles and rod lengths of the closed chain.

"Biological linkages frequently are compliant. Often one or more bars are formed by ligaments, and often the linkages are three-dimensional. Couple linkage systems are known, as well as five, six and even seven-bar linkages. Four-bar linkages are by far the most common though."[30]

In biology, many creatures favour a closed kinematic chain structural arrangement based on four-bar linkage, such as the jaw dynamics of many fish. D'Arcy Wentworth Thompson[31] showed this as the basis of variation in species, in his work *On Growth and Form*.[32]

A perfect and obvious example (one of many) in our bodies is the knee joint, which attaches the upper leg bone (femur) to the lower leg bone (tibia) by the cruciate ligaments. These are referred to as an X-bar arrangement.[33] (See Figs 10.1–10.4 in Chapter 10, The Elastic Body.)

A linkage designed as a network, such as our body matrix, models a closed kinematic chain. As referred to earlier, one bar in such a system is fixed; from this the closed chain can move as a whole. Our fixed bar is the ground. We ourselves are not fixed. We are indeed compliant, but we can change our whole arrangement from moment to moment by incorporating the ground differently as we move (see Fig. 9.8). Effectively, we take the ground with us wherever we go on earth, using it under and between the parts of us on its surface, as we need to at the time. As Gracovetsky suggests, we exploit gravity to our energetic advantage.

Dynamic and Whole

Wherever we are and whatever poses we are in, we form a closed linkage system **including the ground as one of the bars**: i.e. the *temporary fixed* one. The simple recognition of our curved structures begins to account for how we might see whole movement (as it is performed) and recognise that (1) we are closed chains and (2) there are no levers in our non-linear biologic systems.

The dynamic arrangements of bones, myofascial continuities and dynaments (Jaap van der Wal's term for dynamic ligaments) form webs, linkages and cross-links throughout our tissues. Lattices are literally everywhere. Obviously, they are all joined up; as we are. Human biomechanics are far more sophisticated than levers, although we can include lever-like movements. We incorporate many more options in our three-dimensional compliance, naturally integrating fascia throughout our form, joining (in complete and relentless continuity) every joint in our limbs and spines. The closed kinematic chain might begin to redefine what we generally consider functional movement in the classical sense.

Intrinsically Biphasic Movements

Moving one part always influences another part. Figure 9.9 is taken as a moment in time and space. In the joined-up moment-by-moment sequence of their living performance these shapes incorporate "biphasic movement". This is a feature of the body as a tensional matrix, in a closed chain. Each movement automatically triggers a corresponding bar. Two useful examples of this can be offered: the first is a bicycle wheel, the second is the children's toy known as a Jacob's ladder.

This is a key to safe practice and appropriate adjustment.

As teachers, it is important for us to understand this, particularly in the context of adjustment. If we are moving someone's limb as if it were a lever when it is poised and active, we might be unaware of the impact on the "joined-up" nature of the whole form. Change one part and you are inevitably provoking a countermove elsewhere in the chain. If you work from a view that reduces living form to a two-dimensional diagram or if you treat one part as if it is only related via the next joint, you can disturb balance rather than confirm it. Effectively, if you touch one part, you are affecting all of it mechanically, if we recognise this model. Once we consider the fascial network as a subtle and sensitive body-wide, architectural system, it is seen as even more sophisticated.

A bicycle wheel (minimum 12 spokes) is a tensegrity[34] structure in the round. The hub and the rim are the compression members, while the spokes provide the tensioning members. Imagine if the whole wheel is twisted (it resembles a Möbius strip). As soon as you attempt to untwist it, it goes past the mid-point and twists the other way. It naturally counter-twists; you cannot stop it with your hands, because that is how closed-chain mechanisms work. This is an example of biphasic motion; we might consider the pelvis as a ring that holds its volumes under such laws as this.

Move into the squat position, then stand up into Mountain Pose (Tadasana). Then repeat. Any move of any part of the leg, from a standing position, causes

In a Jacob's ladder toy, if you hold it under tensional balance, every movement countermoves the next block. The parts are organised by the ribbons as a closed kinematic chain (see Fig. 9.9 A&B). There is a particular balancing point, on the other side of which the whole structure click-clacks its way naturally through a series of moves and countermoves *biphasically*. The structural organisation automatically responds by changing the dynamics of the whole structure, because they are all linked as a *closed chain*. You only hold the "engine" of the movement (under tension); or you could say, you offer the compression counterforce that is transmitted through the whole in reaction.

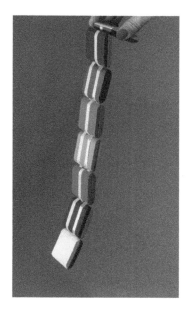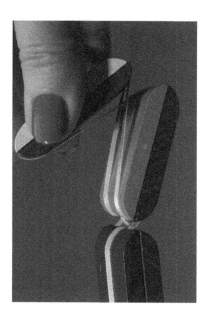

Figure 9.9

Jacob's ladder toy, showing poised tensional balance before the biphasic movements "click clack" through the length of the chain.

a corresponding move in the next segment (see Fig. 9.7 – of Squat). You cannot bend the knee without the hip and/or ankle bending too. It is the basis of our design, i.e. *biphasic movement in a closed kinematic chain*. That chain includes the ground under and between the feet as the fixed bar.

These are technical descriptions of joined-up movements we naturally master, in yoga sequences and in everyday life. Just by walking, climbing stairs, sitting down or standing up we activate these principles of functional movement. Try moving your forearm without moving any aspect of your wrist, hand or upper arm, or your lower leg without affecting the ankle, foot or upper leg. They are part of a closed chain and it is not possible.

Multi-bar Movement in the Round

The ball in Figure 9.10 represents the kinematics of our biotensegrity architecture as we see and experience it. There is no need to imagine a vertical line in the body. This happens as a curved, containing, contained, three-dimensional structure, actively occupying three-dimensional mobility and moving in time, still frame after still frame in close transition, whole and complete throughout, as a scale-free model where cell, lung, bladder and body perform under the same physical spherical and helical rules of biological volumes. It is much more sophisticated than levers (open chain mechanisms) can describe. The sum of the parts behaves very differently when it is united into one whole enclosed system (as a closed chain) inside a tensioned "skin pocket". We seem to include various types of link (joining or folding patterns) to enable range at each so-called "bar" in our systems but our movements (particularly in the yoga classroom) are clearly not restricted to balancing levers and sticks in purely horizontal and vertical flat planes, or lines.

Gliding Motion

Gliding motion is worth emphasising here as a fundamental tenet of our structure and its fascial integrity. The ability to glide between the textures of the fascial compartments and between the forms is crucial to our movement functions everywhere in the body: at the joints (so that they are frictionless), between the skin (superficial fascia) and muscles (deep fascia) and around the organs (so that we can move around without compromising them). The same ability allows the vessels *within* us to move *with* us. The serous fluid around the lungs, for example, is fundamentally designed for frictionless glide at every breath, contained by the visceral fascial laminae and containers. Where are the levers in the lungs? The idea that they can be described as separate functional systems to movement is difficult to make sense of.

A Universal Pattern

The pattern of a lattice is another kind of four-bar system. The lattice is a universal pattern throughout the body, a basis of fascial tubing. It forms around vessels, muscles and muscle fibres (Fig. 9.11).[35] The layered tunicae of the blood vessels, for example, spiral around each other and these overlapping spiraling tubes, in cross-section, form a lattice arrangement (Fig. 9.12).[22]

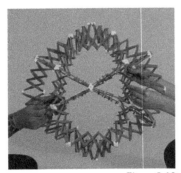

Figure 9.10

This multi-bar linkage ball expands and contracts kinematically as a closed chain. It represents the linked system of breathing motion as a possibility for a biotensegrity architecture.

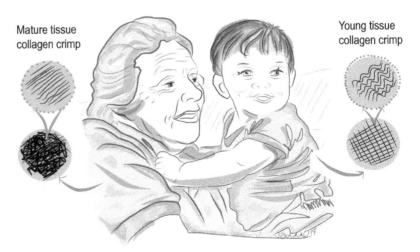

Mature tissue collagen crimp

Young tissue collagen crimp

Figure 9.11

In young mobile tissue, the folds and depths of fascia appear to be laid down in alternating directions, with a crimp feature. Ageing or sedentary tissues can show a more matted configuration. There really are no straight lines in the body matrix.

The geometry of these patterns is the same on every scale and common throughout biologic forms. Chirality in trees, for example, is a part of the repertoire for tree merchants and the industry concerned with forestry. Tree growth rings are known to occur in counter-chiral patterns,[36] although it is not known whether they are genetically determined or based upon environmental responses through the growth period of a specific tree. It is known, however, that if a log cabin is made from a tree that does not counter-chiral its growth rings (to grow straight), it will appear straight at first but twist when it dries out.[37]

Multi-bar Mobility

What all this information adds up to is a complex, self-contained organism designed for mobility via the ground, as we use it. It affects both ends of a given limb, as a feedback system under constant tension–compression forces, wrapped in the bodysuit of our skin.

Thinking about the variety of yoga postures, and of the body parts we place on the ground to do them, from head to toes, draws us towards a very compelling explanation of whole body movements. The common denominator becomes the ground and responsive-spine relationship, via the girdles and the limbs, however we choose to use them, seen as a whole organising shape, including the head (if not initiated by it). According to Leonid Blyum: "…actually I should say this statement more emphatically – head control is not simply important for walking and so on – head control is the single most important factor, the absolutely necessary condition and pre-requisite of ANY controlled locomotion where a human body is in the contact with the ground!"[38]

We have the "motioning" ability to change which angle we move in and which parts of us create the "joint" with the fixed bar (the ground), given the various lengths of the bars (i.e. the bones of our limbs and torso) and the curvature of the whole spine (Fig. 9.13).

This suggests our relationship to the ground is as profound and responsive as many a yoga guru would have us believe. Certainly, the yoga matriarch Vanda Scaravelli,[39] for example, attributes integrated movement to exactly that relationship, of breath and spinal wave, responding to the earth. Whatever shape we are making, if we include the ground in the wholeness of the posture, we begin to see how we use it constantly and even unconsciously.

When you next do yoga or watch a class, observe each pose as if it is part of a multi-bar chain. Include the changing invisible "joint" at the ground and notice how the whole system moves every bar in the "chain" from (and including) the "ground bar" or "ground print" (see Ch. 17). It could be the heels, but equally it might be the toes, the heels of the hands, the sitting bones, the elbows, and so on, depending upon the pose.

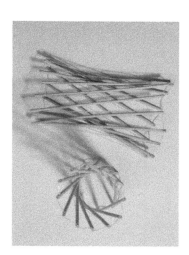

Figure 9.12

This model was made by Graham Scarr using tensegrity principles; the arrangement shows a spiral structure (see Fig. 6.21). Note that the pattern of spiral and counter-spiral in cross-section is a lattice. This structure holds itself open.

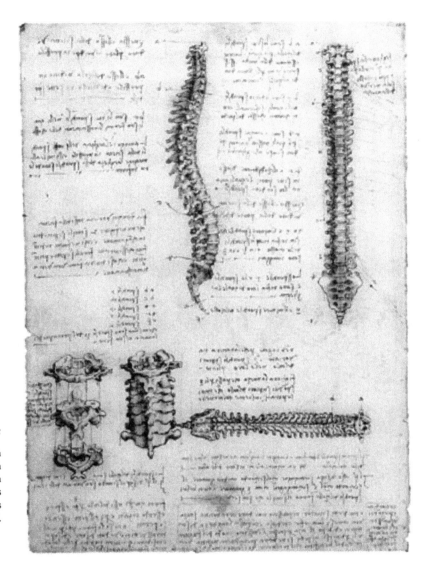

Figure 9.13

The S-shape of the spine in this sketch by Leonardo da Vinci arises even on a classroom model from the design and shape of the interlocking spaces between the vertebrae that the somites originally prescribed.

Finding Stillness

"In many postures, the adult human spine does not function as a column or even a simple beam. When the spine is horizontal, the sacrum is not a base of a column but the connecting element that ties the beam to the pelvic ring."[40]

Do closed kinematic chains and spinal engines begin to invite us into realms of biomechanics that make sense of yoga? If biotensegrity architectures account for whole, multidimensional structures such as we appear to be in

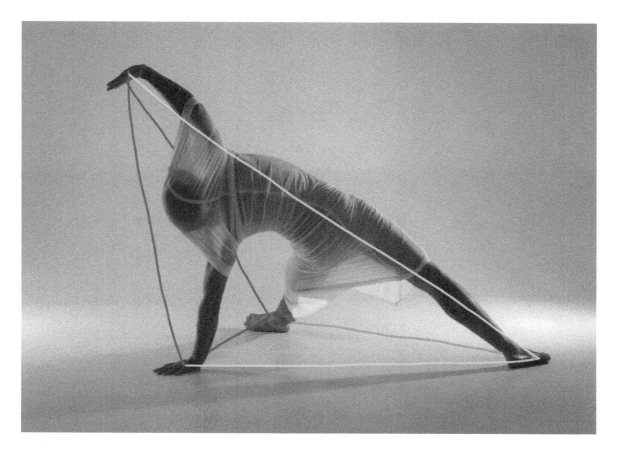

Figure 9.14

The geometry of form – recognising the whole posture in space, as a multi-bar linkage system using the ground, can be worked with any pose, as a way of seeing the whole. This was a moment in time, captured as part of a sequence throughout which Wibbs experienced and expressed balance. (At no time was his spine like an upright or straight pole.) This image is a moment of suspended animation, showing the body in a three-point wheel pose (Chakrasana). This posture can be shown as part of a multi-bar linkage system from toes to hand, where Wibbs is naturally balancing and counterbalancing the movements. The sleeve provides a visual metaphor for the balancing of forces within the tension–compression architecture of his body structure; balancing itself.

Reproduced with kind permission from the Art of Contemporary Yoga Ltd. Model Wibbs Coulson. Photographer Amy Very.

every yoga classroom, does it draw us towards more holistic explanations of how we interpret this (and any other) movement art?

We begin to see a picture emerging that is worthy of further exploration. While Table 9.1 compares the difference between the classical and contemporary models, it is worth noting that the contemporary one represents a paradox. In a way it goes full circle to the ancient knowledge of the Vedic sages (see

Table 9.1

Classical model	Contemporary model
Parts (cogs – bio-mechanical)	Whole (re-cog-nise – bio-motional)
Compression	Biotensegrity (tension–compression)
2D diagrams (duality)	3D holograms (triunity)
Two-bar levers and pendulums	Four-bar and multi-bar linkages
Open chain mechanisms	Closed kinematic chains
Divided down into planes	Multiplied up into containers
Linear biomechanical systems	Non-linear biologic systems

Ch. 12) and can be found in the drawings of the Sacred Geometry studied by philosophers and architects referred to in Chapter 2. Perhaps we are exploring a unifying process beyond the limits of dualistic thinking, the rebirth of what yoga actually stands for and a return to a deeper understanding of ancient wisdom.

Further Reading

The spinal engine theory put forward by Serge Gracovetsky, PhD, is explained and illustrated in very accessible form in Erik Dalton's book *The Dynamic Body* (Erik Dalton, *The Dynamic Body*, Freedom from Pain Institute, Oklahoma, 2011; http://erikdalton.com/). Gracovetsky originally published his theory in 1987 and updated it in 2008. See also Appendices 6 and 7 of his 2010 publication *Non-Invasive Assessment Of Spinal Function Automatizing The Physical Examination: An Application Of The Theory Of The Spinal Engine*. Appendix Six discusses the concept of stability, an issue of importance for the determination of best posture, including the role of the sacroiliac joint. Appendix Seven explores the importance of the coupled motion of the spine and its application to sports medicine. The book is available from the author (gracovetsky@videotron.ca); from Amazon; or from the publisher (www.lulu.com). Space does not permit reproduction of any of it here but it is well worth further research by the reader. See also https://sites.google.com/site/gracovetsky/home for details of other publications by Serge Gracovetsky.

Stephen M. Levin's website (www.biotensegrity.com) contains various articles examining the logic of closed kinematic chains and how our bodies elaborate this model.

Graham Scarr's website (www.tensegrityinbiology.co.uk) is full of highly informative articles and illustrations. It also includes models of the geometry behind the forms, referred to as Geodesic Geometry: see *Biotensegrity - The Structural Basis of Life*, Handspring Publishing, Edinburgh, 2014.

Theo Jansen is from Holland. In 1990, he began building large mechanisms based on closed kinematic chain principles, made out of PVC (and more recently 3D printed on a smaller scale) that are able to move on their own propelled by the wind, or the shape of the land. They are called (collectively) Strandbeest. They are kinetic sculptures that appear to "walk". The original designs are hand built on a large scale by the Dutch artist, based on closed kinematic chain movement principles. www.strandbeest.com. Smaller ones have been made in 3D printing.

See also papers referenced below in specific links, in the text.

Notes

1. Stephen Levin, http://www.biotensegrity.com/resources/tensegrity-truss-spine.pdf: "The Tensegrity-truss as a Model for Spine Mechanics".
2. This is a phrase used powerfully by one of my mentors, Caroline Myss, PhD. It actually comes from the era in which Julius Caesar defied orders and "crossed the (river) Rubicon" back into Rome, to form what became the Roman Empire. The word Rubicon comes from the same root as "ruby" referring to the red soil of the region. Needless to say it is a symbolic reference to a huge sea-change in motif and motivation.
3. http://www.fasciacongress.org/2007/. Serge Gracovetsky, Fascia Congress Part #1 of 3, Boston 2009.wmv. Available on You Tube (with parts #2 of 3 and #3 of 3).
4. Serge Gracovetsky (1997) Linking the spinal engine with the legs: a theory of human gait. *Movement, Stability and Low Back Pain - The Essential Role of the Pelvis*.
5. Stephen Levin (2008) Human resting muscle tone (HRMT): narrative, introduction and modern concepts. *Journal of Bodywork and Movement Therapies* 12:320–332.
6. Serge Gracovetsky: his presentation on the spinal engine theory given in Brighton, England, in September 2011.
7. See Chapter 6 for detailed explanation of *ground reaction force*, equal to the body's mass.
8. Ibid.
9. See Appendix A, *Bone is Fascia* by Stephen Levin.

10. John Sharkey (2019) Regarding: Update on fascial nomenclature-an additional proposal by John Sharkey MSc, Clinical Anatomist. *Journal of Bodywork & Movement Therapies* 23(1):6–8.

11. Chris Jarmey and John Sharkey, *The Concise Book of Muscles*, Third Edition. "Biotensegrity – Biomechanics for the 21st Century", J. Sharkey and Stephen Levin, p. 50

12. A.T.Masi, J. Hannon (2008) Human resting muscle tone (HRMT): Narrative introduction and modern concepts. *Journal of Bodywork & Movement Therapies* 12(4), 320–332.

13. Vanda Scaravelli, *Awakening the Spine*, 2nd Edition, Piner and Martin, London, 2011.

14. Stephen Levin: www.biotensegrity.com

15. Serge Gracovetsky; see suggestions for further reading. See also https://sites.google.com/site/gracovetsky/home.

16. Ibid.

17. Stephen Levin, et al (2017) The significance of closed kinematic chains to biological movement and dynamic stability. *Journal of Bodywork & Movement Therapies* 21(3):664–672.

18. Serge Gracovetsky's spinal engine theory; see suggestions for further reading, below, and https://sites.google.com/site/gracovetsky/home.

19. Leonid Blyum (www.abrtherapy.com/team-member/leonid-blyum/) refers to the secondary parts of the upright "S" as "super curves" rather than demoting them to the term "secondary". Since they give rise to a much greater range and articulacy of movement, it honours the advantage the spinal engine theory elaborates. Rather than suggesting they are less important, or secondary, this elevates the curvature at the neck and waist to the assets it bestows on our range, elasticity and natural style of motion.

20. Graham Scarr, www.tensegrityinbiology.co.uk, article: "Geodesic". See also: *Biotensegrity: The Structural Basis of Life*, Handspring Publishing Ltd., Pencaitland, 2014.

21. Stephen Levin, et al (2017) The significance of closed kinematic chains to biological movement and dynamic stability. *Journal of Bodywork & Movement Therapies* 21(3):664–672.

22. John Sharkey (2018) Biotensegrity-Anatomy for the 21st Century Informing Yoga and Physiotherapy Concerning New Findings in Fascia Research. *J Yoga & Physio* 6(1):555680.

23. Karen Kirkness, MFA, MSc, *Spiral Bound: Integrated Anatomy for Yoga*. Handspring Publishing Ltd, Pencaitland. In press – due 2021.

24. Centre for Anatomy and Human Identification, School of Life Sciences, University of Dundee, Scotland. John Sharkey Keynote Speech at the Massage & Myotherapy Australia National Conference at the Gold Coast in June 2018. Excerpt from: *Massage & Myotherapy Australia* (Summer 2017), "Myths and realities: The only word? The last word? Musings and 'biotensegrity-informed' opinions from Clinical Anatomist John Sharkey MSc (BACA) concerning human anatomy and physiology."

25. Stephen Levin, personal communication, 2013.

26. Stephen Levin (2005) "The scapula is a sesamoid bone": www.biotensegrity.com. Letter to the Editor, published in the *Journal of Biomechanics* 38(8):1733–1734.

27. D'Arcy Wentworth Thompson, *On Growth and Form*. Cambridge, Cambridge University Press, 1961.

28. See Further Reading for links and website

29. Kenneth Snelson, http://kennethsnelson.net/.

30. Wikipedia, Biological Linkages, Linkage (mechanical).

31. Sir D'Arcy Wentworth Thompson CB FRS FRSE was a Scottish biologist, mathematician and classics scholar 1860–1948, Education: University of Dundee, Trinity College, The University of Edinburgh, University of Cambridge.

32. D'Arcy Wentworth Thompson, *On Growth and Form*. Cambridge, Cambridge University Press, 1961.

33. X-bar linkage reference in N. Farhat, V. Mata, D. Rosa and J. Fayos (2010) A procedure for estimating the relevant forces in the human knee using a four-bar mechanism. *Computer Methods in Biomechanics and Biomedical Engineering* 13(5):577–587.

34. *The Ease of Motion*. pp. 77–79.

35. R. Schleip, W. Klingler and F. Lehmann-Horn, "Active Contraction of the Thoracolumbar Fascia: Indications of a New Factor in Low Back Pain Research with Implications for Manual Therapy". In: A. Vleeming, V. Mooney and P. Hodges (eds), *The Proceedings of the Fifth Interdisciplinary World Congress on Low Back and Pelvic Pain, Melbourne, 2004*. T.A.H. Järvinen, T.L.N. Järvinen, P. Kannus, L. Józsa and M. Järvinen (2004) Collagen fibres of the spontaneously ruptured human tendons display decreased thickness and crimp angle. *Journal of Orthopaedic Research* 22(6):1303–1309.

36. Jian-Shan Wang, Gang Wang, Xi-Qiao Feng, Takayuki Kitamura, Yi-Lan Kang, Shou-Wen Yu and Qing-Hua Qin (2013) Hierarchical chirality transfer in the growth of Towel Gourd tendrils. *Scientific Reports* 3:3102.

37. Hans Kubler (1991) Function of spiral grain in trees. *Trees* 5:125–135.

38. Leonid Blyum (www.abrtherapy.com/team-member/leonid-blyum/) is the director of Advanced Biomechanical Rehabilitation (ABR). His extensive work and research in the practical application of biomechanical principles is richly documented through clinical experience and an advanced education in mathematics. He translates complex models into practical applications for practitioners and parents of children where rehabilitation is required and in the rehabilitation of complex syndromes where biomechanical function is impaired.

39. Vanda Scaravelli, *Awakening the Spine*, 2nd edition, Pinter and Martin, London, 2012.

40. Stephen Levin, http://www.biotensegrity.com/resources/tensegrity-truss-spine.pdf: "The Tensegrity-truss as a Model for Spine Mechanics".

10

The Elastic Body

"...First discovered by studies of the calf tissues of kangaroos, antelopes and later of horses, modern ultrasound studies have revealed that fascial recoil plays in fact a similarly impressive role in many of our human movements. How far you can throw a stone, how high you can jump, how long you can run, depends not only the contraction of your muscle fibres; it also depends to a large degree on how well the elastic recoil properties of your fascial network are supporting these movements."[1]

Robert Schleip

Since the first edition of this book, I have enjoyed the privilege of working with John Sharkey[3] and joining faculty at the private college run in Dublin, Ireland; the original centre for European Neuromuscular Therapy. I learned a new word from him, that he in turn attributes to Michael Shea,[4] with whom he studied embryology. The word is "quiescence" – a beautiful way of describing stillness, when the innate elasticity of the body is recognised as an asset of multidimensional awareness, co-ordination and biomotional integrity. Gratefully noted.

Everyone has a motion pattern that we could call their movement signature. In the yoga classroom, it is tempting to think that good form matters more when we are *in a pose*, officially "doing yoga". The real test or value might be in what we can *accumulate* to improve our posture when we are doing the transitions between poses and beyond, to times when we are not doing yoga, or even just standing still in a balanced way.[2] It is still a unique movement signature, but can we sign it with vitality and a flourish, or do we struggle to find relative ease and balance in ordinary, everyday movements, before we get to the yoga classroom? How comfortably do we relax in our own skin? Understanding fascial architecture opens a new context for fostering the Elastic Body, explaining biomotional integrity and the asset of free energy afforded by appropriate elasticity. That brings with it something we might refer to as "equipoise". It's an asset in the quiet moments, as well as the vigorous ones! It lives alongside *comfortable resting tension* – a term that indicates ease of motion for the Elastic Body. Let us consider what this means, how important it is and that some of the interpretations of this language might contribute to how it is fostered optimally in practice.

Body-writing in Our Own Hand

Every movement signature is a personal hallmark. In yoga classrooms, the general celebrity qualities seem to be flexibility and stretching. Those with naturally bendy bodies can get top marks while the stiff people, who feel they cannot reach, twist and contort with ease, are often considered "not as good" as their naturally flexible companions. "I'm too stiff to touch my toes" is not an uncommon response from people explaining why they think they are *unable* to do yoga.

One of the difficulties in discussing the Elastic Body, is that the word "elasticity" is sometimes considered to be synonymous with bendy, stretchy, flexibility – along with the ability to fold ourselves in half and stretch our joints and tissues sufficiently to wrap our legs around our necks (think Sleeping Yogi Pose – *yoganidrasana*). There is, however, a much more valuable and powerful distinction available, once we appreciate the myofascial, living tensegrity body and its pre-stiffened structure (see Ch. 6) in the context of wholeness. Elasticity really refers to our overall *energy storage capacity*. Once that is understood – and there are a lot of misconceptions around it that we will explore – we have an immeasurably valuable resource for vitality. It is, metabolically, our *free* energy store. It really implies something more like innate or natural "recoil", that invites the ability to move lightly in a self-contained way, on or off the mat. It may or may not have anything to do with being able to reach certain extremes of postures as if that is a worthy goal, for all body types. Although stretching, like elasticity, can be prioritised in the yoga story, it actually invites a multitude of meanings and misunderstandings. In fact, to honour the Elastic Body, stretching could be *exactly the opposite* of what an already super-bendy or hypermobile body needs in order to develop or improve their innate *elastic recoil capacity*. Stretching, when we consider the body as a whole, closed, kinematic-chain mechanism,[5] and learn from our animal friends, might need new definitions. It may even be the last thing we want to do. (See Appendix B.)

STRETCHING closed, kinematic chain patterns. Stretching seems to be one of the most variously described definitions in body work and movement therapy.[6] First however, if we realise that we are non-linear (and what that really means), we can understand that we might over-apply the term semantically (see Appendix B). Somatically, when we use force to go beyond our natural elastic limits, stretching can have a *detrimental* effect. Here are some images of a closed chain pattern to help make sense of this visually. (See example in Figs 10.1–10.4 below.)

Here is a simple lattice (closed chain) arrangement, as a sheet (i.e. area – 2D) representing some of the lattice-like structures of the fascia (see Ch. 6 for detail) showing cross-helical fibres.[7] When we join that lattice to appreciate it *as a tube*, it is still exactly the same size as the original sheet, just forming one *tubular* arrangement (Fig. 10.2). (That brings us from area to volume: 3D.)

When we "stretch" the tube, the *dimensions* of the tubing material *do not change*. We simply "shape-change" the way the whole tube is organised, *everywhere*. (In the body, tubes do not have seams or joins; they are continuous. See Fig. 10.3.)

The hardest part is seeing this in even more continuity, because inside the body, the tubes are continuous. There is no "top end" or base as such (as in the image). Any tubular structure of our tissues, on every scale, is virtually entirely enclosed and even folded in on itself (*invaginated*); see Fig. 10.4.

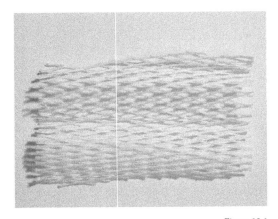

Figure 10.1

Lattice in the flat: 2D, triangular
organisation of the weave.

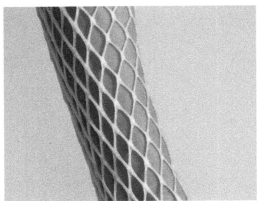

Figure 10.2

Lattice in the round: as a volumetric 3D tubing
of the 2D weave.

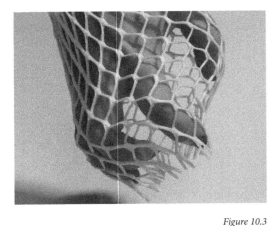

Figure 10.3

Lattice being stretched, or *shape-changed*, as a 3D
volume of a 2D weave

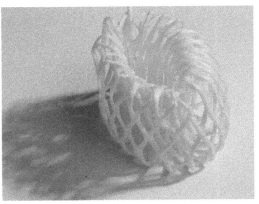

Figure 10.4

Lattice invaginated, which is "moved through itself" from
a 3D volume of a 2D weave and offers new 4D properties,
recapitulating embryonic forming patterns (see Ch. 4).

In this image the tube has been folded in on itself and formed a toroidal shape that resists deformation even more efficiently – because it is *stiffer* and *denser*. This is creating *suitable stiffness* by forming a multi-lamina, tubular ring inside (and out of) a tube. It is technically a 4D version of the original 2D sheet, that has been connected and "moved through itself" using exactly the folding principles by which the embryo self-assembles (you already did that to become you). This stiffer model (made from the original material, but organised architecturally to have higher *energy storage capacity*) has higher *elasticity* than the single lamina tube, that yields more easily.

That, essentially, is how fascia works in the tubular pockets and pouches of the matrix, be it the tunicae of the blood vessels or the wrapping of muscle fibre or the dura of the nerves, or the fascial wrappings around the nerves, given their relative depths and organisations in the body. When we focus only on stretching and flexibility, the difficulty might be (for a given fascia profile, see Ch. 17) in animating *appropriate stiffness* to bring tissue integrity and natural resting tension into elastic body balance. If the tissues do not have sufficient stiffness, they will fold rather than support. This matters in pursuit of Elastic Body integrity.

Flexibility? It Depends

We can all intuitively read movement signatures. It is part of recognising a friend walking towards you by their rhythm and pattern, gait and style of gesture. As yoga teachers we foster this aspect of our proprioceptive awareness in body reading and assessment (see practical section, Part C, Ch. 17 for examples). Identifying elasticity, once we distinguish its true definition, is an extremely valuable teaching tool and part of an important "kinaesthetic dictionary" to build and refer to, in action.

In order to foster *structural integrity*, "stretching" (in certain meanings) can of course be valuable (see later for different definitions) but useful practice is by no means limited to (or defined by) it. Elastic *integrity* is the asset – not necessarily bendiness, however popular it is in the yoga classroom! It may not be useful to everyone if "stretching" takes us beyond our *own* tissue limits, if one person's "stretch" is another person's "tear" or *disorganisation*. For some people, focus on flexibility can actually compromise their natural elastic body balance, particularly if they are naturally (or too) flexible anyway. Elasticity is a feature of fascia in terms of its innate recoil properties[8] and our resting architecture, our natural *personal posture profile* (see Ch. 17). Because of the way we are organised, as living tensegrities, the body benefits from the value of elasticity, in dynamic stillness, just as much sitting on a meditation cushion, as it does when springing through an Ashtanga series. **This is a crucial point in understanding the elasticity of the living tensegrity architecture of the fascial system.**

"Human resting muscle (myofascial) tone (HRMT) is the passive tonus or tension of skeletal muscle that derives from its intrinsic (EMG-silent) molecular viscoelastic properties. The word tone has been used to convey varying clinical and physiological features that have led to confusion and controversy. HRMT is the vital low-level, passive tension, and resistance to stretch that contributes importantly to maintain postural stability in balanced equilibrium positions. In contrast, co-contraction of muscle is an active neuromotor control that provides greater levels of tonus for increased stabilization.

Functionally, HRMT is integrated with other passive fascial and ligamentous tensional networks of the body to form a biotensegrity system. This review aims to achieve better understandings of HRMT and its functional roles."[9]

Even at rest, a muscle is a pre-tensioned part of the *tension–compression properties* of *all* the tissues, whether or not it is participating in a specific, measurable action.[10,11] When we are sitting in meditation, for example, muscles would be "EMG-silent" but they are still actively contracting; that is all they can do. This is one of a number of ways measuring systems have affected how we attribute movement to specific muscle units; but we don't move "in units"[12] (see Ch. 8) and muscles are active, just by holding us up, in shape *as a volume.* John Sharkey, Exercise Physiologist and Clinical Anatomist, points out another cogent reason why the way we measure "muscle activity" may influence our understanding of this complex issue:

"There is always a level of tension within the myofascial (or neuromuscular) system. Unfortunately, scientific endeavours investigating muscle tone seldom, if ever, take bone into consideration. [Living] Bones are malleable, bending and rotating. Concerning bones, this point is crucial as the very points researchers are using to calculate the contractile elements and the elastic (i.e. tendinous) element would obviously move. Points of reference, in this regard, would not be ideal for such measurements and any conclusions derived would fall short of the true reality. There are no resting muscles in living human anatomy and physiology."[13]

Tension, stiffness and strain deserve to be presented, free of their negative connotations, as values on a graph or scale of physical attributes that, switched on appropriately at the time, allow us to fine-tune and foster overall *elastic*

What Does Elasticity Mean?

integrity. It is essentially the spring in our step and the ability to contain our tissues in close-packed organisation and precision, such as a yogi, ballet dancer or gymnast can enjoy, holding a pose. If we focus only on stretching, then elasticity can get lost in translation and pain and fatigue enter the story if there is insufficient stiffness for a given

The distinction of elasticity relates closely to muscle tone; however, we are not using the term here, in order to establish "whole body awareness" and encourage thinking in terms of the entire organism (bones, skin and tissues) rather than the parts (as if they are separate, which they *never* are in living bodies). There are difficulties in finding new definitions.

Understanding and recognising innate elasticity is made more complex by the many different meanings we have for the word "elasticity" itself. There is a general perception in yoga that it is associated with **bendiness, stretchiness** and **flexibility** (the archetypal heroes in our yoga movement story). The enemies in this story might be seen as **tension, stiffness** and **strain** or stress. They are much maligned! We need new and more favourable terms for these so-called "bad guys" because they are vastly misunderstood. Far from being the enemy, they are often guardians in disguise. We are designed to "stiffen up" to *resist deformation,* or to manage a movement that requires high tensional integrity – like reaching and holding a posture (especially into movement signature. Elasticity is a neutral and powerful resource of *free energy* that the body can exploit and preserve to save metabolic energy, whatever our age and stage of fitness.

a balanced Headstand or Handstand). We want the body to do (and hold) these postures without damage in the short or long term; we have to know, sense and contain our limits *in action*, globally and locally, in the round – and it is unique to us all!

Exploring New Terms

In order to see this as a general and global distinction for movement integrity and overall vitality (at rest), we can include the four main attributes of elastic integrity on a "soft graph" of Stiffness to Suppleness (x-axis), from Speed to Stillness (y-axis) (Fig. 10.5). At first glance we could be forgiven for asking what stiffness is doing on a chart for yoga and assuming that we should err

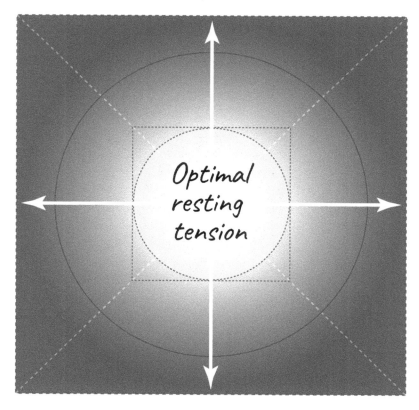

Speed

Stiffness

Optimal resting tension

Suppleness

Stillness

Figure 10.5

Graph from Speed to Stillness. Different types and styles of movement can be placed here for their emphasis on different aspects. This schema can be used in many ways, informing the diagram in Figure 10.13 as a context that can be taken into assessment of optimum fascia types/matching movement types.

towards the bottom right-hand corner of the figure. Fascial stiffness, however, has a whole other meaning and without it we can experience difficulties. In the absence of suitable stiffness, it profoundly affects our range and elastic vitality. For an extreme example of this point, to demonstrate why *suitable stiffness* is offered as a valuable asset of our structure, see the syndrome known as "swimming-puppy" syndrome.[14]

The Middle Way

The schematic in Figure 10.5 is deceptively simple. Balance and access come from the centre; it is a balance of suitable stiffness, which means *suitable resistance to deformation*, **at the time**. In fact, "Bendy Wendy" (see Fig. 10.16) might need more stiffness (which in this instance correlates to training for a "spring" in the step, i.e. higher tonus), *not more stretching*.

The terminology needs some reframing and the idea that yoga is *synonymous with stretching* might be a disservice to its nonetheless powerful contribution to *elastic integrity*. Elastic energy is very low cost metabolically; it is the essence of healthy, vital movement, on or off the mat. To fully appreciate *living* tensegrity as the basis for suitable balance between stiffness and compliance in the fascial tissues, the two versions of the same tensegrity model in Figure 10.6 make a useful point.

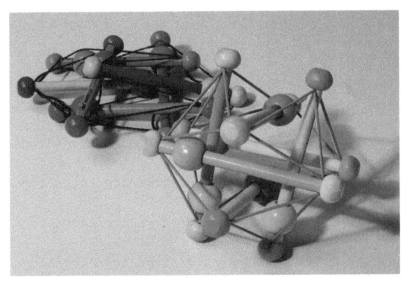

Figure 10.6

These are two Tensegritoys[50] of the same size and dimension. It shows the different *volumetric morphology* between a suitably stiffened (right) and an *overstretched* version (left) of the same model. The toy on the left is "soggy"; it has very low tension, or stiffness. The one on the right can bounce more. These "Tensegritoys" have elasticated tension members and "compression" shafts made of wood. They make the point, however, because they are identical in size, but the left-hand toy has lost its tensile integrity and is more collapsed. It has low stiffness.

General misunderstandings in using tensegrity models to explain the elastic body

- Confusion is created by the use of *elastic bands* in building tensegrity models. This is partly because they represent the *forces of tension and compression* rather than the *forms of muscles and bones*, which is the primary mistake people make in using them as a pedagogic tool to explain tensegrity as a living body model (see Ch. 6).

- The next misunderstanding tends to be between elasticity as a property of any material and "*elasticated*" bands. Classroom models are made for ease of assembly. Tensegrity models are actually optimised using *non-elasticated* materials, which *do* have suitable stiffness to *resist deformation*. Non-elasticated tensegrity masts demonstrate spring (with sufficient stiffness) and accurate examples of how collagen behaves in our body architecture, containing our elastic recoil capacity. It is different everywhere *in our form* depending on the texture of the fascial matrix at any given location in our body (see Ch. 7). This can be demonstrated with the models in Figures 10.6 and 10.7.

- Another issue is that (as John Sharkey points out): "*...the models are made of two materials; elastic cord that has a knot in it, to join it and the solid struts together. In the human body there is only one material: i.e., fascia.*"[5]

- Another issue is time and yet another is flux. We can change our tension–compression relationships constantly. In effect, that is the essence of an adaptable, flowing yoga practice. Models represent a moment in time of our elastic integrity – and as we know from doing yoga, that changes: within a practice and over years of practice and depending on the age and stage of health and mobility at the time.

- While the tissue itself has recoil properties, a common misunderstanding is that the balance of *elastin* and collagen in the fascial fibres gives rise to our *elasticity*. That would be an inaccurate assumption from the way the fibres are described, collapsing the distinctions of "elastin" and "elastic". They relate,

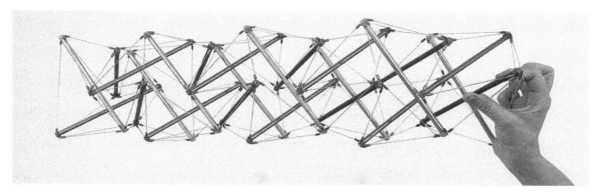

Figure 10.7

This tensegrity mast has no *elasticated* components. It demonstrates high elasticity because it has suitable stiffness. (Model designed and supplied by Bruce Hamilton, http://www.tensiondesigns.com, and final construction by the author.)

but structurally the body has its innate architectural organisation, designed to maintain and preserve energy. Elastin fibres can elongate up to 150% of their length and then restore (*reformation*). It is, in fact, one of the suite of tissues the body calls upon in, for example, specific, specialised circumstances, such as wound healing.[16] Suitable tension–compression balance (or ideal elastic properties in our tissues) and overall *elastic integrity* rely upon the *stiffness of the collagen matrix* (as in the steel mast in Fig. 10.7), which is essentially *low in deformation* and relatively *high in resistance to it* (i.e. stiffness). (It stretches only up to about 5%.) In other words, it is more like steel (high elasticity). This, in balance with our architecture, creates and contains overall *energy storage capacity*. If we were too "elasticated" we could not function. It can look like a soggy structure that (*if we describe it as over-tensioned*) needs a stiffer texture (*more compressive-based training*) to support it or *hold itself (or its shape)* up in space as an integral volume. This can be the result of insult, injury, inertia or sedentary living due to illness or lack of motion. Whatever the reason, it has a profound impact on our structural integrity. (Think of a marquee, made with soft jersey T-shirt fabric instead of strong, inelastic canvas – and elasticated guy wires, instead of steel cables. It will give you a visual as to why that internal volume would be soft and unsuitable, draping and folding and flapping in the wind, instead of sustaining its shape or volume-in-space as a marquee is designed to do).

Defining Elasticity

We are in constant phase-change; one moment the arms in Warrior have to be held out in mid-air, the next we ask them to weight-bear in Downward Dog, then we ask them to softly fold in Prayer Position, or Eagle Pose and Child Pose it is different again. All those *tension–compression expressions* are different patterns of shape changing, self-regulating balances in constant flux. If we can't make those changes *at the speed of a Vinyasa Flow* class, we consider ourselves "not very good at it". In time, with practice, it develops through our soft-tissue, innate, global and local ability to phase-change *within the tension–compression, biomotional integrity* of our own (suitably stiffened-to-spring) movement signature. No two are alike – neither practice sessions, nor participants! What we call "getting stronger" or "progress" may in fact be our developing Elastic Body recoil – essentially we get to spring better!

Elasticity can be helpfully considered as one side of a coin. The other side of that coin is **stiffness**. Stiffness is the *resistance to deformation* of any material. (All materials have elasticity.) Elasticity is the ability for reformation (spring-back). The literal definition is "stored energy capacity" which is a function of elasticity and stiffness *in balance*. **This is crucial in yoga practice, or any movement discipline.** The true amount of *stored energy capacity* is relative to the stiffness and elasticity of a material, which in body terms is the fascia.

Viscoelasticity. This is the term generally used for elasticity in liquids; the same principle is measured in viscosity (thickness). Honey is more viscous than (bulk) water because it *resists deformation* when you stir it. Bulk or free water has relatively *lower viscosity* and is *less resistant* to deformation (i.e. it is more likely to deform and take the shape of the container). Egg white has higher viscosity than water; it is slower to deform. These are time-dependent rates of change (think liquid crystal; see Ch. 7) that are slower due to their crystaline formation. Viscoelasticity acts as a "damper" – it *slows down the rate* of deformation. It may be a *time-dependent* way of regulating elastic "spring-back" or recoil. Another difficulty arises here, because there are no *liquids* (like running water, for example) in the living body, except for urine (see margin note). The language for the quality of the tissues is distinct from that describing the properties those tissues can exhibit under certain circumstances.

Poroelasticity (see margin note for definition) may also be relevant and takes us into a feature of geology and biology (more specifically rheology) that may relate to the structure of ground substance in the extracellular matrix.[17] The combination of our tissues and contained fluids includes some of these

On this basis, steel has higher energy storage capacity (elasticity) than rubber. That may seem counter-intuitive, as we think of a rubber ball bouncing more than we imagine steel bouncing; however, steel ball-bearings (for example) technically have higher elasticity, which makes sense if you know it means "higher ability to

characteristics as essential ingredients of the "in-between" in our architectural form, from embryo to elder (see Ch. 7). However, the research suggesting that the tissue of the in-between is also the fascia[18] is relatively recent and the terms for describing it are perhaps calling in new questions and definitions of how the body naturally moves in the round, filled as it is with extra-cellular matrix, as the in-between. There are no "empty spaces", as such, inside the living body. They are described as "virtual spaces".

Suitable Stiffness as an Attribute of Living Tensegrity Architecture

"The tensional forces that are generated in contractile acto-myosin filaments in the cytoskeleton are resisted by the cell's external tethers to the ECM, and by other cytoskeletal filaments that resist being compressed (e.g., microtubules, cross-linked actin filament bundles) by these inward-directed forces. For this reason, all cells in our tissues also exist in a state of isometric tension, and it is because of this internal prestress that surgeons need to suture together wounds when they incise living organs. Thus, tensegrity is used to stabilize the shape of living cells, tissues and organs, as well as our whole bodies."[19]

resist deformation". That also depends upon its density and its arrangement, or structure. For example: a steel car spring has high stiffness, while a Slinky™ toy has low stiffness. *Both have elasticity.* The car spring (higher stiffness and therefore higher elasticity) is better able to *resist deformation* and therefore to be supportive. You would go nowhere with a Slinky™ toy support-ing the forces your car has to transmit to stay in one structure as you drive it around over uneven surfaces at differ-ent speeds. If, however, your car spring is too stiff (or *brittle*), it will break for a different reason. It is a fine balance in both hard and soft matter – which is not always easily described.

The water in our bodies (see Ch. 7) is *bound water.* That is, bound with protein – so the viscoelastic aspect is that of a liquid crystal, which offers the time-dependent changes that perhaps hallmark our ability to perform, deform, reform as we move around and retain our overall shape at rest – but they cannot be reduced to these essentially "hard matter"-based

Whatever direction you pull or push a tensegrity model in, the structure nat-urally resists deformation because of its structural (tensegral) organisation, if it has sufficient stiffness.

- the force is transmitted throughout the structure
- the architecture resists you, whether you pull, push, bend or twist
- it naturally counters any movement by stiffening more
- the whole structure can bounce (exhibit recoil) in any plane
- it is independent of gravity, needing no external support to hold it up or out
- it can move in any direction (assuming it is not torn or broken)
- it reforms immediately from deformation within its resilience range
- it conforms to the geometry of a tensegrity icosahedral model (and many other shapes besides) within the pre-stiffened tensegrity matrix
- any change anywhere in the structure affects the whole
- these properties are multi- and omni-directional

In the models, the "soggiest" one (see Fig. 10.6) of the two Tensegritoys (left), is the most *stretched*, which makes it the *weakest*; its self-sustainable structural energy leaks. **Stretching is an ingredient of biomotional integrity, but only in balance with suitable stiffness.** The mast (see Fig. 10.7), with no elasticated fabric, retains its elasticity when it is still, just as we can. (The mast is hard matter, so it is static. We are living soft matter, so even when we are still, it is a dynamic, liquid-crystal state – *even in stillness!*)

Stretching: New Definitions

definitions. Even after an hour or more of shapeshifting throughout a vigorous (or slow) yoga class, we can bounce back into our shape and release the postures; we don't get stuck in Eagle Pose very often, nor do we spread into a puddle when we sit in Lotus! (See Fig. 3.12 cartoon in Ch. 3.)

Definition: see Note 17 for source of this definition: "*Poroelasticity is the term used to describe the interaction between fluid flow and solids; deformation within a porous medium. As their name indicates, porous materials are solid structures comprised of pores or voids. This type of material is typically associated with natural objects, such as rocks and solids, as well as biological tissues, foams, ceramics, and paper products.*

As we are discovering, there is stretching and stretching. We have suggested above that when you are working with a closed-kinematic chain architecture, what appears to be a "stretch" is technically a *shape-change*. To put it simplistically, if you lengthen *someplace*, there has to be a reciprocal shortening *someplace else* to co-create balance. Technically, to really *stretch* tissue is to pull it beyond its natural integrity, to a point where it can no longer naturally resist deformation. It's a complex issue,[20] but in overall terms it helps to understand why stretching isn't necessarily the best term, or the primary goal, in a successful yoga practice.

Once "stretched" beyond the point of elastic reformation, the tissue can *retain the deformity*, which is called *plastic deformation* (see below). It can also be a tissue tear, to reach or exceed that point. We need enough stiffness to hold our structure together, poised under active conditions and retain our shape! When the body can "flop" and "fold" into postures like the splits (Hanumanasana), for example, or the knees naturally hyperextend, there is not a basis for congratulations, but rather a concern for *low elastic recoil capacity* – and a need for more stiffness. That person's movement signature may need less stretching (tensioning) and more containment (compression). It is the reverse to some ways of thinking.

When Stretching Works:

When an external load is applied to a porous medium, the volume fraction of the pores is affected. The fluid-filled pores experience a change in pressure under this mechanical stress, which, in turn, leads to fluid motion. As a reaction to this change in pore volume, the solid material shifts and deforms elastically.

Here we are not saying that stretching is not valuable, in the sense of exploring *within* our natural range (uniquely defined by our own movement signature). Rather, we are placing it in a specific context. Exploring stretching and elasticity in animals provides some interesting clues as to the value of certain types of stretching. It also provides insight into different profiles (Ch. 17), or movement signatures. Fascia research is also reframing notions of stretching as preparation for action, in peak performance, for example.[21] In our search for some of the common denominators of what might work, and when and why, we are invited to see through a different lens as we learn about pandiculation,[22] and the specific value of *yawning stretches* to our fascial system. They have a different quality, of reaching with a contractile squeeze to dampen and slow down the rate of reach, rather than just reaching for the sake of it. Yawning is something animals naturally do, but when?

"It is now recognized that the myofascial system is integrative, linking body parts, as the force of a muscle is transmitted via the fascial structures well beyond the tendinous attachments of the muscle itself (Huijing and Jaspers, 2005[23]). It is argued here that pandiculation might preserve the integrative role of the myofascial system by (a) developing and maintaining appropriate physiological fascial interconnections and (b) modulating the pre-stress state of the myofascial system by regularly activating the tonic musculature."[24]

Is this indeed Nature's way of maintaining the functional integrity and elastic recoil properties of the myofascial system?[25]

Animal Stretching

Big cats. Consider the cheetah, for example (Fig. 10.8). All cats can soften, rest and relax, stretch at a suitable time and move at great speed when they need to. To chase or pounce on their prey, they can stiffen, stalk, sprint, leap and spring, deploying their powerful elastic recoil abilities in action, at varying speeds. When they rest, they become languid and serene. After they have rested, they yawn-stretch (*pandiculate*) their whole body to wake up their tissues. That period of rest effectively *released the suitable, or optimal, tensional stiffness* for a length of time. (It is quite distinct from the "warm up" or "cool down" we employ in practice. Animals tend to walk/stalk and stiffen themselves into readiness for hunting.)

When a cheetah anticipates prey (think in terms of preparing for a peak performance), the last thing it appears to do is *stretch*. (Can you imagine a cheetah turning to its cub-in-training and saying: "keep an eye on that stray wildebeest while I stretch, won't be long …"). Quite the contrary, they compress their tissues by actively stiffening them. They *stalk* their prey and seem to draw their bodies *in* – the opposite of stretching: *compressing*. It is a global

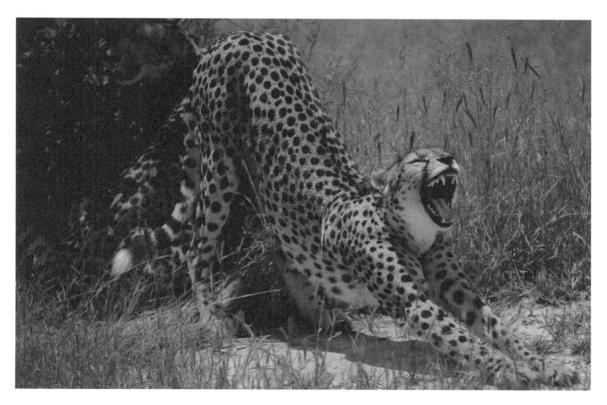

Figure 10.8

This is a yawning stretch or pandiculation (see text). A wild cheetah in Up–Down Dog Pose, its own version of Adho Urdhva Muhka Svanasana.

(Reproduced with kind permission from Shane McDermott, http://www.shanemcdermottphotography.com)

Springboks. On this theme of priming and tightening tissues to elaborate their recoil properties, springboks provide another detail that is of interest. If you watch them, even at play, they seem to practice "pinging" up in the air, from standing, for the sake of it. Are they training their internal force transmission and priming their tissues *for springing?*

When you look at a large cat and a springbok together, one chasing the other, you see two very different means of deploying elastic recoil. *Each depends on their particular movement signature to survive.* The cat, as we have pointed out, spring-loads to sprint and pounce, leaping in long strides at high speed, in clear directions. (Their velocity is their advantage, not their turning circles.) Now the springbok no longer pings upwards "for fun" but uses its ability to ping and run and leap in many different directions to evade capture. It darts and gallops in anything but a straight line, using short,

action that can reduce the space they occupy! They shape-shift their volume, containing (in-drawing) all their tissues, globally.

This compression (or global in-drawing), which seems to be part of priming their bodies, makes the animal ready to deploy the potential to pounce or sprint as required – *springing and reaching into their maximum stride, to meet the new demand for speed and breath.* It seems they maximise their catapult capacity by compressing the whole matrix, to spring-load it in the round. Even their fur stands on end, perhaps for super-sensitivity to the task. Cheetahs, like many other mammals, focus and draw their tissues *centripetally* to make them fit for purpose, globally. Then they spring *centrifugally* to leap. There is a time and a place, a dose and degree for them to stretch – and it is not before, or during, peak performance.

Note also the distinct and different resting tension of the two animals. The springbok has long, stiff, highly tensioned legs and does not appear to indulge in the languid serenity of a cat very much, even at rest. The bodies of springboks are geared for tightly contained, ready-to-rebound, "potential catapult" structure. The cat, on the other hand, has a distinctive state of "resting tension" that seems to occupy a much bigger range between rest or release and stiffened animation or spring. Although they are designed for considerable speed, like most cats they have an almost meditative ability to rest, which compared to the spring-loaded signature of the springbok places them on different ends of the spectrum. Do springboks yawn and stretch as much as cats?

How Does this Translate into Practice?

sharp turning angles (even mid-air) to confuse and tire the cat. Both types of animal speak their own kinaesthetic language as a survival mechanism, with both dependent upon *species-specific elastic integrity.*

Recent research suggests[27] that optimal preparation for peak performance in elite athletes does not include stretching as part of their warm-up period, as it can deplete strength just before a sprint, for example. Priming the tissues with short, elastic-type recoil or rebound movements, such as jumping on the spot or springing in various ways, is reminiscent of what we see in the animal kingdom. (This may be a personal, signature/occasion-dependent issue![28]) It does not necessarily mean stretching is wrong, although we may need to redefine what it means. It brings us closer to refining the dose, degree and timing (and time and place) of how and when we use it.

New Strategies

Bears. At the other end of the active scale, a research project on Grouse Mountain in British Columbia studied how hibernating bears survive a winter of sleep without experiencing osteoporosis or degenerative conditions in their muscles even after months of inertia. The hidden camera in their

This research suggests that "post rest" is generally a good time for natural (yawn-type) stretching, while preparation for peak performance at least might better include micro-movements of the tissues and "mini" versions of the work being prepared for, at low amplitudes (e.g. walking before running, playing before training, and so on). Gradually increasing the amplitude towards performance is worthy of consideration.

Before we consider the implications in (or applications to) yoga, just in terms of everyday life, we might ask ourselves how often we remember to yawn-stretch after a period of relative inertia? Given the many hours we spend den revealed an interesting instinctive habit. They get up around midday every day and do 20–40 minutes of movement. They do gentle yoga-like stretches in all directions, yawning and wriggling and pacing around, reanimating the tissues, before they settle back and sleep (hibernate) for the next 24 hours. They do this in the lowest state of energetic demand and vitality.

in cars, in beds or sitting at desks and tables, could this be quite an important consideration for health? Do we counterbalance these periods of sitting with yawning stretches to reanimate and maintain our tissues? No cat, dog or bear would "forget" to do this after a period of inactivity.

We, on the other hand, will consider forcing ourselves to stretch to reach the most extraordinary shapes as if that is the purpose of yoga. Our fascial matrix is actually designed as a profoundly sensitive system to transmit and respond to movement forces, *as distinct from forced movements*. For some people who are already at the stretchy end of the scale, stiffening or tightening their tissues may be more valuable than spending too long focused on stretching for its own sake. Let us establish why this whole principle of elasticity relies so heavily on suitable stiffness and why it is also important to understand it as a feature of our bodies at rest.

Elastic Integrity as a New Value

New measuring equipment is changing the accepted biomechanical assumptions about how muscles work to move us. A useful example regarding new ways of understanding elasticity is in research on the Achilles tendon. Classical kinesiological models suggest that in jumping, for instance, the Achilles tendon is the strong, supportive, relatively less mobile binding, connecting the calf (*gastrocnemius*) muscle to the heel bone (*calcaneus*) at the back of the ankle joint. The "movement" has been classically assigned to the calf muscle (*gastrocnemius*), assuming it actively contracts and releases (i.e. based on the action assigned to that particular muscle, one of its attachments being the Achilles tendon) (Fig. 10.9A).

Using modern ultrasound equipment supported by force-plates capable of measuring the force production of muscles fibres *and fascial tissues in vivo (40% of the maximal voluntary force)*, researchers were surprised to discover that in oscillatory movement, the muscle fibres contract, or stiffen, isometrically (without changing length) and the Achilles tendon in fact acts like a strong elastic spring (Fig. 10.9B).[29] This would mean the muscle can behave more like a brake on the spring-loaded (predisposed) recoil of the Achilles under such circumstances. This might suggest the muscle units have a role in *modifying or regulating stiffness and elasticity in appropriate length to tension–compression balance,* depending on the occasion and loading.

This all, however, presumes a linear function of the tissues as a lever-based system, as if the gastrocnemii (could) move on their own. The movement of the leg cannot be easily assigned to *only* the Achilles tendon, as if it functions in isolation. The limb is a rounded volume, in continuity with the rest of the body and the surrounding tissues to which it is directly connected. Those tissues form a closed kinematic chain which suggests new parameters for research questions.

Over recent decades, the accumulation of research investigating the various and subtle roles of the tissues has given rise to the very paradigm shift we are now in. It even highlights different *qualities* of stretching to include classical stretching and the difference of actively loaded stretching (Fig. 10.10).

The article from which the quotation below is taken[30] points to the important role of tendon behaviour, relating to *lack of stiffness* and the subsequent impact on adaptability and elastic storage capacity. The researchers also considered the different roles of tendons and tendinous sheets (aponeuroses) mediating our responses:

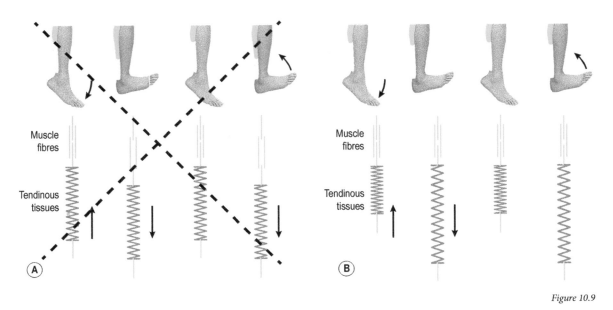

Figure 10.9

Images of research by Kawakami and colleagues (see note 29), after Schleip, showing the cooperation of muscles and fascial tissues. Effectively this suggests that the muscles act more like brakes, while the tendinous tissues lengthen and shorten like springs. (A) is classical assumption. (B) shows findings (after Kawakami).

"During low tensile loading or with passive lengthening not only the muscle is elongated, but also the tendon undergoes significant length changes, which may have implications for reflex responses. During active loading, the length change of the tendon far exceeds that of the aponeurosis, indicating that the aponeurosis may more effectively transfer force onto the tendon, which lengthens and stores elastic energy subsequently released during unloading, in a spring-like manner."[31]

This, in fact, endorses the foundational principles of biotensegrity, since it explains these complex force transmission responses that the body can vary according to load, circumstances and rate or range of motion. Magnusson and colleagues go on to elaborate the significant role of the fascia in maintaining adaptability where there is a suitable balance of stiffness or appropriate tension–compression. They show that far from playing a passive role in our structure, there is remarkably high metabolic activity in human tendon which *"affords the tendon the ability to adapt to changing demands"*:

"With ageing and disuse there is a reduction in tendon stiffness, which can be mitigated with resistance exercises. Such adaptations seem advantageous for maintaining movement rapidity, reducing tendon stress and risk of injury, and possibly, for enabling muscles to operate closer to the optimum region of the length–tension relationship."[32]

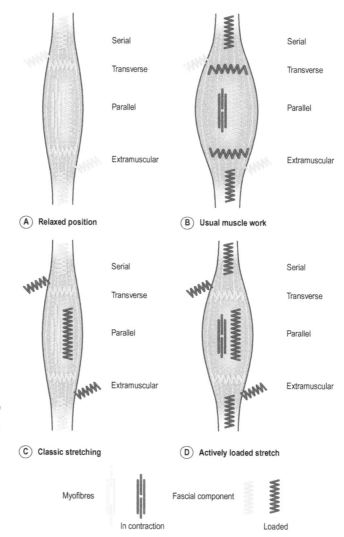

Figure 10.10

"In an 'Actively loaded stretch' the muscle is both active and also loaded at the long end of its range; it includes long myofascial chains. Most of the fascial components are being stretched and stimulated in that loading pattern."

(After Robert Schleip, *Terra Rosa* e-magazine, Issue 7, April 2010.)

Auxesis, in Greek, means "increase". Auxetic properties refer to the fact that tendons can in fact *increase* in size when stretched – which is completely counter-intuitive to the standard assumptions that they get thinner when we pull on them or "stretch" them. Graham Scarr elaborates on this point, in detail, in his book.

This suggests that it is the appropriate *stiffness* that affords the tendon suitable adaptability and "spring". While there is purpose in fostering flexibility, suitable stiffness may be an aspect that deserves consideration with a more heroic ranking in the yoga classroom!

More recent research into tendinous behaviour implies that the classical understanding of muscles changing length and tendons remaining the same is even more complex than we think! According to Sharkey[33] "*recent research (Gatt et al 2015)[34] reports auxetic properties of not just the Achilles tendon, but in fact all tendons. An unexpected mechanical property shows that they get fatter, rather than thinner when they are stretched, which is in fact a first principle of tensegrity structures, confirming their soft-matter emergent properties.*"

We are invited by various research projects into the fascial matrix[36] to view the muscles as part of the continuity of myofascial balance throughout the tensional web of our architecture; think back to Chapter 4, where we learn how it forms in its entirety. If the fascial matrix, as Jaap van der Wal suggests, is the primary tissue, then all others emerge from it, or from within its organisation. The tissues clearly participate in the subtle translation and mediation of all types of forces, through movement. While research might focus on different specific (types of) tendinous organisations, we must remember that the body itself does not go about getting agreement from each separate part. It organises and acts *as an instinctive whole* and if the fascial matrix is the original unifying (or unified) medium within which these specialisations occur, then its role as a whole tensegrity-based network makes sense of what we witness in movement classrooms.

We have to expand our view to include the whole body to get a sense of why the bones play such an important role in creating suitable tensioning, or stiffness, in our tension–compression form, thus contributing to our elastic integrity. They are living aspects of the whole matrix too; they simply change in a different time frame to the more superficial tissues. This is the quantum leap, from muscles as separate structures, acting as levers, to muscles as moderators of stiffness and softness (or tension and compression), in the weave of our three-dimensional architecture. That leap can be made, with the right language to support us.

This important distinction is to define this essential scale of elastic recoil as a predisposing property of our resting tension and its innate pre-tensioned design. The bones are the stiffest aspect, the softest soft tissues (of the interstitium perhaps) and the most supple. In between their respective ends of the spectrum we have the myotendinous organisations and aponeuroses, moderating the orchestration of appropriate stiffness to softness at the time. It will learn to do that one way, to complete a Vinyasa Flow class, while doing so quite differently to undertake a Restorative Practice or a Power Yoga Hour or an Iyengar style class. Each one is valuable, in its own way, according to the movement signature of the participant. Arguably, the more variability we can include, the better – however, that is a matter of time and place and personal preference. The point is that the body is fine tuning *itself*. Do we help matters by being so focused on stretching? Or strengthening? As if they are the movement goals. Is overall tone, adaptability and variability more of an asset?

The Foundation Stones of Balanced Structure

Understanding some fundamental tenets of elastic integrity might provide some clues about these foundation stones of our balanced structure, as we search for a context for all the postures and our respective ways of interpreting them. There are four main themes:

1. the ability to globally expand and reduce overall size (think of the prowling cat, drawing in its tissues, to stalk its prey – and the active exhale)
2. low-cost energy resource (aka energy storage capacity)

3. the basis of compliance and communication throughout the fascia; its pre-stiffened nature
4. what do we mean by springs and suitable stiffness?

1. The Global Ability to Expand and Reduce

We can appear to expand our chest when we inhale. We may have to expand our thinking in a similar way (see Fig. 10.1). Moving from area to volume is from "circles to spheres" and we breathe in the round (see Ch. 11). Tensional integrity works in a non-linear tension–compression system with 360° of movement potentials, as a global volume. Although we can do all sorts of things with our bodies, they rely on this particular biological architecture for one very fundamental feature: we can globally expand (into tension) and globally in-draw (into compression) to stiffen *as a whole* – and part by part (i.e. globally and locally). An example of this kind of movement pattern can be seen in a creature such as a puffer fish[37] (globally) or the ability of an elephant to swing its trunk (soften) or stiffen and straighten it to reach a branch above its head and pluck the leaves (locally). It is an attribute of human structure; we constantly use it everywhere in our physiology. (We can hang an arm by our side or hold it stiffly, parallel to the ground in Warrior Pose (*Virabhadrasana*) – we can expand our torso with an in-breath, and reduce the tissues into compression, with the squeezing out of the active exhale (see Ch. 11). That is the distinction here – all of which is *in the round* – so for every motion there is a counter-motion somewhere in the body. It doesn't add material. It just shape-changes it.

Simple examples of this are found in various parts and functions of the body, from breathing to giving birth, from emptying the bladder to the movement of food through the gut via *peristalsis*. Although digestion operates along a tube, the method is a long-evolved, rhythmical ability to appear to expand the shape of the tissues outward and reduce the shape inward (tension and compression) in the gut tube. The tissues rest in the "middle state", so that drawing inwardly or expanding outwardly are available as natural resting potentials, from the middle state or resting tension.

2. Low-Cost Energy Animation

In the last chapter we elaborated upon the body's primary concern for energy conservation. It starts with a pre-stiffened state of poise.

Demonstration

Take hold of a strong elastic band (Fig. 10.11) and place a finger at each end inside its loop, to hold it open but untensioned. Then pull your fingers apart to the halfway point. Then stretch it to its full limit. You have just demonstrated three stages of stiffness: (1) resting tension, (2) semi-tensioned, (3) fully tensioned. Beyond the third stage is the "elastic limit", past which the band either tears or breaks.

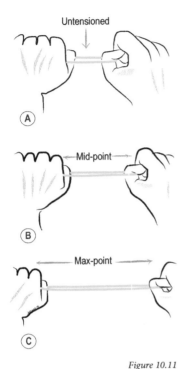

Untensioned

(A)

Mid-point

(B)

Max-point

(C)

Figure 10.11

Demonstration of pre-stiffening.

Imagine flicking a paper pellet with a
metal school ruler. Within its elastic
limit, the ruler would catapult the
pellet across the room (high elastic –
free – energy storage capacity in the
metal). If, however, you pulled the ruler
back too far and exceeded its elastic
limit, it would bend and stay there (it
is non-reversible, no reformation). It
would fail to "ping" the pellet. This is
a demonstration of its *plasticity*. The
exact boundary between plasticity and
breaking point depends on the ruler's
bendiness (ductility) or brittleness.*
Rulers made of different materials
would exhibit different plasticity and
elasticity. The ruler will effectively tire
until it breaks, at the plastic limit. A
plastic ruler, which has properties of
high brittleness and low ductility, will
break at a point of much less strain than
a metal one. A wooden one will behave
differently again. *Each texture of material has different emergent properties.*

When you tension the elastic band and stretch it, you are sensing its *resistance
to deformation* – that is, its *stiffness*. When you release it, you are demonstrating its *elasticity* – that is, its ability to return/*reformation*. Several important
facts arise from doing this exercise, which are:

- You need sufficient resistance to deformation (stiffness) or the band is floppy
  and pulled out of shape too readily.

- By fully releasing the band you **do not** demonstrate *resting tension* in the
  human body.

- It is the *halfway point of the elastic band*, the semi-tensioned stage B (see
  Fig. 10.11), that demonstrates *resting tension* in the human body.

We are "pre-stiffened" or "pre-tensioned" – *we do not deflate*. We do not experience the state represented by the elastic band lying untensioned on the table,
ever (we are always a volume). In the demonstration above, we would start
at the second stage, the middle way, which is our *default elasticity*. We find
appropriate balance in life, essentially around the middle way. **It is a key to
vitality – and understanding human structure.**

We know from experience in the yoga classroom that stillness takes as
much focused attention as movement. Holding postures is a skill in itself.
Holding an elastic band at the mid-point of tension–compression balance
shows precisely why. We live between stages B and C in our demonstration
(Fig. 10.11B & C) in terms of living elastic integrity. If we go beyond C,
however, and venture beyond our elastic limit, we can enter one of two
states: these are *plasticity* (permanent irreversible change) and injury.
Plasticity can be an advantage or a disadvantage, depending on the material and reason for changing it. Like elasticity, it is a property rather than
a value. It can mark improvement or injury, depending on whether the
change it presents is valuable on that occasion, at that time, for that individual – or not.

Beyond the elastic limit of a material is a state called plasticity. Plasticity
means that there is no ability to reform. Between elasticity and stiffness, deformation has reversibility, i.e. a capacity for reformation. The moment that natural limit is exceeded, deformation is no longer reversible. The material retains
the deformation.

Elasticity, plasticity, brittleness, ductility, etc., are properties of *all materials*; however, they are measured on a linear stress–strain graph in hard-matter materials. More confusion therefore arises for human bodies, since we
"don't do" linear stress–strain graphs, because we come under the different
subset, of soft-matter, non-linear materials. Our tissues have to be *continually stretched and strained repeatedly* over time, if we want them to *retain
deformation*.

If the elastic limit is reached too rapidly (these are time-dependent features), then damage can occur in the form of a tear, a break or the snapping
of a tendon. Our tissues are sensitive to temperature, hydration, range and
chemistry as well as *rate of change* (see Ch. 7).

Consider, for example, the practice of ear stretching, using ear plugs to expand the ear lobe gradually over time, but permanently, once the tissue has gone beyond its elastic limit and reached a state of plastic deformation. A graph of this viscoelastic deformation has what is called a "J-shaped, curved, stress–strain pattern". It is "non-linear" because we are non-linear systems and it never goes to zero because we are pre-tensioned." We never start at nothing: we always start at something (because we begin

One of the values of warming up before exercise (besides all the known benefits of stimulating circulation and preparing the body) is to wake up the tissues and activate their elastic potential and "interfascial glide" after rest. They can become adhered and insufficiently stiffened. Elasticity is an energy asset throughout many forms of our internal and locomotive structure; all the tissues are under tension, not just the muscles: the tendons, ligaments, blood and nerve vessels and viscera – it is the nature of our formation. Even the diaphragm demonstrates a continuous, tensioned myofascial membrane (recapitulated in the images of yoga practitioners inside fabric tubes throughout the book) that relies on pre-stiffening to hold its structure so we can breathe. It is innate to our structural integrity.

"The visco-resilient nerves are under a constant internal tension. The strength of these forces is seen in ruptured nerves. Simply because of their tremendous elasticity, the two severed nerve stumps shorten by several millimeters. In repair procedures, the surgeon has to use a considerable amount of strength to bring the two nerve ends together again … It is elasticity that allows nerves to adjust to the movement of a joint without loss of function."[40]

pre-stressed). J-shaped stress–strain curves demonstrate lower energy cost which nature is predisposed to preserve. Note the same principle can apply if we wish to improve our abilities by repeatedly practising new, useful patterns. The time-dependency aspect of this principle of viscoelasticity can be to our advantage.

There are many aspects of our anatomy and physiology and biomotional congruency that rely on elastic integrity. These include, and are not limited to, the nerves, blood vessels, lungs, bladder, digestive system and locomoting tissues (Fig. 10.12[41]). There is good reason to consider, particularly in terms of the living tensegrity architecture, that it is a feature of the whole system.

"The collagen molecule exists in many different configurations and is a major component of the extracellular matrix (ECM) that surrounds virtually every cell. The matrix attaches to the cellular cytoskeleton through adhesion molecules in the cell membrane and forms a structural framework that extends through the fascia to every level in the body."[42]

3. The Basis of Compliance and Communication Throughout the Fascia

If we become overstretched, over time we can lose that "spring-back" facility if tissues are repeatedly forced to exceed their natural elastic limit (or tensegral envelope). Plastic deformation then becomes irreversible (as in the use of the ear plugs/extenders).

Watching a flowing yoga class, for example, the body clearly has the ability to distribute forces throughout the system, changing the fulcrums and managing the form transitions seamlessly from the crown to the ground. The classical models rely on levers and inverted pendulums to explain human motion. However, we have established that two-bar (lever) mechanics fail to explain fully how we can achieve the fabulous forms of yoga practice without shearing, breaking or falling off our own structural parts (as we explored in the last chapter).

Further study[43] reveals the powerful potential of the living tensegrity model as an explanation of our natural elastic movements. What we do see, from the outside, is in fact relatively integrated movements that, over time, become

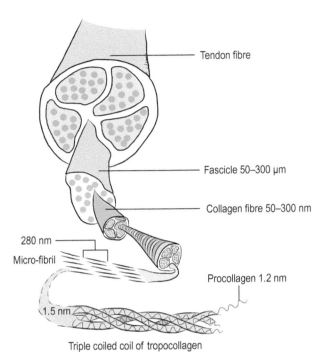

Tendon fibre

Fascicle 50–300 μm

Collagen fibre 50–300 nm

280 nm

Micro-fibril

Procollagen 1.2 nm

1.5 nm

Triple coiled coil of tropocollagen

Figure 10.12

Graham Scarr (see note 42) provides detailed explanation of how the geometric principles of biotensegrity translate into a recognisable model of capillary formation, bone formation, "musculo-skeleto-fascia" formation and many other aspects of our form.

(Modified after Graham Scarr, www.tensegrity.co.uk)

more and more refined as we practise them and train (or tune) our tissues *on every scale* to become more naturally resistant to deformation, while retaining their compliant ability to shape-shift. The research that is accumulating on the study of "fasciategrity" is perhaps so compelling because it suggests a scale-free explanation of these local and global movements, with principles that apply from the microscopic organelles within a cell to the whole organism. We recapitulate at the cellular level the same micro-patterns as whole bodies performing macro-movements, on a continuum from embryo to elder. This is simplified, but nevertheless honoured, if we recognise the whole "volume control" between stiffness and compliance (suppleness), cross-referenced by speed to stillness. Altogether it forms a platform for guiding refinement towards elastic integrity, in the round. The focus on only one or other aspect of this crucial context of our form can be at the expense of the whole balance we seek throughout the practice of yoga.

All different types of yoga can be placed here for their emphasis on different styles/types of movement. This schema can also include many ways, or pathways, for a given individual (see Fig. 10.5).

4. What Do We Mean by Springs and Stiffness?

Between the pathways from speed to stillness, rhythm and direction also play a role in optimising balancing forces, under the heading of elastic integrity (see Ch. 7 for why rhythm may play a meaningful, basic role in all the emergent properties of the body).

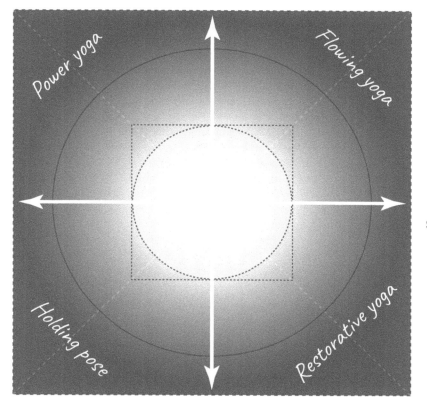

**Fast flowing
Focus on speed**

Power yoga

Flowing yoga

**Focus on
strength**

**Focus on
suppleness**

Holding pose

Restorative yoga

**Meditative
Focus on stillness**

Figure 10.13

All different types of yoga can be placed here for their emphasis on different styles/types of movement. This schema can also include many ways, or pathways, for a given individual.

"The neuronal circuit controlling the rhythmic movements in animal locomotion is called the central pattern generator (CPG). The biological control mechanism appears to exploit mechanical resonance to achieve efficient locomotion."[44]

Once we understand that appropriate stiffness is an asset of organised motion, one of the issues that comes up in class, teaching the value of the spring-loaded Elastic Body, is that people have different ideas of "springs". The difficulty in translating tensegrity models into the living body is that they vary in stiffness, just as we do. What we have to remember is that the softer

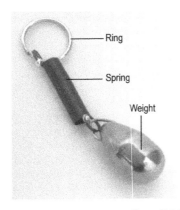

Figure 10.14

This is an example of how the fascia can behave, to help appreciate rhythm and rate as well as how little muscular effort (represented by the finger holding the ring) is required to release elastic energy to move the weight.

the spring, the more metabolic work the body has to do to stiffen (appropriately) and guide the movement. The tauter the spring, the more innate the elastic recoil – which represents the free elastic energy to the elastic body. However – as always, there is an appropriate limit in any direction on the spectrum. Too strong a spring (which builds strength) can provide so much resistance to deformation that it moves towards immobility and brittleness. Too weak a spring (which allows more extreme suppleness) can provide so little resistance to deformation that it moves towards sogginess and insufficient containment. Like everything, it is a question of balance.

It seems that the sensory feedback of our subtle patterns is also profoundly linked to rhythm and resonance. What happens when we find and build our own rhythms, *appropriate* to the task, is that they reflect natural energy conservation patterns; in other words, the more efficient the rhythm, the more naturally spring-loaded and apparently effortless the motion appears. (There is value in practicing both rhythmical and arrhythmical motion; they have different effects on the tissues and can be used – given dose and degree – to guide and foster individual movement signatures towards optimal adaptive patterns to support them.)

This principle of the elastic body, in finding rhythmical motion, is naturally fostered by the yoga sequences that integrate rhythmical breathing as part of the practice. Practice being the operative word:

"Not all methods of postural yoga practice harness rhythm in the same way. Breathing gives us an inbuilt metronome, which can be driven with the same virtuosity as a musician brings to their instrument. Regular, random, progressive, flowing, or alternating patterns give variety to the shape of rhythm in music.

Likewise, variety in movement-breath coordination give us access to a spectrum of vibration amplified by the pace and intensity with which we might choose to interact with the ground. The choice to move with some speed comes with the potential to rebound, inviting the "bounce" of our landing to reverberate within us and to further direct that energy as breath into the refrain."

Karen Kirkness[45]

What Level of Elastic Integrity Are You Voting For?

"A recognised characteristic of connective tissue is its impressive adaptability. When regularly put under increasing physiological strain, it changes its architectural properties to meet the increasing demand."[46]

We tend to vote with our feet in the yoga classroom. There are so many different forms, each focusing on one or other aspect as primary – from power yoga to restorative yoga, to meditative or dream practices – with all sorts of

Pilates and Gyrotonic® teachers are very familiar with this principle working with machines and weighted cables. The reformer (as one example) tends to help a new student by adding stronger springs to give them more external resistance. As they develop their own ability towards coordinated, appropriate stillness, they can generate a more coherent performance with less external resistance, i.e. softer springs. They have built their internal resistance to deformation; in other words, they have improved their Elastic Body structural integrity. It seems counter-intuitive, however it makes perfect sense, when we recognise the spectrum from stiffness to suppleness is precisely that – and we can change it, with practice, to the point of balance for each individual, from within their Elastic Body.

variations of focus in between. While we are alive, we do not get to abstain from this choice to find optimum resting tension. The "vote" for inertia sets up its own strain (or lack of strain) patterns. What is crucial is the timing of how our strain patterns are accumulated. Training at speed or training in stillness is not just about joining an Ashtanga class, or Power Yoga and doing it seven days a week or, at the other extreme, taking up meditation full-time.

Our bodies self-regulate in very intelligent and subtle ways and variability is perhaps the key. There is a case for suggesting the benefits from occasionally sampling a practice that includes some of everything. Whichever way we do yoga we are looking for a place of *elastic integrity*, and adaptability wherever we are (at the time) in terms of resting tension. The different qualities of pre-stiffened fascial tissues work in concert to modify stiffness and elasticity *in balance* (on and off the mat). Each aspect of our tissues responds in different time frames and at different times and rates.

Temporal Tissues

If you find/make a spring like the one in Figure 10.14 and bounce it in a gentle, rhythmical way, you are being the "metabolic energy" in this example, to activate motion. The spring begins to gather momentum and will gradually begin to express its spring-loadedness with minimal energy input from you (i.e. natural elastic momentum, which is the free part). However, if you move the spring in a staccato way, or in many directions, arrhythmically, it loses the rhythm and bends and folds readily and randomly, *leaking energy as it does so*. The bounce, or integrity of the springiness, is lost without establishing momentum.

The easiest way to imagine the muscles as "turn-buckles" is to think of the keys on a string instrument that tune it. A harp, for example, is a tension–compression instrument. So is any string instrument or any percussion instrument that has a diaphragm-like skin over a container. The keys, or ties, that tighten the tension in the drumskin, or the strings of the harp or cello (or piano) and so on, make the string more taught

In Chapter 7, we talked about temporality and tempo as two key emergent properties in working with a liquid crystal matrix. These become key elements in working intelligently to find and foster our own movement signature, congruently for our own fascial matrix. From a tensegrity point of view, every web of fascia is connected and interconnected. The muscle aspect acts like a "turn-buckle" on the web; as the muscles, or myofascia, become strengthened or organised (through different styles of practice), they can build the variability, over time, of a responsive, relaxed Elastic Body; primarily because *it has practised responsive, variability* and relaxation!

The training focus on the "myo(fascial) meat" tends to react to training rapidly and thus the general experience of weight training, for example, is to see a fairly steep graph of improvement over a relatively short period of time (weeks or a few months) at first. This is based on the time-dependent adaptability rate of muscle protein in resistance training that focuses on so-called "isolated muscles" in the upper and lower body. (Nothing is isolated; from a fascial integration point of view, it still affects the rest of the web however we describe it). By doing this, the myo part of the myofascia is the focus and the effect is one of stiffening the matrix. The tissues move towards the "muscle-bound" end of the spectrum.

The pattern, in the most general terms, is a six- to twelve-week rapid change and then a steadier plateau. If you stop training, the linear graph also tends to drop fairly rapidly. Typically, a body builder who leaves the gym for a two-month holiday knows it can cost them their "peak form". It is a high-maintenance, metabolically demanding training. The frequency is usually advocated at alternate days.

By contrast, the fascial aspect of the myofascia responds to the duration and timing of training in a very different way. In the short term it and more highly tuned (and "highly strung"). There is an appropriate balance of length–tension tuning that denotes a perfect tone in any instrument. (The harp is strung inside the frame, the guitar over it – they are variations on a tension–compression theme) (n.b. they are not tensegrity structures, but they are tension–compression designs). This language correlates closely with the body's architecture. Muscle-focused training tends to make the strings taut and move the body towards the STRENGTH end of that spectrum, away from the SUPPLENESS end. Flexibility and mobility-based training tend to move the body the other way. There is an argument to suggest that we can all do with a little of what is at the other end of our spectrum, to bring balance to the body and grant it the range and potential of the middle way!

takes time to "deconstruct and reconstruct" after a period of intense movement/training. This process of reorganisation is called *collagen synthesis*. Research[47] shows that before this stage can be reached, the body requires a period of time during which it enters a phase called *collagen degradation* (Fig. 10.15). The collagen degradation period is optimal resting phase.

In the long term, including the short-term repetitions, the soft-tissue training graph takes six to twenty-four months to facilitate collagen transformation.[48] This supports the value of working at less frequent intervals, over a longer period of time, to see the steady accumulation of balance and optimal training in the fascia. Schleip recommends we take the approach of a "bamboo gardener" who nurtures and waters his seedlings for many months, until they grow into healthy resilient plants that can reach their full potential.[49] This takes years, not weeks.

As far as yoga is concerned, this perhaps confirms an aspect of the difference between a twenty-four day (consecutive days) intensive training programme and the same number of days incorporated over two years, once per month. The total hours may add up to the same on paper, but not to the body. While we can definitely say "use it or lose it" we might add something about "gradually trained for change sustained".

Fascia-inclusive Training

This points to why the concept of training the fascial matrix is a valuable addition to many fitness approaches – although we have to recognise, it plays a role in all of them. The traditional main aspects of training focus are *neuromuscular coordination*, *strength and conditioning*, and *cardiovascular and endurance training*. These are completed and complemented by attending to the elastic component of our structural integrity. It includes working at a different pace, with a specific focus on the fascia and its elastic recoil and rebound properties. However, it requires sufficient and suitable *rest*.

Yoga can and does enhance this complementary quadrant, if it includes (or completes) a balance of all four aspects on the scale of stiffness to suppleness and speed to stillness. Meditation is aware and conscious resting of the dynamically still body, quite different from sedentary non-activity, slump or sleep. It offers deep and suitable counterbalance to high levels of activity that allows the mind, body and being to enjoy all aspects of elastic integrity.

Once we start to examine how tensegrity applies to a three-dimensional architectural model (as a basis of our elastic integrity), it invites us to consider that elasticity is actually fundamental, in varying degrees, to every part of our healthy mobility and internal motility at rest. All these tissues (cells, organs and us) are organised by the connective tissue matrix as tension–compression (or *pre-stiffened*) force transmission systems in three dimensions, even when we are in seated meditation. We could perhaps define our living tensegrity *architecture* as "elasticity incorporated" to varying degrees. Think about the elastic band we stretched to position (B) (see Fig. 10.11). This position is the most difficult to hold. This is our resting tension, designed for mobility and poised for it, in all directions. In a body that is held together

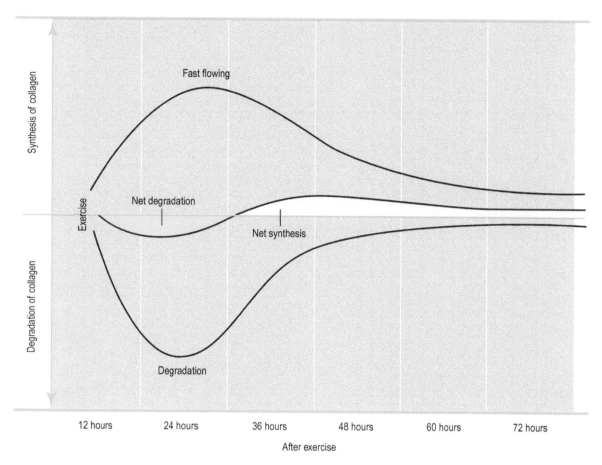

Figure 10.15

Perhaps this begins to explain why most injuries in athletics, sports and exercise are soft-tissue injuries. Whatever the training, if it is intensely pursued without sufficient time to rest and restore the body, then the collagen matrix is in a phase of degradation and has not necessarily reached synthesis before the next training session. It is a clear indication of why forced movement and overtraining can conflict with elastic integrity.

(Modified after Magnusson[30].)

by a tissue continuum in which muscles arise and live in active contraction (coordinated by a neural net, designed to appropriately inhibit contraction), *all within the net*, we begin to make sense of our sophisticated *biomotional integrity* and how it moves itself around – and uses rest and restoration as a deliberate and conscious advantage, given appropriate dose and degree and rhythm.

It begins to explain motion in 360 degrees and the bigger question of life's rhythm, in which sufficient "rest and restore" is so essential.

Body Reading Elastic Integrity – a useful tool

Posture Profiling* (see Part C, Ch. 17, where we will explore this as a teaching aid) compares different body types to what we might call the "movement archetypes" that we have addressed here (i.e. speed, stillness, suppleness and stiffness). Fascial body types are linked closely to the ability to express elastic integrity. The questions to take with us are (1) "Does this individual's elastic integrity serve them optimally?" and (2) "Is there a yoga practice they could do, over time, to enhance and preserve it?" This skill of recognition together with your experience can serve as a fast-track guide to optimum practice, one that can embrace everyone, and not just the "Bendy Wendy types" (Fig. 10.16)!

The dog in Figure 10.17 is not actually stretching in the technical sense to reach the pool and drink, even though it is "a stretch" to get there. In order to do so without falling in or swimming, it is actually *stiffening* its tissues throughout the length of the whole form, to balance from the tip of its tail to the end of its nose. In fact, it even reaches out its tongue very carefully to avoid disturbing the whole-body balancing act required to reach the water. Every part of its structure is engaged in coordinating the task it intends to complete. It is the perfect balance, at the time, of an integrally coordinated elastic body; organised and precisely fit for purpose. The "downward dog" is a balancing performance in progress.

This can obviously also be said of doing any yogasana practice!

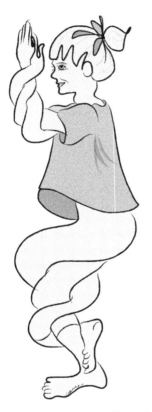

Figure 10.16

Super "Bendy Wendy" types might not always have the best advantage for elastic integrity!

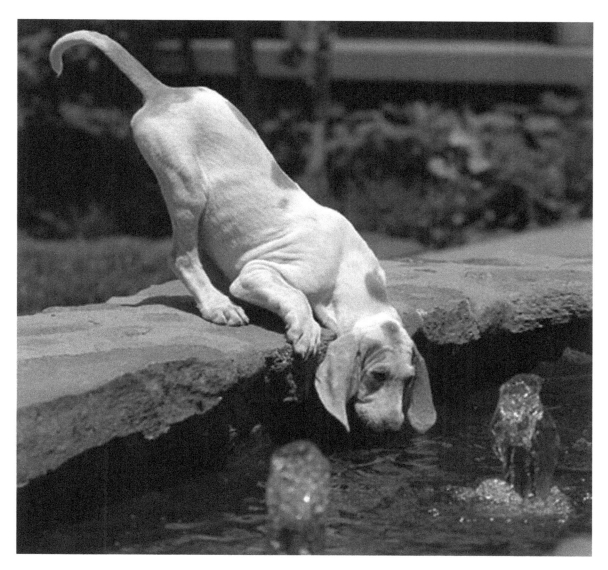

Figure 10.17

This is a wonderful image of biotensegrity in action as a global aspect of functioning form. Perhaps, apart from its ears, this basset hound is containing its whole architecture in a focused balancing act to avoid tipping.

(Reproduced with kind permission from Shane McDermott, http://www.shanemcdermottphotography.com.)

Notes

1. Robert Schleip, "Foreword", in Luigi Stecco and Carla Stecco, *Fascial Manipulation: Practical Part*, English edition by Julie Ann Day, foreword by Robert Schleip, Piccin, Padua, 2009.

2. Kazuya Takeda et al (2020) The effects of combined static and dynamic stretching of anti-gravitational muscles on body flexibility and standing balance: A preliminary study of healthy young participants. *Journal of Bodywork and Movement Therapies* 24(1):221–227.

3. John Sharkey, Clinical Anatomist and Exercise Physiologist. www.NTC.ie in Dublin Ireland, home of European Neuromuscular Therapy (NMT). Published by Lotus & North Atlantic Press: *The Concise Book of Neuromuscular Therapy* (ISBN: 1556436734), *The Concise Book of Dry Needling* (ISBN: 1623170834), *Healing through Trigger Point Therapy*, John Sharkey & Devin Starlanyl (ISBN: 1583946098).

4. Michael Shea: https://www.sheaheart.com. Home of biodynamic craniosacral work and embryology.

5. S. Levin, et al (2017) The significance of closed kinematic chains to biological movement and dynamic stability. *Journal of Bodywork & Movement Therapies* 21(3):664–672.

6. In 2007, Dr Leon Chaitow invited several renowned authorities, worldwide, in bodywork and movement therapies to consider this question and why there seems to be a need to redefine it, as the research develops in the field of fascia. (This is the same year as the first International Fascia Research Congress.) This research was an article in the *Journal of Bodywork and Movement Therapies*. Leon Chaitow (2003) The stretching debate. *Journal of Bodywork and Movement Therapies* 7(2):80.

7. Graham Scarr: *Biotensegrity: The Structural Basis of Life*, Handspring Publishing Ltd., Pencaitland, 2014. 2nd Edition. Ch 4 The Twist in the Tale, p 65–68: The Crossed Helical Tube.

8. Robert Schleip, "Foreword", in Luigi Stecco and Carla Stecco, *Fascial Manipulation: Practical Part*, English edition by Julie Ann Day, foreword by Robert Schleip, Piccin, Padua, 2009.

9. Alfonse Masi et al (2008) Human resting muscle tone (HRMT): Narrative introduction and modern concepts. *Journal of Bodywork and Movement Therapies* 12(4):320–332.

10. Chris Jarmey and John Sharkey, *The Concise Book of Muscles*, Third Edition. Biotensegrity – Biomechanics for the 21st Century, John Sharkey and Stephen Levin, p. 50.

11. A.T. Masi, J. Hannon (2008) Human resting muscle tone (HRMT): Narrative introduction and modern concepts. *Journal of Bodywork and Movement Therapies* 12(4):320–332.

12. Robert Schleip, "Foreword", in Luigi Stecco and Carla Stecco, *Fascial Manipulation: Practical Part*, English edition by Julie Ann Day, foreword by Robert Schleip, Piccin, Padua, 2009.

13. John Sharkey, Centre for Anatomy and Human Identification, School of Life Sciences, University of Dundee, Scotland. Keynote at the Massage & Myotherapy Australia National Conference at the Gold Coast in June 2018. *Myotherapy* magazine: Summer 2017 'Massage & Myotherapy Australia' is a brand of the Australian Association of Massage Therapists Ltd. pp. 12–17.

14. S.A. Kim, K.J. Na, J.K. Cho, N.S. Shin (2013) Home-care treatment of swimmer syndrome in a miniature schnauzer dog. *Can Vet J* 54(9):869–72.

15. John Sharkey, Biotensegrity Interest Group, Private Summit, Ghent, Belgium, 2018.

16. Adjo Zorn and Kai Hodeck; Erik Dalton, *The Dynamic Body*, Freedom from Pain Institute, Oklahoma, 2010; http://erikdalton.com/.

17. Defined as https://uk.comsol.com/multiphysics/poroelasticity

18. P.C. Benias, R.G. Wells, B. Sackey-Aboagye, et al (2018) Structure and distribution of an unrecognized interstitium in human tissues. *Sci Rep* 8:4947.

19. Donald E. Ingber (2008) Tensegrity and mechanotransduction. *Journal of Bodywork and Movement Therapies* 12(3):198–200.

20. In 2007, Dr Leon Chaitow invited several renowned authorities, worldwide, in bodywork and movement therapies to consider this question and why there seems to be a need to redefine it, as the research develops in the field of fascia. (This is the same year as the first International Fascia Research Congress). This research was an article in the *Journal of Bodywork and Movement Therapies*. John Sharkey (2003) *Journal of Bodywork and Movement Therapies* 7(2):90–92.

21. A.G. Nelson, N.M. Driscoll, D.K. Landin, M.A. Young and I.C. Schexnayder (2005) Acute effects of passive muscle stretching on sprint performance. *Journal of Sports Sciences* 23(5):449–454.

22. Luiz Fernando Bertolucci (2010) Pandiculation: nature's way of maintaining the functional integrity of the myofascial system? *Journal of Bodywork and Movement Therapies* 15(3):268–280.

23. Peter A. Huijing, R.T. Jaspers (2005) Adaptation of muscle size and myofascial force transmission: a review and some new experimental results. *Scandinavian Journal of Medicine & Science in Sports* 15(6).

24. Luiz Fernando Bertolucci (2010) Pandiculation: nature's way of maintaining the functional integrity of the myofascial system? *Journal of Bodywork and Movement Therapies* 15(3):268–280.

25. Ibid.

26. Grouse Mountain in Vancouver: http://www.grousemountain.com/wildlife-refuge. There is a "BearCam" facility and it is possible to watch bears Coola and Grinder in hibernation. Researchers and rangers in the park run a blog and show films about the bears (and other wildlife at the reserve) and their hibernating habits.

27. A.G. Nelson, N.M. Driscoll, D.K. Landin, M.A. Young and I.C. Schexnayder (2005) Acute effects of passive muscle stretching on sprint performance. *Journal of Sports Sciences* 23(5):449–454.

28. See Note 2

29. Y. Kawakami, T. Muraoka, S. Ito, H. Kanehisa and T. Fukunaga (2002) In vivo muscle fibre behaviour during counter-movement exercise in humans reveals a significant role for tendon elasticity. *Journal of Physiology* 540: 635–646.

30. S.P. Magnusson, M.V. Narici, C.N. Maganaris and M. Kjaer (2008) Human tendon behaviour and adaptation, in vivo. *Journal of Physiology* 586:71–81.

31. Ibid.

32. Ibid.

33. John Sharkey, Clinical Anatomist, Centre for Anatomy and Human Identification, School of Life Sciences, University of Dundee, Scotland, Biotensegrity Influenced Dissection Programme, June 2019.

34. R. Gatt, et al (2015) Negative Poisson's ratios in tendons: an unexpected mechanical response. *Acta Biomater* 24:201–208.

35. Graham Scarr. *Biotensegrity: The Structural Basis of Life*, Handspring Publishing Ltd., Pencaitland, 2014. 2nd Edition. Ch 4 The Problem with Mechanics, p. 40: Non-linearity and Auxetics.

36. Robert Schleip, Thomas W. Findley, Leon Chaitow and Peter A. Huijing, *Fascia: The Tensional Network of the Human Body*, Churchill Livingstone/Elsevier, Edinburgh, 2012.

37. Stephen Levin: www.biotensegrity.com; lecture at the University of Leuven, Belgium, October 2013.

38. Scott Ramsay, University of Toronto. *Ductility, toughness and resilience.* https://edtech.engineering.utoronto.ca/object/ductility-toughness-and-resilience https://www.youtube.com/watch?v=CMuBpazobwE&feature=youtu.be

39. Stephen Levin, www.biotensegrity.com: "Tensegrity: The New Biomechanics"; Fig. 18. Published in M. Hutson and R. Ellis (eds), *Textbook of Musculoskeletal Medicine*, Oxford University Press, Oxford, 2006.

40. Jean-Pierre Barral and Alain Croibier, *Manual Therapy for the Peripheral Nerves*, Churchill Livingstone, Edinburgh, 2007.

41. Graham Scarr. *Biotensegrity: The Structural Basis of Life*, Handspring Publishing Ltd., Pencaitland, 2014. 2nd Edition. Ch. 6 A Twist in the Tale. p. 63 Figure 6.5

42. Graham Scarr's website (www.tensegrityinbiology.co.uk) offers a range of explanatory pages with well-referenced material written in clear and concise terms. It includes various links to current research as well as a wide range of applications of these principles. See also: *Biotensegrity: The Structural Basis of Life*, Handspring Publishing Ltd., Pencaitland, 2014. 2nd Edition.

43. Ibid.

44. Y.I. Futakata and T. Iwasaki (2008) Formal analysis of resonance entrainment by central pattern generator. *Journal of Mathematical Biology* 57(2):183–207.

45. Karen Kirkness, MFA, MSc Human Anatomy. *Spiral Bound: Integrated Anatomy for Yoga*, Handspring Publishing, 2020. Founder, Meadowlark Yoga (karenkirkness.com).

46. Robert Schleip, Thomas W. Findley, Leon Chaitow and Peter A. Huijing, *Fascia: The Tensional Network of the Human Body*, Churchill Livingstone/Elsevier, Edinburgh, 2012.

47. S.P. Magnusson, H. Langberg and M. Kjaer (2010) The pathogenesis of tendinopathy: balancing the response to loading. *Nature Reviews Rheumatology* 6:262–268.

48. Robert Schleip, Thomas W. Findley, Leon Chaitow and Peter A. Huijing, *Fascia: The Tensional Network of the Human Body*, Churchill Livingstone/Elsevier, Edinburgh, 2012.

49. R. Schleip, D.G. Müller (2013) Training principles for fascial connective tissues: scientific foundation and suggested practical applications. *Journal of Bodywork and Movement Therapies* 17:103–105.

50. Tom Flemons made and sold toys designed on tensegrity principles for many years. His "Skwish" toys were licensed to a local company to manufacture in 1987. Manhattan Toys subsequently bought that company and the licensing rights in 1995. (See also Ch. 6.)

11

The Elastic Breath

"There is an intimate connection between the breath, nerve currents and control of the inner prana or vital forces. Prana becomes visible on the physical plane as motion and action and on the mental plane as thought. Pranayama is the means by which a yogi tries to realise within his individual body the whole cosmic nature."[1]

Swami Sivananda

The Breath is Round

Much like the original cell (of us) and the planet upon which we breathe, the breath occurs naturally in 360 degrees of roundness. However we describe it, it somehow helps to remember this in practice. It is important in understanding the biotensegrity of the breath.

Lengthy descriptions of the anatomy and biomechanics of breathing function may provide useful information. However, lest we forget in our hunger for naming parts, the breath is round and we survive because the air *surrounding* us is alchemised into something we call Life Force. Yoga calls it Prana. Martial arts call it Chi or Qi or Ki. Whatever it is, it animates our form and functions.

It is more than "the breath". It accounts for the integration and transfiguration of the resource that air provides into the living energy that everything alive on this planet requires to survive and thrive. Access to oxygen, through water and air, via all the maths, physics and chemistry of our biologic forms, relies on our structural *volume* – our geometry, to proceed. We live and breathe in the round.

That roundness is essential and it is that essential roundness that we take for granted and forget in classical, hard-matter physics-based explanations of breath and motion. It takes us back to the chapters on the embryo (Ch. 4), on biotensegrity (Ch. 6) and on the Elastic Body, preceding this one. The Hoberman's Sphere is a valuable asset for setting this context of wholeness before we go into finer explanations of the breath as a functional mechanism – or the more subtle categories and sub-categories that yogic practice of pranayama invites us to consider in more detail.

The bones do not touch each other, but "float" like the bones of a corset, within the weave of the fascial matrix; its closed kinematic chain structure acts similarly to the Hoberman's sphere. That doesn't mean we have a Hoberman's sphere inside our thorax; it means the pattern of the torso matrix is organised under CKC rules; we are rounded, not spherical – the model is an example of force transmission patterns. See Figure 11.2 for the CKC fascial pattern.

John Sharkey has pointed out in various educational settings that the word "contraction" means "to shrink". We don't shrink when we exhale, or when we inhale. Furthermore, as we saw in Chapter 5 and continue to recognise throughout this work, muscles don't relax (or shrink for that matter). It bears repeating that muscles only know how to contract. Like every neuro-myo-osseo-fascial integration of movement (not to exclude the viscera), breathing includes the ability of our volume to *appear* to fill up and empty. That does not mean "collapse" or "shrink" in any way; it means to harness the elastic recoil mechanism that animates the entire tide of the breath. In truth, we appear to "expand" and to "in-draw" as a reciprocal dance of the torso's volumetric ability to tension and compress globally, with a wonderful symphony of movements included, as we will explore.

Breath is synonymous with aspects of spirit in many languages: "Allah" means the Great Breath; Atman (Hindu) mean Eternal Self, "Atmen" (German) means "breath", inspira (Spanish), inspirer (French) mean both inhale and inspire; in English "respiration" comes from "re-spiriting" or bringing spirit in, as inspiration implies illumination. We can be inspired by a new idea, a new pose or a new project. It is the spirit of life itself, expressed uniquely in each one of us, whatever path we take in life. We all have to breathe.

The first image shows the ball at its smallest, never reduced to zero, modelling the in-drawing of the full or active exhalation represented by the left hand side of Figure 11.1. The second image shows the same structure towards the mid-point. It begins to represent the middle phase of the breath, which is neither expanded nor in-drawn: our resting tension. This is the place of natural dynamic stability, poised for movement (we are at rest, with the lungs semi-inflated; they are invariably pre-tensioned). This is approximating the middle phase in Figure 11.1. In the third image the ball is almost expanded, modelling the movement of the fuller inhalation. The last shows the ball fully expanded, modelling the full, active inhalation. Together these links enclose a space. If you were to add fabric and tension it, connected to and spaced by floating compression members, you would have something resembling the architecture of our torso responding in the range in which we breathe.

This "opening and closing" of a closed, kinematic chain mechanism that is whole and complete (in the round) will be referred to here as the "expansion and in-drawing" motions of breathing. It is an important distinction that deliberately avoids "contraction and relaxation" of muscles (see Ch. 5).

The "expansion and in-drawing" capability is the essence of the breathing mechanism (if we have to refer to it as that). The maths of it (pressure gradients), the physics (soft-matter and electro-magnetic impulses), the chemistry (gaseous exchange), the anatomy (of various structures) and the biomechanics (see Chs 6 and 8) are all subject to the recognition of roundness as a simple but significant foundation to this enquiry. There is NOTHING linear about the breath, EVER. It is based entirely on volume; the expansion and in-drawing to appropriate constraints of a closed kinematic chain *volume*tric architecture. That volume is in biotensegral balance of the lung pockets to the thorax, of the lateral diaphragms to the torso, or the in-breath to the out-breath. Analyse it as you like, it is the source of our life force. No breath; no life. The end.

Then there is that metaphysical notion of spirit. Interestingly (given my primary fascination with language) the word for "breathing" in many languages is associated with "spirit"; that invisible force that breathes us in spite of ourselves. It is the exceptional system of the body that is both voluntary and involuntary; the one we can learn to control to some extent, however we cannot hold our own breath to the point of asphyxiation. Nature (or some force greater than us), it seems, has the last word on that matter!

Round things form themselves into pockets, tubes, pouches and soft-matter organisations, which (at their finest) form (and are formed by) threads (*nadis*) that can then weave themselves into tubular, lattice-like arrangements (see Ch 10). (This is along the structural notion, of weaving a closed basket out of woven, triple-helical strings – see Ch. 10, Fig 10.12.) Examples of this are the gut tube, the bronchi and the vessels of neurovascular tracts, lymphatics and so on. The torso itself is a tube, so this system of closed kinematic chains (elongated and integrated as they invariably

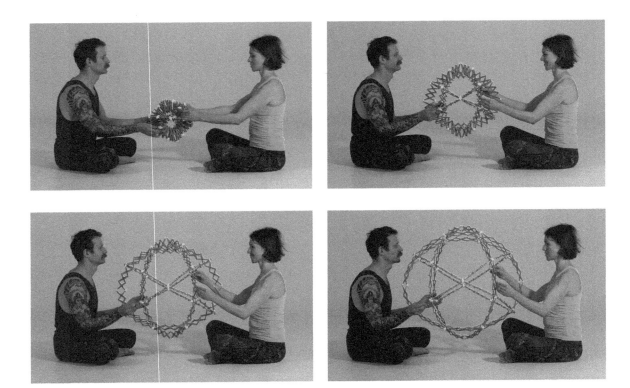

Figure 11.1

Hoberman's Sphere. People pick up this model and instinctively recognise it as representative of the breathing motion. Its roundness invites that recognition and echoes our structure.

become) moves everything else on the basis of biotensegrity. It is moved *by* everything else moving, on every scale; all aspects operate under the same structural laws.

A background metronome by which the rest of the bodily systems syncopate, with the heart-rate and other rhythms, is the breath. Whatever the symphony being conducted at the time, the breath precedes and performs and proceeds from it. The yogis consider this a super-subtle, integrated suite of subtle energies, motions and performances. They have names and distinctions for all of them. (Sanskrit tends to be a very poetic and subtly nuanced language that we simply cannot match with Western linguistic equivalents.) We can't make *any* sense of all that detail within our own *felt sense* or haptic perception or proprioception, from learning intellectual lists of named parts. Whether that is the classical Western anatomical attachments of the variously named primary and secondary breathing muscles or the Eastern somatic categories and sub-categories of the pranas and vayus (and so on), *we experience breath as a volume*. That is, in the round, wrapped in the intricate webbing

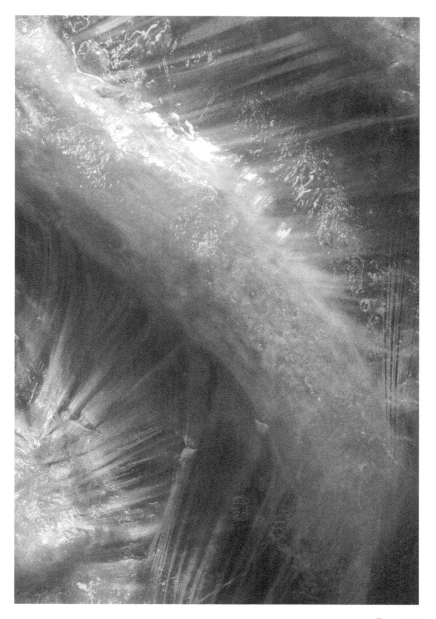

Figure 11.2

This beautiful image of a section of one rib in the rib-basket makes this point visually. The fascial wrappings of the intercostal myofascial web weave in a lattice-like arrangement around the entire structure. The torso is a tube, the wrappings and counter-wrappings (chirals and counter-chiral tubular weaves) of the torso can respond continuously to all the pressure differentials and senses of breathing motion *as a whole* – to modify an *appropriate response at the time*. The lattice-like organisation is ubiquitous.

(Reproduced with kind permission from John Sharkey.)

Pranayama

When we become conscious of
the breath it feels like an expansive
expression of the spirit-of-life force:
a deepening of presence and awareness. Pranayama is also a key feature
of conscious self-regulation: you can
gauge instantly, by the breath, how you
are doing. We know that stillness is an
attribute of an integrating nervous
system or, we could say, neuro-myo-
osseo-viscero-fascial integrity! (See
Ch. 5.) Perhaps the ancient yogic sages
understood this profoundly (without
naming it as such!). They introduced
Vipassana[2] to help us learn how to
harness and nourish the values of
stillness to our physical, emotional and
animated bodies, fostering our ability
to self-regulate, without over-thinking.
Whatever you believe spiritually, this
was a larger foundation of learning
various ways of mastering the physical
realm, through our awareness of it *as
distinct*. The purpose of performing
asana, was to explore and foster a more
powerful Pranayama practice and

of all the fascial matrix, as a whole; all the time we are breathing in a natural,
non-pathological way.

In the yoga classroom, we generally classify the breathing "techniques" as Pranayama practice. The word prana translates as "life force" and ayama means
"extension or expansion". We could say it is the expansion of life force in the
body. That is a function of reciprocal in-drawing; it is how we breathe from a
living tensegrity point of view.

We can recall from Chapter 2 that these subtle aspects, or invisible forces,
of the human spirit, or emotions, had been segregated from the domain of
functional anatomy when early science began to develop four centuries ago.
Yoga wasn't created from quite such reductionist principles. Its origins in
Ayurvedic Medicine are very different.

Pranayama is sometimes thought, in the West, to mean "breath control".
The yogic path is considered to include the "ways" known as "yamas" and
"niyamas" (**yamas:** *ways;* **niyamas:** *personal ways or observances*) followed by
devotees of yoga. Sometimes associated with "ways of controlling" the senses
or mind, for example, Pranayama, can be *misinterpreted* as prana+yama; i.e.
breath control. It actually derives from *prana + ayama* (meaning *expansion*),
so it invites us to subtly extend our selves beyond the physical domain, to the
benefits of expanding *awareness*. It does not actually mean imposing correct
actions (i.e. breathing techniques) upon the body. Its true meaning invites us
to expand into a fuller potential or possibility, rather than be constrained by
a method of control. It can become a very simple and rewarding practice. We
might hold it as "pre-position" rather than "im-position" as a valuable way to
become familiar with being aware of where we are in space and how we are
at the time as a body: a deepening of our proprioceptive sense, one breath at
a time.

"Although breathing is mainly an unconscious process, conscious control of it may be taken at any
time. Consequently, it forms a bridge between the conscious and unconscious areas of the mind.
Through the practice of Pranayama, the energy trapped in neurotic, unconscious mental patterns
may be released for use in more creative and joyful activity"[3]

develop meditative studies to transcend the physical aspects of the being,
to enhance the energetic subtleties,
beyond the bodily sensations. This
state of formlessness is not a "thing",
nor can language do it justice; let's
just say, it lives beyond the intellectual
descriptions of breathing mechanics or
machinery!

Perhaps this speaks to the Medial and Lateral Lemniscus pathways we referred
to in Chapter 5. For sure, the body of work in yoga based upon the values
of developing a breathing practice is one of the distinguishing features of
yoga and possibly its therapeutic values.[4] Valuable research is currently being
undertaken regarding the "respiratory pace-maker" of the breath,[5] governing
many aspects of interoception and the limbic system. According to practitioners like Ben Wolff,[6] the rhythmical pacing of the breath has far reaching
consequence to the biomotional being. Adult humans breathe 21,600 times
per day[7] and for many of us this breathing can be local and shallow, rapid

and rushed, especially when we are under pressure to meet daily demands. Our full capacity to bring life-giving oxygen into the body, for all its myriad functions (allowing waste gases to be efficiently released and recycled), seems linked to much more than the obvious physiological functions. In the early 1900s, the average healthy breathing rhythm was considered to be 6–8 breaths per minute.[8] That is somewhere in the region of an eight-to-ten-second inhale and an eight-to-ten-second exhale. The average breathing rhythm of an adult human being in the 2000s, a century later, is somewhere nearer 18–22 breaths per minute. That is between two and three times faster, approximately 3 seconds per inhale and per exhale, as a Resting Breathing Rate.

That is an interesting indicator of cultural change and it is worth considering if that is progress, since we haven't had much evolutionary time to establish the ability to adapt to live at a pace our Great-Great-Grandparents might have considered a daily 24-hour sprint. In an age where information is faster than instant (it somehow even precedes our need sometimes), our ancestors would arguably be stunned on several counts.

It seems we don't always use the extra time afforded us (by rapid acquisition of information), to relax and savour it. We use it to manipulate more information in a shorter time, so we are almost holding our breath to complete tasks – as if we were in a fairly common state of what our ancestors would have considered an emergency. What this effectively does is lose our optimal Resting Tension, or natural homeostasis (or allostasis); something that the Elastic Breath Cycle teaches very simply and accessibly. It can support anyone, in or out of a yoga classroom. It can be done anywhere, easily and it serves as a reminder on many levels that presence (of mind, body and being) is a valuable asset! Let's consider the contemporary and yogic models.

Elastic Breath Cycle

Classical anatomy addresses individual breathing muscles, such as the diaphragm, the intercostals, the scalenes, quadratus lumborum and so on, as separate entities. The body does not experience breathing in this way, however, although we are capable of focusing our attention on a single area of the body at a time as an exercise. From a biotensegrity point of view, the connective tissues account for the geometry of our breathing architecture in 360 degrees. If we remember, the embryo forms the spine and the cavities of the torso in continuity, growing them around and down (head towards tail) from folding and enfolding spaces to form the various pockets they enclose (see Ch. 4). We might reasonably consider that our bodies do not separate its breathing muscles into categories (as embryos or adults). We have established it does not function as individual muscles, but as *incorporated* bio-*motion*. We breathe as a whole, amplifying the rhythm according to requirement, echoed throughout the force transmission system that is the fascial matrix. Levers are difficult to find in our breathing apparatus; largely, perhaps, because they don't exist.

The multi-bar ball, the Hoberman's Sphere that we first examined in Chapter 9, is clearly representative of a breathing model in three-dimensional form,

What is key here is that understanding the breath as a crucial subliminal rhythm provider (see Ch. 6) is another of the biotensegral properties that affect the nature and emergent properties of liquid crystal forms – like us. The rate at which we expand and in-draw the torso and body has an impact on the degree and style to which we can. Breathing rapidly can tend towards a shallower depth in order to meet a faster demand, especially if we are physically sitting at a desk, moving little more than our fingers at a keyboard, if that. Our ancestors would have had to move to get information (go to a library or lift a book or visit an exhibition). We can acquire masses of information with only a mobile smartphone and an active thumb.

in the round. It demonstrates how the body seeks compliance, not permission, from each coordinating muscle (or myofascial) group in the torso. An example of this type of multi-bar structure can be seen in Figure 11.1.

A great mini-model of the breathing torso is the Chinese Finger Puzzle (Fig. 11.4). The weave of our tissues around the thorax is formed in the embryonic pulses of our most primitive development (see Ch. 4). The forming cavities work as a whole and in reciprocal responses between the diaphragms (pelvic floor, respiratory diaphragm, thoracic inlet and so on). Before we consider the yogic forms and formalities of Pranayama (or exercising the bandhas individually), there is value in recognising a model of how all these diaphragms work in a united rhythm as a completely enfolded, enclosed form. The basis of the exercises associated with them is to improve elastic compliance throughout.

"In biotensegrity, the 'four-bar' is a 3-D vector equilibrium tensegrity icosahedron. It naturally oscillates. The rate can be changed by changing tension (tone) in the system. At any instant, there may be a phase change, and tension may become compression and vice versa. The models we make are only an instant in time and only exist in our imagination. Even when 'paused', movement is present at some scale."[9]

As John Sharkey points out: *"in the models we have two materials, in the body we have only one"*. It is almost impossible to represent this in two dimensions but in your hands, by opening and closing (pulsing) a multi-bar structure (illustrated in Fig. 11.1), you sense the rhythm of your pulse, the breath and the oscillation of the whole body as a part of the expression of the elastic breath, in the round. All the "linkage" points of this model conform to the biotensegral geometries of a living structure, or overlap of tissue organisation in the body. The principles of biphasic movement and elasticity are held in the midpoint balance that represents our **resting tension** (see Ch. 10 and Fig. 11.3). This effectively means we balance and counterbalance every breath we take. We live in poised potential; our resting tension is balanced between extremes, breathing (in and out) from the mid-point of the semi-tensioned elastic band in Chapter 10.

Natural Breathing Rhythm

Many yogic breathing practices are designed to animate and strengthen different aspects of the breath. If we consider them from the perspective of biotensegrity, however, the fundamental theme of enhancing elasticity, rhythm and compliance runs through them all.

In class, whatever the ability or age of the group, this one value (of elastic compliance) can provide potent access to breathing well. The elastic breath cycle is designed as an exercise to be done consciously for a few minutes, at most twice a day. The breathing body is instinctive and it is not designed for us to think it through the day's activities. In healthy bodies we can, for the most part, sense our own breathing rhythm.

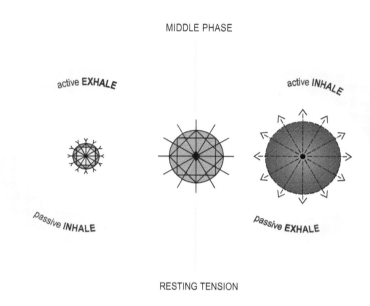

ELASTIC BREATH CYCLE

MIDDLE PHASE

active **EXHALE**

active **INHALE**

passive **INHALE**

passive **EXHALE**

RESTING TENSION

Figure 11.3

The Elastic Breath Cycle provides a simplified structural breathing exercise (and visual reference) for a biologically, biomotionally integrated breath as a resource. It works on the fundamental principles of living tensegrity patterns, in practical application. (Exercise below.) The practice elaborates the biotensegrity architecture of our fascial form in breathing. It works in practice as a simple foundation, recognising the middle phase as our relaxed state.

(Reproduced with kind permission from Art of Contemporary Yoga Ltd. Artwork by Bex Hawkins.)

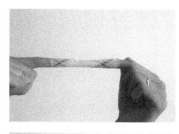

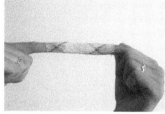

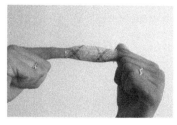

Figure 11.4

Chinese finger puzzle.

Intensive Pranayama sessions can cause distress if people change their breathing patterns too rapidly or hold them to an imposed rhythm that does not suit their body. It is possible to over-breathe. It is important to start from wherever the person is at the time, making small incremental changes.

This subtle and simple practice can, over time, lead to improved regulation of the breath and more refined and expansive utilisation of the full breathing capacity. This in turn, from the fascial perspective, balances the polarities of elasticity and stiffness (i.e. in service to compliance). It can expand our sense of life force and our sense of being present in the body, which can have far reaching psychosomatic and subtle benefits.

"So the physical and the breathing components are actually facilitating this central process, which is the meditative process. And the meditative process is not just a cognitive technique; you're actually changing brain function. When you change brain function you change brain physiology you change brain anatomy. Literally the brain is plastic, so as you do different tasks mentally, the brain will actually change in that direction, so this ends up being very profound.

Even though many people are thinking 'well it's just a mental game', but it's actually changing brain structure and function."[8,10]

As far as the anatomy is concerned, it raises interesting questions. If you accept biotensegrity as the basis of our architecture and include the fascial matrix as a body-wide tensional system that is literally everywhere, then what myofascia is not involved in breathing? The breath itself must be a primary

Foundation Work

signaling motion, communicated throughout the architecture: moment by moment and breath by breath. Breath is universally accepted as a sign of life force. Placing value on elasticity (i.e. energy storage capacity) as an important feature of its architecture is a global gesture towards every local aspect of our vitality. You do not have to be a yogi to

Respiratory Tensional Integrity

appreciate this notion (or to enjoy the benefits of breathing well and being able to respond accordingly to life's circumstances). Elastic energy is free; a labored breath is a metabolically expensive one. So the more natural compliance, the more light and efficient the breath.

This is one of the reasons it is important to learn to sit optimally (see Part C, Ch. 13), so that breathing practice can be done without compromise to the elastic integrity of the spine and breathing motion, throughout the body. Using support to maintain ease in the spine is preferable to forcing "uprightness" for its own sake, with muscular effort. The reason for practising breath work in sitting is to work with attentiveness without falling asleep! (It is also recommended to practice this, or any Pranayama techniques, on an empty stomach so that the body is not preoccupied with digestion.) The practice itself can improve the ability to sit at ease. They are mutually beneficial.

In essence these exercises are not designed to impose "right ways" of breathing on the body. Rather, they train the breathing movements for enhanced compliance and expand the capacity to vary the breathing rate and elasticity naturally, neutrally to meet a fuller range of possibilities. They improve the natural function of one of our most primitive, original biomotional rhythms; closely related as breathing is to the heart. The lungs grow around the heart (Ch. 4), intimately relating their cooperating structures.

The practice of these very simple exercises begins to develop awareness of this life-giving resource we happily ignore (because it generally works pretty well whether we think about it or not). This is foundation work, ideal before going on to more advanced practices, so that changes can be naturally incorporated without any adverse or extreme reactions. Fascia responds to its loading history and, as it takes a long time to develop a sub-optimal breathing pattern, it may take a while to gradually develop a new, more optimal one. It is rewarding to take any new breathing practices slowly, almost imperceptibly, through a gradual journey of incremental improvement, over time.

The lungs rest semi-inflated, at about 50% full (or 50% empty, depending on your point of view). That is their **resting tension**: technically termed the *pre-stiffened*, or *pre-tensioned* state of our *resting architecture*. Compliance relies on this feature for the ability to expand from it (towards fullness, exceeding 50%) and in-draw from it (towards emptiness, less than 50%).

The initial purpose of the breathing practices is to strengthen and enhance capacity of the breathing-related tissues in their entirety, including the lungs and surrounding architectures, to optimise healthy range and responsiveness. This can improve balance between the various related systems of the body (all of which could be considered to benefit from cardio-respiratory efficiency). In tension–compression balance, this full range of capacity between full exhale and full inhale (between which extremes we find resting tension at the mid-point) could be considered as biotensegrity regulation of the whole breathing apparatus.

This is how tensional integrity can work in 360 degrees. If the spine is able to relax and restore its natural curvature without undue strain (i.e. you can sit curved-upright in comfort), then it follows that the morphology of our integrated breathing apparatus is less compromised and more optimised (i.e. the primary curve of the ribs is in place and the secondary curves of the waist and neck allow for the exercises to be done in optimal positions for the head and tail (see Ch. 13).

Elastic Breath Exercise

Find a comfortable seated position. (Initially it may be useful to work supine to establish the rhythm, or in a comfortable supportive chair or on cushions with the back supported by a wall; use support until it becomes a more natural posture.)

The active inhale (expansion)

Let the breath settle at the natural mid-point. Softly inhale, experiencing the breath through the nostrils and into the body with a feeling of expansion. Inhale as far as possible, with a sense of tensioning (filling) the whole torso and all the details of the tissues between the ribs, under the arms, throughout the back, front and sides, the upper and lower parts of the body. Pause to observe the "peak" of the inhale for a moment.

The passive exhale (release)

Let the breath release gradually and it will naturally find the mid-point of "resting tension" as the exhale is releasing. The breathing action continues *through* this point. It does not stop there. (A shallow breathing pattern can be observed in people who inhale and exhale to and from this point only; they are using only the right side of the schema in the illustration (see Fig. 11.1).) The exercise asks us to continue through the middle phase, in smooth transition.

The active exhale

As smoothly as possible, begin to activate and "squeeze" the exhale, effectively compressing the rib basket in the round. The tissues that were tensioned on the inhale are now being drawn together. Keep squeezing them until the whole torso is gently compressed, along the length of the spine. This is an active sense of drawing inward of the ribs and abdomen, tightening all the tissues of the body wall toward the spine. Observe the end-point of this active exhale when all the breath feels squeezed out of the body, without collapse. The torso is tensioned and stiffened by squeezing, into temporary compression.

Passive inhale (release)

Let the breath release gradually and the body will naturally find the mid-point again, only this time it is a passive inhale as release (see Fig. 11.1). This is one whole breathing cycle. In smooth transition, it elaborates expansion into tension and squeeze into compression, at both ends of the elasticity scale. A healthy body with a naturally compliant breathing pattern will do this anyway. A less compliant pattern can be observed using only one side of the chart. In either case, there is value in observing the breath and extending gently and consciously through the full cycle.

Repeat the exercise quietly, without overworking the breath, simply becoming aware of the torso's ability to expand globally and squeeze globally, through the "middle way" or mid-point of the resting tension. The lungs rest here at about 50% inflated when we are relaxed. Pause between cycles if required.

Transitions become the key. After five rounds, rest and return to normal breathing. Over time, this exercise can be increased in small increments: more rounds and slightly greater range. It is designed to train elastic integrity and the meditative ability to observe the breath. It eventually becomes instinctive.

This is a Basic Technique to animate a healthy neutral breathing pattern. Rhythm is personal. This is a foundation practice to all other Pranayama techniques. There are many and various Pranayama practices in yoga, originally designed for a variety of reasons, bodies and circumstances. Kapalabhati, for example (Skull Shining), focuses on strengthening the elastic recoil of the *in-drawing phase* (exhale), the left side of the schema in Figure 11.3 and thereby contributes powerfully to elastic integrity. The elastic breath exercise is not designed to replace established ancient and valuable yoga practices. It is offered as a relatively simple foundation practice; a way to prepare for more advanced work with the yogic bandhas and traditional Pranayama techniques. Skull Shining (Kapalabhati) is a metaphor for "polishing" the inner pathways; it is a cleansing, illuminating breath. The cleansing practices are the Kriyas, designed to purify the body. In this

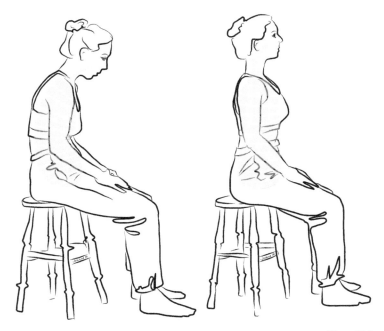

Figure 11.5

The breath fills the deepest part of us; it provides a rhythm that is shaped by our posture and, in turn, shapes it (see margin note).

Transitions

case the Kapalabhati serves the central nerve pathways, hence the reference to illuminating the being – making the skull shiny. (We engage a similar idea in phrases such as "her face lit up" when describing someone feeling *inspired*.) Indeed, after doing the Kriyas, people often do look brighter, or shiny! They are lit up with the effect of the deeper benefits of yogic practice. *N.B. It is advisable to be guided in the Pranayama practices by an experienced teacher. Understanding how to work with Bandhas, Kriyas and advanced Pranayama practices is not a list of*

The essence of this exercise is the smoothness of *gliding between transitions*. Through mastering the quality of transitions, the flow of the breath can become rhythmical and harmonious at various rates. The stillness of meditation and the speed of a Vinyasa Flow class with the variations in between can all eventually be readily and instinctively accommodated without needing to overstrain the body; it's a valuable and gentle purpose.

By reinforcing the natural elasticity of breathing compliance, the quality of rebound of elastic energy storage capacity accumulates it. Eventually it renders these movements relatively effortless. While the breathing becomes more efficient and acquires more range, so the elastic balance of the tissues improves and demands less metabolically expensive muscular effort and retains more natural spring. It can impact everything on a body-wide basis, because a yoga practice pays such specific attention to breathing for its own sake. It is capable of endorsing the benefits of breath containment, and just by carrying out this small practice on a regular basis,

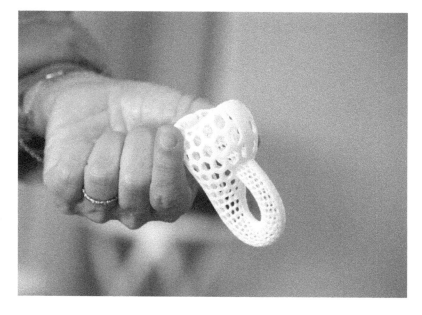

Figure 11.6

This shape is effectively a 4D Möbius strip; a shape that has enclosed and moved through itself in complete continuity. The inside becomes the outside in a continuum.

in appropriate dose and degree, the tissues of your whole fascial matrix can become cumulatively more responsive, with the smallest incremental changes. Imagine saving a tiny dot of energy (remember elastic energy is free) more than 21,000 times per day *anyway* just because you are enjoying a more naturally Elastic Breath; it *has* to become a valuable investment over time!

The Pranic Body

A Möbius is the name given to a shape, like a figure-of-eight, with a particular quality. If you take a strip of paper and join the two ends to form a circle, but add a twist to the paper first, it forms a Möbius strip in which the outside becomes the inside; they unite as the one form. If you trace the outside of the shape with your finger you will find yourself on the inside (and vice versa) as you go around it. It becomes a useful metaphor/visualisation in this practice. It is one of the foundations of biotensegrity, since many myofascial aspects of the body incorporate elaborate folds and follow this geometric progression. In multi-dimensions, this forms a shape called a Klein bottle, a volume where the inside and outside are in complete continuity. Scarr

Yoga considers the body in very subtle ways, including our energetic field, or something that might relate to the "kinesphere" and "innersphere" we alluded to in previous chapters. Compared to Western anatomy and physiology, it includes different aspects of our being and our functions in its subtle but important distinctions. Considered to be the most vital process of the body, and closely related to all the others, Pranayama influences and nourishes every part of us; however, it is understood as more than just functional breathing. It represents an essentially qualitative aspect of quality in our movement practice. Like the hub of a biotensegrity wheel, it is believed to give us access to health in psyche and soma, in all directions.

Yogis believe that if Prana does not flow through the channels (the nadis, considered as threads or meridians throughout the body and limbs), or if it becomes blocked (possibly at the region of, or in relation to, a particular chakra), it is a reason for disease or dysfunction. (The nadis are possibly synonymous at the microscopic scale, with the tubular network of the fascial matrix.)

This can be observed at the physical level of non-compliance in the tissues. In this case, rather than breathing with natural elastic integrity, the body recruits extra muscular effort to "fund" these otherwise natural rhythms when suggests this pattern may belong to the body in terms of several myofascial organisations.

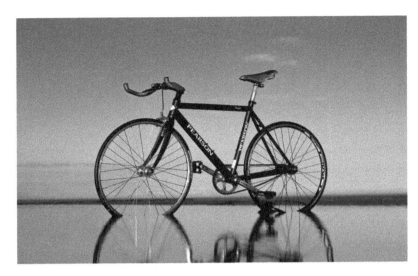

Figure 11.7

A bicycle wheel is a tensegrity structure. A wheel, in yoga, is a "Chakra". The Chakras denote energy centres, with specific frequencies, which tend to be part of the more metaphysical aspects of our individual movement signatures.

(Photo by Zoltan Tasi on Unsplash.)

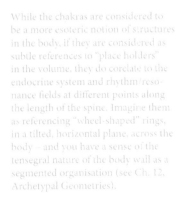

While the chakras are considered to be a more esoteric notion of structures in the body, if they are considered as subtle references to "place holders" in the volume, they do corelate to the endocrine system and rhythm/resonance fields at different points along the length of the spine. Imagine them as referencing "wheel-shaped" rings, in a tilted, horizontal plane, across the body – and you have a sense of the tensegral nature of the body wall as a segmented organisation (see Ch. 12, Archetypal Geometries).

they are structurally or emotionally blocked or disturbed, or adhered. It does this autonomically and it can directly link or accumulate to the dis-ease and distress that ill health or injury can cause. Relentless or unresolved stress, poor diet, sedentary activities or overexertion and other features of a lifestyle that is not in balance, can obstruct pranic flow and deplete vital energy. (This correlates with depletion of energy storage and therefore elasticity.) The practice of Pranayama is considered to be restorative and revitalising if the "pranas" can be brought into balance. However, this is not a set of "symptoms" for which a "pill" can be administered. It is more akin to a series of events or even feedback loops that may seem stuck and can be restored through these simple practices. Needless to say it is not an intellectual process of the reasoning mind. We have to do it; participate in animating it consciously to begin uncovering these benefits.

Fascia responds to its loading history; subtly accumulated in the motion of breathing just as it is in the movements of the postures. In animated real life, on the mat, we can effectively restore shallow or irregular breathing patterns to more optimal ones. Eventually, they can be managed and organised in a more healthy way so that they allow the breath to respond in more instinctive and adaptable compliance, naturally expressive of elastic integrity. As teachers we can guide and facilitate this process, but this is an area where forcefulness (self-imposed or otherwise) seems to fail. The participant must want to participate. We are working to enhance and recognise (or even reveal) the most profound and subtle forces that are already there. The purpose is to accumulate valuable *default* breathing patterns rather than learn breathing techniques, if they are imposed. It is a subtle but important distinction.

The Vital Energy Body

Yoga considers the human framework to consist of (and operate in) several dimensions, including the material body, the mental body, the vital energy body, the psychic body and the transcendental body.[13] This is a different vital anatomy based on living beings (as distinct from that generally inferred from the evidence of cadavers in classical Western medicine). It is not necessarily more right or wrong but it does lend itself to a more sophisticated possibility for how we experience ourselves as humans breathing. It speaks to a subtlety and variability found in soft matter, distinct from the hard-matter-based physics of classical biomechanical descriptions of respiratory function.

In yoga, these pranic bodies organise together to form an integral whole. **It is their mutual congruency that yoga seeks to reflect in our body.** It is the vital energy body (Pranamaya Kosha) to which the main practices of Pranayama refer. These are known as the five Pranas (capital "P") including: prana, apana, samana, udana and vyana. Between them they allow an interesting and subtle context for our balanced breathing patterns. These qualitative distinctions are more recognisable in terms of our earliest expression of life, in embryogenesis (Ch. 4).

"The techniques of pranayama provide the method whereby the life force can be activated and regulated in order to go beyond one's normal boundaries or limitations and attain a higher state of vibratory energy and awareness."[5]

Prana (that is Prana with a capital "P") is all-pervading life force (global). The five pranas (small "p" – see Table 11.1) are within the body and express Prana in relation to its location and related functions (local). They are called the five vayus, or "inner winds". They imply direction; for example, apana is associated with the eliminative organs. The movement associated with it is through the skin, via the urogenital system (birth and excretion) and through the mouth (as exhalation or regurgitation). Within these classifications are five "sub-pranas" which include hiccoughing, sneezing, and so on. It is a different *quality* of classification that nevertheless accounts for all our bodily functions. As we would describe the weather in terms of perhaps a light breeze, or a strong wind, or a gale, the yogis use similar distinctions to denote different levels of energy and quality of energy flow or current, through physical expressions of the living body. These are expressed as different *pranic states*.

The direction is also relevant, as the appropriate flow of prana in the nadis (energy channels throughout the body) is considered paramount. When one of the pranas is "out" it throws the subtle and interrelated network off balance. This is expressed as "dis-ease" or imbalance in the body. When the flow, quality and direction of the pranas are appropriate, they are thought to express health and vitality. These are what we refer to as "autonomic" functions as when they function naturally and congruently they do so without us having to think about it – they are involuntary. The breath, however, is both involuntary and voluntary. Thus it can be considered as a portal to animating and even illuminating life force (Prana) within us, if we consciously practice Pranayama.

Table 11.1

The pranas

prana refers, in this context, to the flow of energy governing the cavity of the thorax from the thoracic inlet to the diaphragm (pleural and pericardial cavities). It includes the heart and main organs of respiration together with the nerves and all the tissues that directly activate them. The fabric and forces that draw the breath into the body are included here. (The animation of the inhale and the mesodermal features of the embryonic forming.)

apana refers to the flow of energy governing the cavity between the diaphragm and the pelvic floor (peritoneal cavity), including the large intestine, kidneys and urogenital system. These animate the fabric and forces that fully release the breath out of the body. (Exhalation, relating to the endodermal layer in the embryo.)

samana is between the heart and the navel, activating the digestive system and associated with transformation (solar plexus and umbilicus; the original embryonic connection to the nutritive maternal source). Literally this is the transformation of food into nourishing nutrients. It can also symbolise the transformation of the conceptus to the embryo (of birth and expansion of consciousness).

udana refers to the neck and head, including the sensory platform (of eyes, ears, nose, tongue) harmonising the sensory tissues, skin, nerves and joints of the limbs and spine. It activates efficient, easy spinal posture and responsiveness to the outside world. It refers to and governs sensory awareness. We might consider it inclusive of, but not separate from, the original organisation of the ectodermal layer in the embryo.

vyana is everywhere in the body, regulating all movement and orchestrating the other pranas. It is described as their "reserve force". We might relate this to the role of mesenchyme in the embryo, being everywhere, and the extracellular matrix in the adult.

The Purpose of Pranayama Practice

Each different style of yoga explores different ways of utilizing the breathing techniques. They are universal; however, they can be misused if knowledge is inadequate or sufficient attention is not paid to their subtleties and power and the individual learning them. A yoga therapist or a Kundalini Master understands the nuanced qualities and abilities associated with the different techniques and the appropriate times for teaching and animating them in an individual. It is recommended that they should not be used without appropriate knowledge, guidance and respect.

Whether you stick to the simplest of conscious breathing exercises, or develop the more specific practices of Pranayama techniques, one of the many valuable assets of this work is fostering the ability to be still at will. As we considered in Chapter 5 (Sensory Architecture), the ability to be still is an expression of a coordinated, healthy system. It means the nervous system can inhibit random movement, at choice. We tend to focus on what we can do and how "well" (by whatever standards) we can do it. However, there is much to be said for the ability to choose to "not" be in action, but in "active" or "dynamic stillness".

The purpose of yoga, before the organisation and order of postures was formalized in the West, was to prepare the body for sitting in meditation, to transcend the needs of the physical domain. Ultimately, the yogi learns to acquire complete authority over bodily function. Even with its promise of enlightened practices, the breath work is often used to train the body to be able to sit still in meditation, to simply rest deeply as a counterbalance to activity.

Meditation is beyond the scope of this work, as there are many valuable books on the advantages and various styles of meditative practices. Resting, to breathe well, on a regular basis does not need to be a formal meditation. Its value in simply "pressing the pause button" on a regular basis can provide a profound and cumulative resource in our madly busy, fast-track, rapid-breathing-rate society. Yoga Nidra,[14] for example, can help in calming the system so that an easy breathing rhythm can naturally arise.

Meditative Breathing

A Footnote on Paradoxical Breathing

Once the foundations of the simple breathing exercise, the Elastic Breath, or other Pranayama practices are established, there are various specific practices (particularly for meditation purposes) that are designed to gradually refine Pranayama in the individual. Vipassana is the most well-known of these: a meditative practice that begins with simple observation of the breath. We eventually develop the ability to be still and observe the body from the quiet and calm perspective of the (inner) witness. Using various breathing techniques can improve refinement and the ability to move and balance energy within the body. This is at levels that might not be immediately available to us before developing a foundation practice, along with more extensive and personally guided work in Pranayama. Like any other practice, once it becomes instinctive we do not have to think about it. Its care of both the local and global aspects of the breathing body and being, foster exactly the principles that biotensegrity explains.

When an optimal breathing pattern arises from the elastic breath, a natural flow between transitions of expansion and in-drawing, *the neutral state of resting tension,* becomes more accessible and appears to arise spontaneously without force or effort. In that place, the body is naturally ready to spend a while in reflection, or contemplation, or meditation, whatever kind is enjoyed. Meditation is designed to enhance the possibility of that balance arising and so it is encouraged by the very simple exercise of balancing expansion and in-drawing. The natural and neutral state of resting tension can become a place of rest, within the tidal rhythms of the breath. It translates to a kind of "composure" in the body, the "quiescence" we referred to in Chapter 10.

The purpose is to establish balance in the fascial architecture of the breathing form, as a profound, natural resource. It incorporates the assets of free energy as described in Chapter 10; elasticity is the expression of our energy storage capacity. Springing to life, a spring in the step, are natural states of a pretensioned architecture; which is our default design. This can then become the foundation in other physical disciplines and competitive sports and also more esoteric pursuits, e.g. advanced meditation practices to take us beyond the animation of the physical body to the illumination of the more subtle bodies (koshas) that yoga also respects.

Paradoxical breathing is both common and quite complex; however, it is worth mentioning so that it can at least be recognised. This type of breathing is often associated with trauma and specific pathologies. It involves reverse responses internally to the natural motion and pressure balances between the body cavities in the normal, healthy breath cycle. In practice, the movement of breath behaves as paradoxical to the pressure response of expand (inhale) and in-draw (exhale). It can be in evidence without specific pathologies, and is often part of a picture that includes fatigue.

Working with Paradoxical Breathing

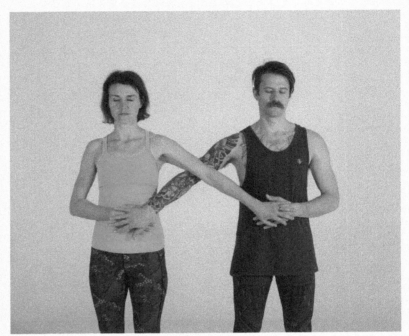

Figure 11.8

Working with
Paradoxical
Breathing.

Exercise for Paradoxical Breathing Pattern (for *you* the practitioner).

This type of breathing is most readily demonstrated in supine or seated position, to focus upon abdominal breathing, without strain. (Harder to do and not recommended in upright Anatomical Position). The participant breathing paradoxically will tend to in-draw (squeeze the abdomen) back towards the spine on the inhalation and expand (or push it out) on the exhalation; which is a reversal of the natural pattern. This is a counter-instinctive pressure response, most clearly understood through demonstration and most easily adjusted the same way. It is a complex phenomenon, because it can involve accumulated compensatory patterns between the thorax and abdomen. However, if it is detected soon and the participant can recognise it before it creates chronic patterns, it can be a rewarding relief that restores balance beyond just breathing pattern.

You, practitioner, sit beside the participant, each in a comfortable chair, or if on the floor, with backs against the wall. (This way you both feel relaxed and supported). Sit on the sitting bones so that the spine is upright, allowing its natural curvatures. Place your (outermost) hand on your abdomen while the participant places their outermost hand (furthest away from you) on their abdomen. Invite them to place their other hand (nearest you) over yours, while you place your free hand (nearest them) over theirs (Fig. 11.8). (This can be done, with client supine and practitioner seated or standing beside them; however, both sitting is recommended.)

You breathe gently in and out, slightly exaggerating the expansion of the inhalation and the release and in-drawing of the exhalation and release. You invite the participant to follow you and do the same. The hands act as guides, slightly emphasising the appropriate direction of the abdominal movement. If the participant is paradoxically breathing there will, at first, be resistance under your hand and they will feel the difference in your breathing movements. In my experience, this works very quickly to re-educate the system kinaesthetically as it does not impose, but invites reorganisation through the felt, proprioceptive senses. It may help to work with eyes closed or it may be preferable to allow the client to see the movement. This is a matter of personal judgement for the practitioner. In any case, it can guide the participant back to a more optimal pattern with ease and rapidly. It may need to be repeated after a rest, a couple of times.

After a short while, the participant is then invited to place their own hands over each other and work alone, using the hands to assist with slight pressure on the belly to animate in-drawing on the exhale, while expanding the breath into the hands on the inhale, letting the abdomen expand. Abdominal breathing is recommended in supine or supported seated pose, so that internal structural support is not compromised. This teaches the participant to become self-regulating.

If left in a paradoxical pattern, the breath often influences posture, inviting a more "collapsed" appearance with the exhalation and an effortful "lift" of the upper body on the inhalation. It can be very relieving to rectify this common pattern.

Notes

1. Swami Sivananda, *The Science of Pranayama*, Divine Life Society, Tehri-Garhwal, Uttar Pradesh, Himalayas, India. First published in 1935. The online (2000) edition is freely available at http://www.dlshq.org/.
2. **Vipassanā** (Pāli) or **vipaśyanā** (Sanskrit) literally means "special-seeing" (Wikipedia) and can also be translated as "insight", relating to observation. It is sometimes translated as "Observation of the Breath" as this tends to be how the practice begins.
3. The Bihar School of Yoga. The teachings of Swami Satyananda.
4. Jonathan Gibson (2019) Mindfulness, interoception, and the body: a contemporary perspective. *Frontiers in Psychology* (https://www.frontiersin.org/articles/10.3389/fpsyg.2019.02012/full)
5. https://med.stanford.edu/news/all-news/2017/03/study-discovers-how-slow-breathing-induces-tranquility.html
6. Ben Wolff, Breath Master and teacher; practicing through the lens of contemporary scientific research in breath work, transmitting that knowledge into one-to-one and group practice.
7. The Bihar School of Yoga. The teachings of Swami Satyananda.
8. The Bihar School of Yoga. The teachings of Swami Satyananda.
9. Stephen Levin, personal communication, 2013.
10. Sat Bir Singh Khalsa, Assistant Professor of Medicine, Harvard Medical School, interview for www.yogaintheshadows.com.
11. Graham Scarr, www.tensegrityinbiology.co.uk/, article: "Geodesic". See also: *Biotensegrity: The Structural Basis of Life*, Handspring Publishing Ltd., Pencaitland, 2014. 2nd Edition; Ch 10, Complex Patterns in Biology, p. 119.
12. Ibid
13. The Bihar School of Yoga. The teachings of Swami Satanyanda.
14. Helen Moss: Yoga Teacher, Yoga therapist (BCYT), specialised qualifications in Yoga Nidra and Restorative and Therapeutic Yoga. A Revolution in Rest can be found at https://nidrarestore.co.uk/

12

Archetypal Geometries

"Unity always preserves the identity of all it encounters. We might say that 'one' waits quietly within each form without stirring, motionless, never mingling yet supporting all. The Monad is the universe's common denominator. The ancient Gnostics called it the 'silence force.' The universe was carved of this primeval silence. Everything strives in one way or another toward unity."[1]

Michael S. Schneider

Any number (or fraction) divided by or multiplied by one, preserves its identity and wholeness. If we go back to considering ancient wisdom in the history of anatomy (Ch. 2), we can view it in a slightly different light. When it comes to understanding yoga at a symbolic and archetypal level, beyond the postures and general practices, we can perhaps begin to see how yoga and fascia provide fascinating pathways towards the unity everything strives for. The common denominator of both is the geometry of form, as a result of force transmission. Together these emergent properties co-create the patterns in the matter of living architectures.

Geometry, lost in significance, to some extent, since the advent of calculus, has profound significance in the study of the fascial matrix. If we could consider geometry as a kind of structural code of nature, it suggests the formulae of forming that living tensegrity architecture is beginning to reveal and explain. As we explore, we discover that each number we use (from 0 to 9) has a symbolic role and an archetypal character, as well as its mathematical meaning.[2]

It is possible that the ancients understood mysteries that the study of fascia is providing new access to, for long before yoga came to the West; the patterns used to symbolise the chakras, for example, were schematised in the architectural designs of sacred sites.[3] While modern technology is supporting our efforts to see new things, it may simply be allowing us to explore new *ways* of seeing things already there, perhaps reuniting us with mysteries that our ancestors understood before the advent of technology. (Indeed they are at the source of the mathematical origins of that technology.)

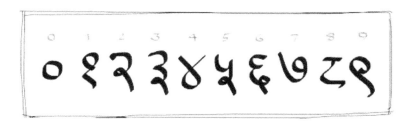

Figure 12.1

The Sanskrit numerals.

Back to the Renaissance

Alongside the other discoveries made at the time of the Renaissance in Europe came the discovery (for Europeans) of civilisations to the east and west, as Christopher Columbus set sail to India and discovered the Americas. The first European to reach the Indian subcontinent was Vasco da Gama, a Portuguese sailor whose journey prescribed the first trading lines – the earliest cultural "connective tissue" pathways between the East and West. Alongside the exotic spices and silks they found in the rich and colourful markets of India, da Gama and the early travelers to India brought back the *concept of zero*. For it was in these markets that the ancient sages had devised the numeric system of symbols we use today (Fig. 12.1).

Zero: Entering Nothing

This concept provided numerical relationships in a way that had not been considered in the West. Zero *as a concept* gave rise to new possibilities of understanding. This is exactly where the state of neutral, referred to throughout this work, resides. The opposites (or polarities) can be united, *through zero*: extending the opposite ends of the line to a triangulated area of a third state. Plus and minus live either side of zero. Together, all three permit paradox but also unite to give each other their relative meaning. It is profoundly symbolic of how fascia unites muscle and bone (as a simple example) and allows them to function, as such, by providing an essential aspect of both – incorporating each in the overall equation of motion.

Zero in Sanskrit: sunya-m "empty place, desert, naught".

"But the next step, the true miracle moment, is to realize that that 'symbol for nothing' that you're using is not just a place-holder, but an actual number: that 'empty' and 'nothing' are one. The null number is as real as '5' and '2,002' – that's when the door blows open and the light blazes forth and numbers come alive. Without that, there's no modern mathematics, no algebra, no modern science. And as far as we know, that has only happened once in human history, somewhere in India, in the intellectual flowering under the Gupta Dynasty, about the 6th century c.e. There was no 'miracle moment,' of course. It was a long, slow process."[4]

–1   0   +1

Figure 12.2

The dot in the decimal system recapitulates the placement either side of zero (i.e. showing whether it is a negative or a positive number) by showing if it is a so-called whole number or a fraction. It is a scaleable whole system.

Negative and positive can only be known mathematically in the context of the existence of zero between them (Fig. 12.2). Plus one and minus one are so because they sit either side of this "non-thing": neither one nor the

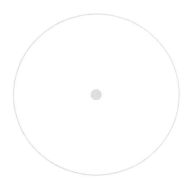

Figure 12.3
The Monad.
(All geometric images by Martin Gordon (www.mothcreative.co.uk).)

other. We call it "nought". It was considered to be "naught". Yoga begins and ends with the circle, the symbol of zero which at the same time represents oneness. It is an aspect of every kind of practice. The symbol for zero is a circle.

The symbol for "one" is the Monad (Fig. 12.3). It is a circle with a dot at the centre. The wonderful saying so often heard in Asia, "same-same but different", applies perfectly here. It is a conundrum that yoga embraces, the one and the all ultimately being (becoming) the same. It symbolises roundness and from that moment on, we develop a new theme of how round things work in their universes, on every scale. Every single circle everywhere, abides by the same rules, ratios and relationships with other circles. We just find it very much harder to "see" when we pop them (icosahedrally) into (high frequency) spheres (Ch. 6). It is harder to see through the spheres to work out how cells organise as a whole; however, it is time!

The Unifying Principle of Zero

During the Renaissance, these Indian symbols came to replace the Roman numerals that were in common usage at the time. The logic of the Roman system was not as elegant and scaleable as the Vedic numerals. It did not include the symbol (or the concept) of zero.

"The Vedic mathematicians had developed the decimal system of tens, hundreds, thousands, etc. where the remainder from one column of numbers is carried over to the next … it has been said that the introduction of zero, or sunya as the Indians called it, in an operational sense as a definite part of a number system, marks one of the most important developments in the entire history of mathematics. The earliest preserved examples of the number system which is still in use today are found on several stone columns erected in India by King Ashoka in about 250 b.c.e.[5] Similar inscriptions are found in caves near Poona (100 b.c.e.) and Nasik (200 c.e.)[6] These earliest Indian numerals appear in a script called brahmi."[7]

In the Roman system of numerals, the number *and the number of digits* have to be translated, added and subtracted. Letters stand for numbers and the placement of a letter (or letters) before or after another indicates whether it should be added or subtracted from the main number (letter). Thus, for example, IV (4) is V (5) minus I (1) (5 – 1 = 4); VI (6) is V (5) plus I (1) (5 + 1 = 6). In the same way, IX is 9, XI is 11, XII is 12, XIII is 13, and so on. One has to count in order to count.

It is apparent from further studies by David Osborn, the writer of the article quoted from above, that the need for numeric reference, the use of algebra and so on, developed in India from the culture honouring its spirituality, rather than simply studying mathematical logic to quantify and measure. By following the phases of the moon, the number of days in cycles in nature, the sages could ensure appropriate timing of ritual and rite in the context of their spiritual culture. Numbers formed part of their devotional expression and poetry. They did not segregate that knowledge and apply one (mathematics) to the other (things to measure) as if the practice of mathematics was separate from the context of nature and devotion to her forms. It was considered part of the means by which those forms express themselves – or we might say, by which Nature expresses them. They used number reverently and symbolically to honour nature, rather than reduce it. Body, mind and spirit were not relegated to separate domains; nor were mathematics, physics and biology separated. The vision remained whole, seeking explanations of differentiations in scale rather than between the components of parts. These ancient sages placed the boundaries in very different ways. They made a distinction between the reasoning mind, the functioning form and the spiritual awareness that were not segregated as separate domains of abstraction. Rather they were distinct, related aspects and stages in developmental awareness, that engaged a student in a devoted, practical lifetime of understanding "the ways" – of life, of nature, of being.

"After 700 c.e. another notation, called by the name "Indian numerals", (which is said to have evolved from the brahmi numerals), assumed common usage, spreading to Arabia and from there around the world. When Arabic numerals (the name they had then become known by) came into common use throughout the Arabian empire (which extended from India to Spain), Europeans called them 'Arabic notations,' because they received them from the Arabians. However, the Arabians themselves called them 'Indian figures' (Al-Arqan-Al-Hindu) and mathematics itself was called 'the Indian art' (hindisat)."[8]

Indian Sanskrit (like Greek and Hebrew and Arabic) is an alphanumeric language. In alphanumeric correspondences a difference of one is allowed. The Greek word "Monad" adds up to 361, symbolising the number of degrees in a circle. One particular Sanskrit verse[9] has a numeric value of 0.314159265358 9793238462643383 2792. That is π (pi), divided by 10, to 32 decimal places. It is unlikely to be pure coincidence that pi is the number derived from dividing the circumference of *any* circle by its diameter. It is an infinite number. The poem is a prayer to the (infinite, eternal) Divine.

In Indian numerals only ten figures were required in a pattern based on numeric archetypes that repeat themselves in a decimal logic. These archetypes incorporate the universal basis of nature's forms, presented in all her geometric mystery. The different numeric values and geometries are found in flowers, plants, snowflakes, trees, growth patterns, features and faces of fish, animals and humans. The patterns of leaves, insects, atoms, molecular arrangements and planetary orbit patterns contain these archetypal designs. Spirals and chirals, forms of wood, flows of water and the structure of crystals all present the variations on a theme represented by each of the different numbers. Everywhere from the cosmos to the microcosmos and back again, including the macrocosmos; these shapes conform to the formulae found in symbolic mathematics. The archetypal one and zero (1,0) brought about what we call the decimal system and the binary system of computer coding that modern technology is founded upon.

"To ancient mathematical philosophers, the circle symbolised the number one. They knew it as the source of all subsequent shapes, the womb in which all geometric patterns develop. The Greek term for the principles represented by the circle was Monad, from the root menien, 'to be stable', and monas, or 'One-ness' … they noted that unity exists in all things yet remains inapparent."[10] (See opening quotation.)

Literal and Symbolic Beginnings

This principle is important to understand in order to appreciate the metaphysical aspects of yoga and recognise how this notion of unity gives it such a significant relationship with the fascia, from the moment of our conception. It lives in the geometry of our form, which is the basis of the living tensegrity model. It is no coincidence that, embryologically, we begin as one conceptus, represented by the Monad (see Fig. 12.3). The fascial matrix arises from the "middle/meso" which emerges from within the one conceptus, symbolised by the circle. (The circle *represents* the sphere that it is; organically and originally. It contains the nucleus – *bindu* – that becomes a tiny part of every part; every single cell in our body derives from this original – one – "Monad"). The actual forming principles of the embryo, from a mystical point of view, conform to the concept zero provides, by giving us one or minus one on either side. It is recapitulated throughout the developmental process. The zero, or null point of axis in three dimensions, is where the notochord (the "non-thing" considered to be a "transient feature" as if it isn't really there) is shown (see Ch. 4 and Fig. 4.10) in cross-section at every stage (Fig. 12.4).

Figure 12.4

This is a sketch, reflecting the symbolic mathematical arrangement, deep to the geometry of embryonic forming. It is taken from Figure 4.9, showing the embryological annotation represented here in the upper (ectodermal) layer, the lower (endodermal) layer and the middle (mesodermal) layer. That middle layer then subdivides three times either side of the "null point" or central axis, notochord, which prescribes the neural tube above it.

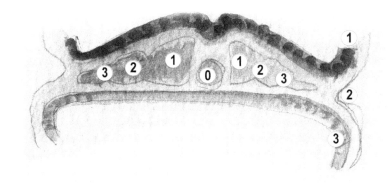

There are three states required for the two to exist, or know themselves as distinct. We can only distinguish muscles from bones because of the connecting tissues differentiating them. It is the context for both of them, yet it is neither of them, *at the same time*. The third aspect connects and unites the other two, coexisting as one whole when they arise together in triune harmony. The same can be said of the meso. From this symbolic point of view, it arises from the "no-thing" between the upper and lower laminae of the bilaminar embryonic disc growing away from each other: *denoting the space between them*. Mystically, it is not a layer, rather a field of "middleness", the essence of which is the in-between, distinguishing and connecting the other laminae (Jaap van der Wal, to respect that, refers to it as "the Meso"[11]). This is what Chapter 14 points to in considering adjustment as a moment of balance between two separate kinespheres (practitioner and participant) joining and creating one balanced shape, or geometry together; it is triune harmony. They connect the "no-thing" between them and form one whole, greater than the sum of the parts. That is, practitioner + participant = their combination. The rules of biotensegrity offer the same opportunity to unify tension and compression into a third facility, resulting from their combination. As soon as they touch each other, their mutual geometries become one multi-bar architecture, using the ground as its fixed bar.

Archetypal Numbering

"Although Vedic mathematicians are known primarily for their computational genius in arithmetic and algebra, the basis and inspiration for the whole of Indian mathematics is geometry. Evidence of geometrical drawing instruments from as early as 2500 b.c.e. has been found in the Indus Valley.[12] *The beginnings of algebra can be traced to the constructional geometry of the Vedic priests, which are preserved in the Shulba Sutras."*[13]

We could say that combination becomes the "steady" part of sthiram, sukham. The sweetness of balance arising is surely the gentle goal of the sensitive teacher, adjusting minimally to assist the form and transform balance for the listening participant. When "tension–compression" is steady, sweetness arises naturally.

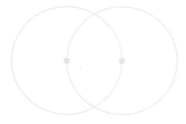

Figure 12.5

The Dyad. There are now three shapes: one, another as a reflection of itself and the Mandorla (almond shape) between them.

Sanskrit was the "higher form" of the Vedic language of India. In his excellent book on the archetypes of numbers, Michael Schneider elaborates on the symbolic and archetypal significance of numbers in every aspect of our lives.[14] He refers to numbers and shapes as the universal language of nature and art.

One (the Monad) (see Fig. 12.3) and Two (the Dyad) (Fig. 12.5) are considered to be the parents of all numbers. Three (the Triad) unifies them and is their first offspring, the eldest of the subsequent six numeric "siblings" that, between them, give rise to the many. The Triad also brings us to "triune harmony", a theme common to many deities and religious cultures (see below and Fig. 12.9).

Four takes us from area to volume: "three points define a flat surface, but it takes a fourth to define depth". The tetrahedron is a volume in space (one of the Platonic Volumes or Solids) that has four identical sides. It provides the four aspects of triangulation that allow us to make tensegrity masts (see Ch. 6).

To get to Five, "beyond the Monad's point, the Dyad's line, the Triad's surface and Tetrad's three-dimensional volume", the Pentad represents "the introduction of life itself".[15] This shape completes the set of the Five Platonic Solids (Fig. 12.6), all drawings of which are derived from within and around the original Monad. Their geometries are deep to the study of motion, when tensegrity structures are being recognised as the fundamental organisation of rounded things, volumes in space in close-packed arrangements (see Ch. 6).

Representing 2 × 3, the Hexad holds the secrets of structure, function and order in the shape of the hexagon, which we saw in Chapter 3 as the basic shape of the endomysium. Double triune harmony gives these three assets to the archetype of "six-ness". The hexagonal shape interlocks exactly and so has stability such as is seen in a honeycomb, for example (which is formed by the bees' bodies moving through it). This is a *tessellated* pattern (where the sides of each shape fit each other). The endomysium is at the microscopic level of

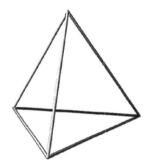

Tetrahedron
4 vertices; 6 edges; 4 faces

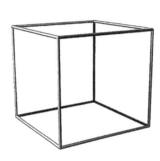

Cube
8 vertices; 12 edges; 6 faces

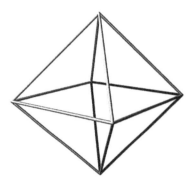

Octahedron
6 vertices; 12 edges; 8 faces

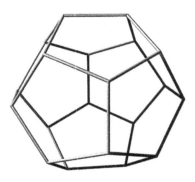

Dodecahedron
20 vertices; 30 edges; 12 faces

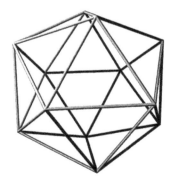

Icosahedron
12 vertices; 30 edges; 20 faces

Figure 12.6

The five Platonic Solids.

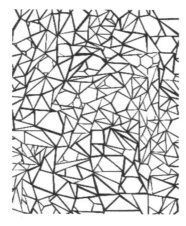

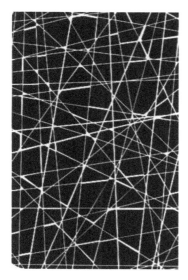

Figure 12.7

The images are inspired by the patterns of the skin above and the fascia under the skin.

(© Victoria Dokas (www.ariadne-creative.com).)

close-fitting structures within the body: the closely organised fibrils and fibres of the muscle bodies within their myofascial matrix. Forms organise in these patterns and, according to Stephen Levin, account for the organisation of our internal world of colloids and emulsions.

There are an infinite number of *irregular* polyhedrons in nature, beautifully depicted, for example, in Jean-Claude Guimberteau's "polyhedral chaos" of the pattern on the skin (Fig. 12.7; see Ch. 3) and the patterns of the fascia under the skin (see below), seen through an endoscopic lens. There are, however, only five *regular* polyhedrons, known collectively as the Five Platonic Solids or Volumes. Others can be derived from these. These form the foundation of questions being explored through tensegrity architectural principles in biologic forms, although it is not limited to them.

The archetype of seven, we learn, is a particular number that does not fit with its siblings. It can only be approximated with the geometer's tools (of a pencil and a pair of compasses). Familiar as the number of notes in a scale and days in the week, the Seventh Day is famous as one of rest – archetypally different from the others. It has unique numeric properties. The ancient philosophers considered there to be only seven numbers, since one, two and ten were the source, or result, of the others. As such, it has a unique place in the system: "Seven represents a complete yet ongoing process, a periodic rhythm of internal relationships"[16]:

"use a calculator to divide the 360 degrees by each of the values one through ten. While every one of the ten, except seven, divides 360 without remainder, only the seven-sided polygon presents an endless decimal and an unmeasurable, elusive angle from its center to its corners."[17]

Eight (from the Sanskrit o-cata-srah meaning "twice four") gives us the Octad, which is about polarity and pulsing cycles (see Ch. 15). The number itself reveals its cyclic nature; it is represented as the Möbius: the continuous nature of the birth–life–death–birth cycle inherent to yogic philosophy (see Ch. 11, the Möbius Breath Cycle).

"Composed of three trinities (9 = 3 × 3), the number nine represents the principles of the sacred Triad taken to their utmost expression"[18]. Such patterns as the magic square (Fig. 12.8) help lend Nine its mystical sense of completion that is the symbol of new beginnings. It gives rise to patterns unique unto itself.

Stepping into Ten represents a recapitulation of the whole. It holds within itself the parents of numbers (zero, one, and two – it is the first having two digits) and their seven children (three through nine). Expressing the properties of all numbers, "Ten" represents a whole greater than the sum of its parts, beyond the number itself. It is the essence of emergent properties, since neither "one" nor "zero" alone can produce offspring; yet with "two" incorporated

4	9	2
3	5	7
8	1	6

Figure 12.8

In a magic square all lines and diagonals add up to 15 in all directions, each square within the square containing a unique digit. Nine in Sanskrit is nava, and was part of the glyphs for the sunrise and the new moon, representing a new cycle. Thereafter is the One and the Zero creating the next whole cycle in a decimal numeric system.

into their triune harmony, the offspring can be birthed, to give rise to the unpredictable sum of the parts, i.e. their emergent property – ten.

One of the difficulties in reconciling symbolic mathematics is that the first three digits are zero, one and two (not one, two and three). One and two are considered to be the parents of subsequent numbers, so three is the first born (and the fourth digit). Symbolically, everything is contained by the wholeness of the next level in the holarchy.

One of the essential bases of the icosahedron, besides its true representation of any sphere (a bubble is a high frequency icosahedron), is that it "approximately" fits together in a close-packing arrangement. That approximation facilitates the properties of the icosahedron, which is the only one of the Five Platonic Volumes that can behave as a liquid crystal. The others can all lock into solid crystalline shapes. These geometries also contain (and amount to) the fluid forms and flows in which they reside (see Ch. 7). The fascia forms the substrate in which the close-packing arrangements are organised (and organise) these transitions. It is profoundly interrelated and so complex; yet paradoxically simplified by understanding the geometry.

We organise in nonlinear ways, motioning through combinations of these various subtle and constantly changing geometric patterns. Each shift in the close-packing arrangement represents what is called a "phase transition". It has far reaching geometrical significance on every scale of our inner and outer worlds. That is the structure of our chemistry, our biology and our movement mathematics; the geometries of motion – of every living thing, everywhere.

From Circles

Every time we draw a circle, we invite these archetypal patterns into our awareness. It is an invocation of creating wholeness. In itself the action of drawing the circle contains the balance of opposites: the stillness of the point (the bindu) and the dynamic movement of the pencil drawing, or spinning, the circumference. That first circle is whole and complete; however, in order to "see" or "know" itself, it has to create "other than" itself.

In order to create a second circle, we keep the compasses exactly as they were, to preserve the exact radius and reverse how we hold them. By placing the point (stillness) of the compass anywhere upon the (dynamic) circumference of the first circle, without changing the radius, we reverse the positions of the two legs and draw an exact reflection (Fig. 12.9). In yoga this is the illusion of Maya. This symbolises the reflection that can only be formed accurately in the presence of itself. (Mirror images are always reversed.) Its circumference passes through the centre point (bindu) of the first one. Thus the first circle has been precisely imitated; it forms the imitation, the illusion of "other" as a mirror image of itself. However, this is to provide the coordinates for three: the triune harmony the two give birth to or cause to arise.

The two circles form an opening between them: the possibility of a third entity. It gives birth, geometrically, to the (coordinates of the) line and provides the pathway, or access, to the third aspect. (These are precisely symbolic of the forming principles of the lamina in the embryonic process of gastrulation.) The ectoderm and the endoderm move away from each other as the space between them becomes the third entity. It emerges from between them *as volume itself.*

Figure 12.9

From the birth of the line, this constructs the triangle, which symbolises area or surface.

(All geometric images by Martin Gordon (www.mothcreative.co.uk).)

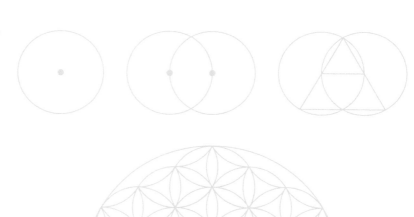

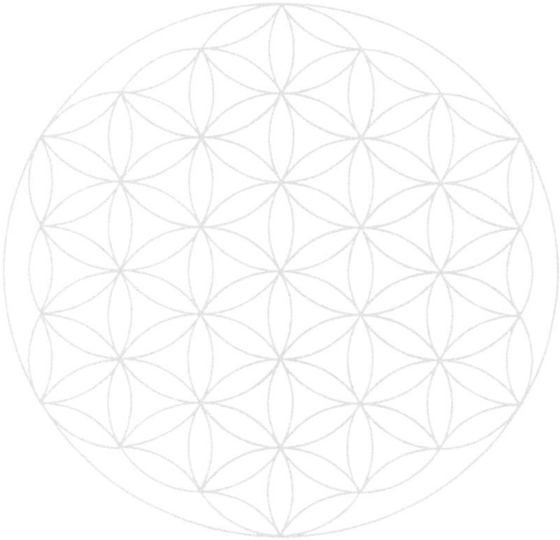

Figure 12.10

Flower of Life.

Every tensegrity model represents a close-packing arrangement of spherical shapes. The "joints" represent the centre points of the overlapping spheres. Imagine a crate of oranges; if you somehow photographed it transparently and turned it into a 2D diagram, you would get overlapping circles. They can close-pack such that each layer sits in the gaps of the layer beneath. Or they can pack by sitting one on top of the other, depending on the boundaries containing them. If you drew lines from centre point to centre point and then "disappeared" the oranges, you would have a geometrical drawing modelled by one kind of tensegrity mast. Our cells are soft biological versions of these moment-by-moment, movement-by-movement geometries-in-motion and dynamic stillness; they oscillate to the rhythm of life force. It is that *force transmission* that tensegrities model – in many variations.

It is the structure of our structure and its implications are both universal and ancient, even if they appear new to us, now that we are seeing this fabric of the "in-between" and appreciating both its volume and its ancient symbolism. (What Jaap van der Wal now refers to as the understanding from "Fabrica to Fabric."[19])

This pattern of circles repeated is the basis of the Flower of Life symbol (Fig. 12.10), within which can be found the Tree of Life (Fig. 12.11), which has profound significance for our form, as it re-iterates the mandorla throughout its pattern. It maps the geometries from which we are formed, the close-packing arrangements of our cells. Originally these are the organisation of the earliest divisions of the conceptus that represent the blastocyst (see Ch. 4).

These geometries all have deep significance in various theologies. They are fundamental to the architecture of the earliest cathedrals and sacred sites. They are fundamental to the patterns of how every cell in our body is "close-packed". They are fundamental to the Golden Ratio, or Divine Proportion which all bodies naturally manifest and conform to, in terms of shape and structure. We are the principles of nature's close-packing geometries, walking around, as conscious creatures.

Once we have drawn two circles, identical to each other, we can join the points and form a cross. From there we have the coordinates to create surface (Fig. 12.13).

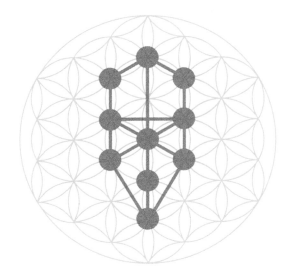

Figure 12.11

Tree of Life symbol in the Kabbalah. Many different traditions and ancient theologies contained and presented knowledge in these geometries through art and symbols.

The Flower of Life

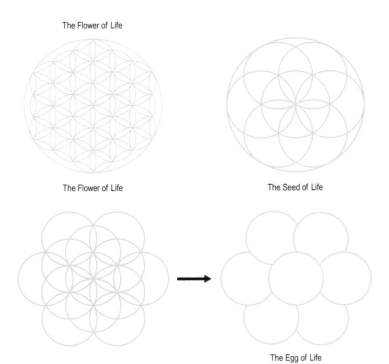

The Flower of Life

The Seed of Life

Figure 12.12

The flower, the seed and the egg of life.

The Egg of Life

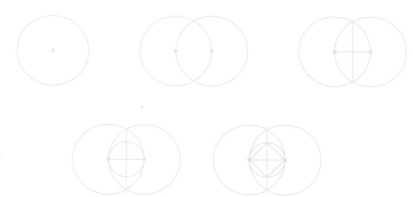

When the two lines are drawn, they provide the possibility of opposite directions. However, they coexist, arising from the same situation or
opening (the Vesica Piscis representing a portal). Symbolically this is the
domain of paradox, the gateway to the next level. These symbolic polarities, represented by the two lines, invite us to unite them by appreciating their differences. Vertical and horizontal can be woven together as if
they are different things, such as warp and weft. When these two aspects
become unified, they combine to form material (weave) and surface (area).
Their combination, working together as opposites, permits the possibility of
something far beyond the sum of their parts. Weaving, according to Kenneth
Snelson, is the mother of tensegrity.[23] Thus we secure two-dimensionality
from which to explore three; by joining three flat triangles, a fourth arises
from the space they leave contained (Fig. 12.14). (Note that this gives rise to a
four-sided shape; each number contains the potential for the next and is held
within it; siblings in the family arising from the original parent numbers.)

The archetype of the parent numbers, one and two, gives birth to the third
form, considered to re-establish the harmony of unity. Combined, two produces three, the essence of creation. The third form can then unite the two.
As we draw the third circle, each individual has access to a reflection of themselves. Between them, acting together they can create "three-ness" and transcend the illusion of Maya (separateness or duality).

This is known as Triune Harmony or Triunity (Fig. 12.15). There are many
literal examples in our bodies, such as the triple helix of the collagen fibres. This
archetypal three-ness is the basis of the field Rumi refers to "out beyond ideas
of right doings and wrong doings". In other words, the duality is united and
transcended by the field containing both; the harmony in which they enter four
dimensions.

Triunity is very familiar as a significant concept from many spiritual practices, for example a triple deity, or triple function of a deity. In this context it
is representative of three levels of awareness that allow us to experience unity.
At this level, mathematics and mythology are symbolic and meaningful. Every
number has its own innate geometries and they all have correlates in our energy

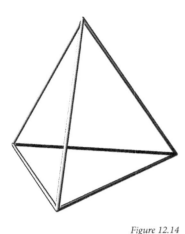

Figure 12.14

Triangles joined form the tetrahedron.

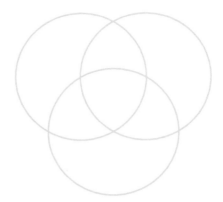

Figure 12.15

Three overlapping circles reunite to create triunity. Each can know itself and be conscious of others.

matrix, which we will see through the "windows" of the chakras as we examine their archetypal geometries, below.

Expanding Awareness

This geometry is symbolic of our approach to meditation. It is a part of the purpose. We sit, literally in reflection, allowing the illusion of duality to dissolve as we learn to observe ourselves witnessing from the place of the witness. We sit still and quiet while the things concerning us, the considerations and judgements and opinions, good and bad, valuable and costly, right and wrong, can be the way they are. We simply observe them coexisting in the circle of silence we create. From that (third) place of observation we become united with our original being. It is always present. We arise from it, or we self-assemble it. So meditation can be seen as a way of temporarily returning to, or remembering the source. It is not complex. It is already listening. We reflect, in order to move through something already deep within us, to the "silence force": the One (or oneness) – the formlessness. Caroline Myss describes the reasoning mind as "an inadequate tool" in this domain of awareness.[24] That does not mean it cannot participate or learn. It just means the logic might require a certain expansion beyond the limits of its usual reasoning, to one that can contain that reasoning. One beautiful expression of this is in the Hoberman's Sphere model. If you pull on *any one* co-ordinate, the whole expands, or compresses. That symbolises the one adjustment, the one change, the one catalyst, that changes the wholeness. Likewise, if you compress one closed joint, the whole sphere "tensions out" in response. It cannot, structurally, do otherwise. In terms of "fasciategrity" it points to the way in which one gesture changes the whole posture or demeanour of the person making it. It even echoes how water functions within the form (Ch. 7), as a liquid crystal.

The fascia, symbolically, begins as a dot (fibroblast) which exudes a thread (spiral) which unites with two other threads to become a triple helical collagen fibril (line). These three can then weave themselves (in complementary directions, which in living organisms tend to form approximately 60 degree angles, not the 90 degree angles of cubes) into fabric (surface) and form shapes (volume) in tensegral organisations, wherein opposing directions unite to form volume. It gets more complex and detailed but if every number is seen as an archetypal possibility of geometric forms, at every one there is a correlated aspect of the fascia.

It is in our ability to draw a circle around ourselves or around others, to create the opportunity of community. Even art and science meet here, in the spiral forms, the shapes of sound waves, light waves and what Mae-Wan Ho[25] calls "quantum coherence", which is a scientific expression for wholeness (see Ch. 7).

Fascia, for its wholeness and active unifying, represents our unity. As John Sharkey points out: "in the models there are two materials. In us there is only one". Fascia is our unity/unifying form. Symbolically it embellishes the purpose of yoga, allowing our anatomy to make sense to us on every level: literal, symbolic and universal. By working with the chakras as symbols of each level of our awareness at ever more refined frequencies, we can correlate the body segments in a way that honours their pre-tensioned nature, from the original forming process and throughout our lives.

Geometry could be considered the language of form, spoken in shapes and profoundly organised, fluid, dynamic relationships. Fascia is our Organ of Form. It expresses itself through geometry – as geometry is fundamental to its every formation. Therein lies the segue that tensegrity seeks to model in three dimensions and reveal in living, conscious iterations of our animated architecture. They reveal our multi-dimensional and innate ability to self-assemble. We can only examine these structural archetypes as models caught in suspended animation. We might not be able to explain them in literal mathematics, any more than we can reason them into submission with intellectual logic (although we can, if we break the traditional spells of levers and segregated, isolated mechanical hard-matter parts). The task is to upgrade to the original symbolism of geometry, without forgetting we *self-organise!!*

Archetypal Geometries of the Chakras

"though we are discussing the subtle body, nadis, samskaras, chakras and the like, as if they are concrete things, we must always be mindful of the fact that this is the result of our language and not their subtle, symbolic true nature. No matter how beautiful or seemingly complete a description you may find in any ancient or modern text, it will always be incomplete … the seeker must always maintain the finest levels of discrimination to properly understand the boundaries between domains."[26]

This, in a way, returns us to where we started. Fascia seems to be about the study of the "boundaries between domains": literally, symbolically and archetypally. In Chapter 2 we suggested that the kinaesthetic realm was lost sight

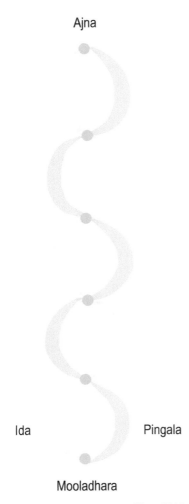

Ajna

Ida   Pingala

Mooladhara

Figure 12.16

The nadis (meaning current, or flow, as in Wind Current) are said to be visible to someone with psychic vision. The Bihar School describes them as "blueprints for physical manifestation". They are considered to be everywhere in the body (72,000 in the psychic body).

of in early Western scientific reasoning. In the East, the sensory aspect of the kinaesthetic was left intact, if only because there was no definite separation of mind, body and being as there was in the West. They were distinguished but they were not dissected or treated as being anything other than whole parts of the one whole being.

The ancient yogic history may not have engaged in the anatomical journey of discovery of Western science, examining the finest details of separate muscles or individual cell tissues in human bodies. However, it did study and describe the most sophisticated detail of the patterns in nature that were common to celestial bodies, human bodies and the bodies of many living phenomena and how they relate in a continuum. In many Eastern cultures, the history behind yoga is a different kind of story to that of the Western study of human beings and human bodies. It has included the aspect of the subtle energy body which is understood in yogic philosophy to form channels, or threads, through which the pranic (life) forces flow.

These flowing currents are brought into balance by the practice of Pawan Muktasana (see Ch. 15). It is designed to "free the inner winds", meaning the flows through these main subtle energy pathways. They are called nadis (through which there is flow or current) and can be related to nerve currents or energy flows, just as we would refer to wind currents and electrical currents, magnetic currents or sound currents, meaning exactly that: *energy flows*.

The three most significant of these nadis, the main ones centring around the spine, are Ida, Pingala and Shushumna, considered to spiral along the length of the spinal axis (echoing the triple helical pattern of the fascia in Ch. 7) (Fig. 12.16) and offering the counter-chiral pattern of opposite forces (masculine and feminine) re-iterated everywhere in our form. Closely related to the crossing points of these subtle energy channels (or nadis), a chakra is located (chakra: meaning wheel or circle). If we think in terms of currents, then each chakra might be understood as a whirlpool or vortex of pranic energy. They are considered to be like an energetic interface, or databank, between the life force and the subtle body animating us and managing the flow of that force – the subtle field, or frequency at each level of the spine. Each chakra is considered to represent what we would call a "psychosomatic" (literally meaning soul-in-the-body) aspect of us and has a particular set of characteristics and a Sanskrit name (Table 12.1). It also represents a geometric pattern, a symbolic quality portrayed in many subtle ways in the letters used, the sounds made by intoning them and the coordinates each chakra represents in the body.

The use of specific sounds of words to describe postures – and mantras to use in meditation – was not arbitrary. They denote forms and particular ways in which the sound waves resonate with certain geometric patterns (musically) or subtle energies. As we have mentioned, even the numeric values of the verses through which the teachings were presented hold significant shapes, just as the energy pattern of a light wave or a sound wave (or a heel strike pulse; see Ch. 9 and the work of Serge Gracovetsky) resonates. Indeed, when we begin to look a little closer at the symbol associated with each of the chakras, it reveals its geometry, through which we enter.

Table 12.1

No.	Theme	Name	Symbol		Yantra	Location	Meaning
9	The Horizon looking out beyond number; new beginnings				Grace Divinity	12-finger point, above the crown	
8	Octad – infinite compassion and continuous cycles	Sahasrara		A shining lotus of 1000 petals	Supreme knowledge or consciousness	Crown of the head	One thousand
7	Septad – approximation	Bindu		A tiny crescent moon on a dark night sky	Awareness	Top of the back of the head	Point or drop
6	Hexad – the cube – structure, function and order – the double triad	Ajna		A silver lotus with two petals; represents the sun (Pingala, positive or active) and the moon (Ida, negative or passive)	Subtle Mind; knowledge and intuition converge: these two pranic flows converge at this chakra with Shushumna, the spiritual force (neutral)	Mid-brain, behind the space between the eyebrows	Also known as the Third Eye; jnana chakshu (the eye of wisdom). Ajna means command; guidance from the higher self or the guide comes through here
5	Pentad – the Pentagonal Geometries; all five regular forms – new life	Vishuddi		A violet lotus with 16 petals	A white circle: the Ether Element	At the back of the neck, behind the throat	Shuddi – purification. It is enhanced by "vi"; a deepening of discernment
4	Tetrad – tetrahedron and Star Tetrahedron – Gaia Metria; when two tetrahedrons (four-sided) combine	Anahata		A blue lotus with 12 petals	A hexagon, formed by two interlacing triangles; the Air Element	In the spine behind the sternum, level with the heart	"Unstruck"; it refers to the soundless sound from which sound manifests
3	The Triad – Triunity or Triune Harmony	Manipura		A bright yellow lotus with 10 petals.	A Red Triangle; the Fire Element	In the spine behind the navel	Mani – gem and pura – city; "City of Jewels"
2	The Dyad – Mandorla or Vesica Piscis – the illusion of Maya	Swadhistana		A crimson lotus with six petals	A White Crescent Moon: the Water Element	Two-fingers width above Mooladhara; the coccyx	"One's own abode"
1	The Monad – circle containing the bindu	Mooladhara		A deep red lotus with four petals	Yellow Square: the Earth Element	The perineum in the male and the cervix in the female	Mool – root, adhara – place. The Root Centre

Sanskrit, the higher form of the Vedic language, is known as a "language in the Wisdom Tradition". In this extremely sophisticated means of expression, each letter in each name has a numeric value. Those correspondences are resonance fields: they represent far more subtle meanings than their spelling appears to denote. Their sounds have specific musical connotations and they unite many aspects of our lives that we might consider separate in the West. We know what sounds we like, in our choice of music, however the ancient philosophers understood the nuance of the sound current at levels of subtlety we find hard to imagine. It included rhythms, harmonies and intonations that are quite distinct from music in the Western hemisphere. Musical scales are profoundly related to all the laws of mathematics and geometry iterated here. Although beyond the scope of this work, the relevance of sound to the resonance of the fascial tissues is literally transforming our understanding of frequency-specific resonance in complementary health care.

Each chakra represents a particular geometry and geometric configuration and place in the body (Fig. 12.17). Once we begin to explore the hidden geometry of all life, we discover that the chakras incorporate specific aspects of it; the numbers, letters, colours, seed sounds and images presenting them all correspond and the mysteries of the energy system are encoded by that geometry. The patterns on our skin – the polyhedral chaos of the fascial matrix seen under endoscopic magnification – all adhere to the laws of Gaia Mater.

We are just beginning to understand the geometry of our structure, through learning about tensegrity architectures. The hidden geometry in every form we know is found on various levels and in all natural forms, be it the chemical structure of an element, the crystalline form of inert rocks, the organisation of petals and leaves on a flower or weed, the dimensions of a snow flake or the structure in fluid arrangements of everything from water to chocolate.

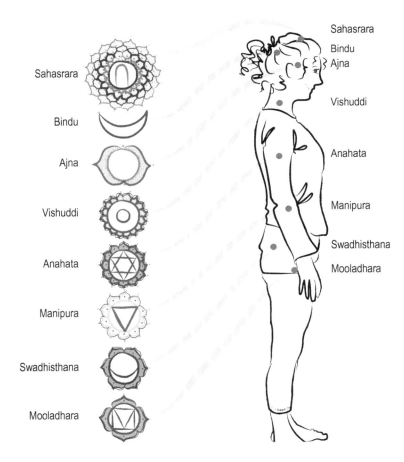

Figure 12.17

Geometry names the field of knowledge that deals with spatial relationships (Greek: geo, meaning earth and metria, meaning measure). Gaia is the Greek Earth Goddess and the origin of the word metria is shared with mater (mother). The word "geometry" incorporates the symbolic meaning: *the measure of Mother Earth.*

The chakra system.

Chakras as Levels or Frequencies

SRI YANTRA is designed as a symbolic geometric *form*. It is an embodiment of the Divine mother *energy*, encapsulating the balance of the masculine (Shiva, upward triangles) and feminine (Shakti, downward triangles). There are 43 small triangles created from the 9 larger intersecting ones, each representing a "loka" (a dimension or world) where a unique deity resides. The spiritual journey and growth (karmic lessons) we go through in our various lives from birth to rebirth is represented from the outer edges of the Yantra (*the manifest*), moving towards the centre (*unmanifest*), to the "Bindu" at the centre (the same as the red dot Hindu women wear between their eyes), which is the point of liberation of the soul. It is considered to be an incredibly powerful meditation tool. It can bring the observer closer to enlightenment, cultivating a deeper connection to the seeking within, the urge to return to Source (the *formless*).

In ancient India, each letter/number holds a resonance field, so each chakra has a series of subtle annotations including its specific name, an image (*yantra*, meaning sacred journey, represented visually by a mandala; see Fig. 12.18) and a sound (*mantra*, meaning sacred sound, represented by a Sanskrit term, designed to be chanted). Each term also has numeric value indicating a specific type of geometry associated with that value. This geometry gives rise to the particular forms and shapes assigned to the specific chakra. Indeed, they each have a corresponding symbol and colour. Bearing in mind the exquisite precision of this metaphysical annotation, the wholeness of each chakra is embodied in the repeated image of the lotus flower. The number of petals at each level has significant links with the "bija mantras" (*seed sounds*) of the Sanskrit alphabet. Like the rules of tensegrity, nothing is redundant and each part is self-contained yet remains an intimate part of the whole. The detail is traceable at every scale and it is universal and intimate at the same time. Besides the *yantra* and the *mantra*, the movements (*tantra*) were the physical manifestations of those references in the body. Regardless of what we have come to make them mean, they were originally designed as a triune harmony of body, mind and being.

At a literal level this is the gross and the subtle, the form and the formless: visible and invisible aspects that unite. When they are in balance, a third state arises, which we are referring to as neutral (as we have throughout this book). In yogic wisdom this third aspect is symbolised in Shushumna: the spontaneous release of energy flowing through a distinct energy channel. This is thought to be at the spinal cord, possibly relating to the original axis defined by the notochord in the embryonic structure.

Shushumna is considered to arise spontaneously as an expression of unity between the other two principal, invisible forces. Thus, together, they can be referred to as "tri-unity" or "triune wholeness". Ida represents the Moon (negative, passive principle) and Pingala represents the Sun (positive, active, principle). Shushumna represents the "zero", the "non-thing" between them that, in triune harmony, allows them all to be *in triunity*.

We could consider that a location of the chakra on the spine is its "*apparent*" manifestation. The energy of that centre, or its frequency, is *inapparent*. Together, however, the chakras themselves provide the *transparency*: the third uniting aspect that allows us a particular view to see through, that is congruent with its colour, sound and symbolism. It also incorporates its subtle relationships to the other chakras. It is a segue into understanding the "anima/animus", the *animated* part of our architecture. Or perhaps we should say: the animated part of us as we express ourselves *through* our architecture – since they cannot be separated!

Opposing Directions

The whole subtle energy system of the body was thought to include more and more subtle or refined frequencies working up the spine, from the first base or Root Chakra (Mooladhara) to the Crown (Sahasrara), upward to the energy centre beyond it. In the other direction, working down the spine, energy becomes more dense and is considered to materialise and manifest from the

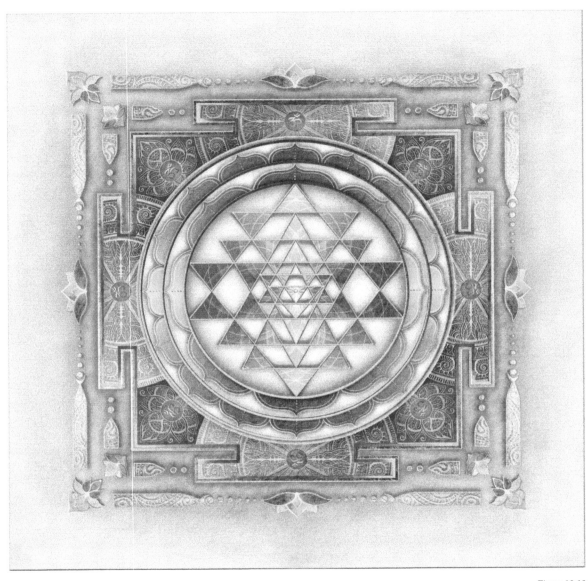

Figure 12.18

Sri Yantra: by Tim Atkins*. This is the sacred "King of Mandalas", the Sri Yantra, which comes from the teachings called the Sri Vidya.

*Tim Atkins can be reached at timothyatkins@btinternet.com for special commissions. Or https://www.redbubble.com/people/digitalzealot/shop. Or you can go to redbubble.com and type in digitalzealot (as one word).

collective consciousness (above) to the individual (downward through to the earth). Divine Inspiration is said to move down from the crown and is then "made real" in the community in the metaphorical sense of "giving birth" to an emerging idea, once it has sufficient gravitas to be manifest.[27]

Throughout this book we have alluded to the unity arising from a third state, the combination of apparently paradoxical ideas creating a third aspect once they can be combined. The third aspect has to be contained by the fourth, and thus each dimension in which we seek to understand living motion is contained by the next. We can only see in 2.5D, but we come to appreciate 4D as the medium in which self-assembly into 3D takes place.

In yogic terms, the ability to move the (Pranic) energy up and down the body is realised as the free flow of the *inner winds*, or currents (see Chs 15 and 17 for classroom sequences that foster this). **Polarities become paired attributes when their sum is unified.** We could say "this is yoga"; uniquely expressed by each of us. Moving energy up and down the body allows for circulatory pathways to remain free and flowing. This is part of the physical and meditational practices of yoga. The directions, or symbolic polarities, unite to become a realm, or field, of neutral possibility combining all possibilities; a sort of observation platform that allows for life to occur precisely as it is.

The notion that we work up from the ground (to the crown and beyond) and then back down from the crown to the ground is recapitulated in all yogic practices. This is in the physical act of balancing in the postures, upright and inverted. In meditation, it is to counterbalance movement itself. If everyday life is mainly about our outward focus (toward the kinesphere) and evolution of our abilities, then meditation could be framed as our opportunity to focus inwardly (toward the innersphere) for the involution of our potentials. We foster balance and counterbalance on every level, by incorporating both, in our practice. We recapitulate these principles with every breath.

In meditation we sometimes begin by focusing on a dot: the centre (or bindu) of the circle. If, for example, that dot is visualised as a stone dropping into a pool of still water, it ripples outward in concentric rings. The stone represents our focused attention and these rings symbolise the larger circles of our expanded awareness. We learn to generate the "witness" in order to observe ourselves seeing the stone and the circles. We explore our own triune harmony through participating in witnessing ourselves witnessing.

An example of the chakra system, representing the different levels of awareness, is found in recognising the different ways we consider what is personal. Figure 12.19 represents a person. We could say that the levels of the chakras as an energy system reflect different aspects of being a person at each level. Working up from the root chakra in this example (presented in reverse order): see Table 12.2.

Symbols of the Chakras

In the system of the chakras, these numeric archetypes are symbolised by levels in the body in relation to the spine. They further correlate to specific levels of awareness on the journey of the self towards so-called enlightenment. That is, the journey from the first chakra (earth) to the highest chakra (heaven) symbolises a journey from denser, earthly levels through the colour spectrum, the musical scales and their related numeric archetypes, to the light (full spectrum) beyond the crown. In *Sacred Contracts*, Caroline Myss[28] suggests that our individual power is expressed in the ability to bring an idea or inspiration back down through these distinct levels of awareness into

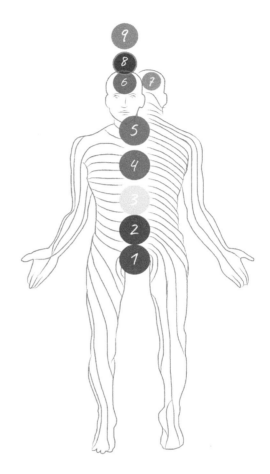

Figure 12.19

The chakras are presented here in relationship to the dermatomes – a purely speculative correlate on the part of the author. The bindu (see Fig. 12.17), shown here on back view, is not included in the main chakras in some references, as it is in the Bihar School of Yoga. This is offered as a way of considering the chakras in a contemporary context.

manifestation, formed in a particular shape that conforms to everyday life and can be birthed into it. The cycle begins again, on every level and in every aspect. Perhaps every time we teach a class, we are in fact "giving birth to" an idea, or an intention to teach and create possibility for our participants. We bring it downward from inspiration (above) to manifestation (below) through a process of transformation and densification. Then we give it away, to have a life of its own in the community.

Thus these geometries can be considered to express different qualities found in our form, correlated directly to our physical well-being and our metaphysical way of being. They relate to the geometry associated with each number. They unite the principles of energy in motion, the vibrations of sound waves and light waves and the geometries of nature's forms. They are not literal, dissectible structures, any more than thoughts or emotions are. Sanskrit, as we have noted, was a language in the Wisdom Tradition. It was the refinement of sounds, expressed by priests, versed in its nuances and very precise expressions of subtle feelings, qualities and metaphysical states and resonance fields. It took lifetimes to learn, experience and teach this work. The flowing of these

Table 12.2

No	Name	Symbol	Chakra Energies At Each Level of Being A Person (Example: from 1–9)
9			Universal Grace: beyond archetypal patterns, this level denotes the realm of pure consciousness from which we emerge, to which we return.
8	Sahasrara		Personae: the eighth chakra denotes the archetypal world of the collective consciousness. Here all manner of personae are present to us as universal archetypes: rich in symbolic patterns we all recognise.
7	Bindu		Transpersonal: the seventh chakra denotes the connection with grace or spirit such as it is for you; representing your own intimate connection with the divine forces that transcends the personal realm, thereby being transpersonal.
6	Ajna		Impersonal; the sixth chakra is symbolic of our knowledge, the intelligence and wisdom we gather from the world around us and our knowing and understanding. If it comes from the heart it can become compassionate knowledge; however, it is not so much "ours" as it is impersonal and shared.
5	Vishuddi		Personality: the fifth chakra is symbolic of our ability to express ourselves, from the heart we "find our voice" as the channel from the heart through the throat chakra to speak directly from it. It is also the central chakra; heart-centred self-expression.
4	Anahata		Inter-personal: the fourth chakra (the heart), symbolising the ability to be in a relationship as a whole and complete person, with another whole and complete person; both self-contained and free to choose. (100 + 100 = 200% here)
3	Manipura		Personal: this is the third chakra (of self-esteem), symbolising the state of individuation. Our sense of who we are becomes personal to each of us.
2	Swadhistana		Co-personal: this the second chakra, symbolising the state of recognition "other than me"; when we become aware of our sibling or parents as separate from us – yet we still depend upon them entirely; we are co-dependent in relationships at this level. (50 + 50 = 100% here)
1	Mooladhara		Pre-personal: this is the first chakra, symbolising the state of entering the world at the level of our tribe. It is "pre-personal" in the sense that we are part of the collective we are born into.

subtle energies was considered paramount to the ability to be at ease with one's self (as distinct from dis-eased). The idea is far from new, but it might be made more accessible by restoring the sense of unity between body, mind and being, and understanding the living, *triumphant* matrix between them.

Perhaps understanding the fascia will unite not only the different aspects of science, such as psychology and physiology, affected by the paradigm shift it is causing, but also the rift between science and art. It invites a pathway – or perhaps a connective tissue network – between mathematics and music, movement and form, anatomy and yoga. (We might hear the echo of "firmitas, utilitas, venustas" from Vitruvius in Chapter 2.)

Hidden Geometry

"The beauty expressed by a flower's hidden geometry is as necessary to the world as its reproductive function is to the plant. How fascinating, though, that their beauty is communicated not by the plant, but by us. It is we who respond to its beauty. It is humanity that has always embedded this geometry

in the world's greatest works of sacred art and architecture, simply because we resonate with these hidden patterns. We, too, are made up of them and, thus, we contain the universe that contains us. Or, as the traditional philosophy for which Keith speaks would phrase it, we are each a microcosm of the macrocosm."[29]

We might add, then, that there is hierarchy, heterarchy and holarchy in the human body. **Hierarchy** means: a system in which members of an organisation or society are ranked according to relative status or authority or order of power or importance (somewhat unlike, if not opposite to, heterarchy). **Heterarchy** means: a system of organisation where the elements of the organisation are unranked (non-hierarchical) or where they possess the potential to be ranked a number of different ways. **Holarchy** means: a connection between holons, where a holon is both a part and a whole."[30]. Each arises from the combination of the other two. It is a beautiful way to consider the human body, symbolically and functionally, so that we can see how tissues work together to allow us to work together.

The world that contains us and the world that we contain expresses the idea of the microcosm in the macrocosm. Understanding the fascia from a view of multiplying up to connect and unite, rather than cutting apart to dissect and divide, is an invitation towards recognising the experience of unifying, as we said at the beginning. That is, unifying mind with body and being, not just unifying the parts of us to become one body. It goes further, to suggest the community (common-unity) of beings together in a universal whole. For the ancient yogis, the metaphysical and the physical are parts of each other. They coexist to form a wholeness, within one another. This is the principle of the embryonic development and the idea introduced in Chapter 4 of a holarchy. A "holarchic structure" is one in which each part is whole and complete, as well as being a part of another (whole and complete) part or wholeness. It drives the mind in circles until it is experienced. Then we can simply recognise it.

We are perhaps beginning to move from the two-dimensional world of the "musculoskeletal" system to a three-dimensional world of the body, where the connectivity is honoured and wholeness and relationships feature (and even take precedence) in the story. When we can allow for something we can't see (but can perform) which is to move through ourselves to incorporate four-dimensionality, we will perhaps expand to see from five. (As described earlier, every number resides in the next.) This is a cultural leap of faith. It takes us by the hand into that field in which the thing that makes us all the same is also what makes us all unique, yet makes us all the same, continuously, like a circle within a circle: the endless cycle of an infinite continuum. Perhaps the greatest gift of yoga is zero, the circle with nothing in it, the symbol of where we begin. From here the only thing to do is create a way – your way, unique in all its glorious forms, whoever you are. Enjoy the field!

Notes

1. Michael S. Schneider, *A Beginner's Guide to Constructing the Universe: The Mathematical Archetypes of Nature, Art, and Science*, HarperCollins, New York, 1994.
2. Ibid
3. http://pearlsofwar.blogspot.co.uk/2011/01/chakras-and-cathedrals.html.
4. © 2001–2013 Douglas Harper.
5. Herbert Meschkowski, *Ways of Thought of Great Mathematicians*, Holden-Day, San Francisco, 1964.
6. Howard Eves, *An Introduction to the History of Mathematics*, Rinehart and Company, New York, 1953.
7. David Osborn (1989) Mathematics and the spiritual dimension. *The Clarion Call* 2(4):36. (This article is now incorporated with illustrations in Narasingha Chaitanya Matha.)
8. Ibid
9. David Osborn (1989) Mathematics and the spiritual dimension. *The Clarion Call* 2(4):36. (This article is now incorporated with illustrations in Narasingha Chaitanya Matha.)
10. Michael S. Schneider, *A Beginner's Guide to Constructing the Universe: The Mathematical Archetypes of Nature, Art, and Science*, HarperCollins, New York, 1994.

11. Jaap van der Wal, private conversation and part of his course in Embryosophy. Please see embryo.nl for further information and Chapter 3 for details of his extensive research.

12. E.J.H. Mackay, *Further Excavations at Mohenjo-daro*, 1938. Reprinted in 1998 by Munshiram Manoharlal Publishers, New Delhi, India.

13. David Osborn (1989) Mathematics and the spiritual dimension. *The Clarion Call* 2(4):36. (This article is now incorporated with illustrations in Narasingha Chaitanya Matha.)

14. Michael S. Schneider, *A Beginner's Guide to Constructing the Universe: The Mathematical Archetypes of Nature, Art, and Science*, HarperCollins, New York, 1994.

15. Ibid.

16. Ibid.

17. Ibid.

18. Michael S. Schneider, *A Beginner's Guide to Constructing the Universe: The Mathematical Archetypes of Nature, Art, and Science*, HarperCollins, New York, 1994.

19. Private correspondence, February 2020.

20. Drumvelo Melchizedek, *The Ancient Secret of the Flower of Life*, books 1 and 2, Clear Life Trust, Flagstaff, AZ, 1990, 2000.

21. Stephen Levin, Biotensegrity Interest Group, September 2013, Ghent, Belgium; www.biotensegrity.com.

22. Graham Scarr, www.tensegrityinbiology.co.uk, article: "Geodesic". See also: *Biotensegrity: The Structural Basis of Life*, Handspring Publishing Ltd., Pencaitland, 2014. 2nd Edition; Ch 2, Simple Geometry in Complex Organisms, pp. 13–24.

23. Kenneth Snelson, http://kennethsnelson.net/.

24. Caroline Myss (www.myss.com), various workshops and trainings.

25. Mae-Wan Ho, *Living Rainbow H2O*, World Scientific Publishing, Singapore, 2012.

26. From *Kundalini Rising: Exploring the Energy of Awakening*, a series of essays brought together by Tami Simon (published by Sounds True, Boulder, CO, 2009). "Kundalini; Her Symbols of Transformation and Freedom" is written by Lawrence Edwards, PhD.

27. Caroline Myss, *Advanced Energy Anatomy*, Sounds True (audio presentation).

28. Caroline Myss, *Sacred Contracts*, Bantam Books, London, 2002.

29.. From the Foreword by HRH The Prince of Wales to *The Hidden Geometry of Flowers*, by Keith Critchlow (K. Critchlow, *The Hidden Geometry of Flowers*, Floris Books, Edinburgh, 2011).

30. This term was coined in Arthur Koestler's 1967 book, *The Ghost in the Machine*, and used by Ken Wilbur.

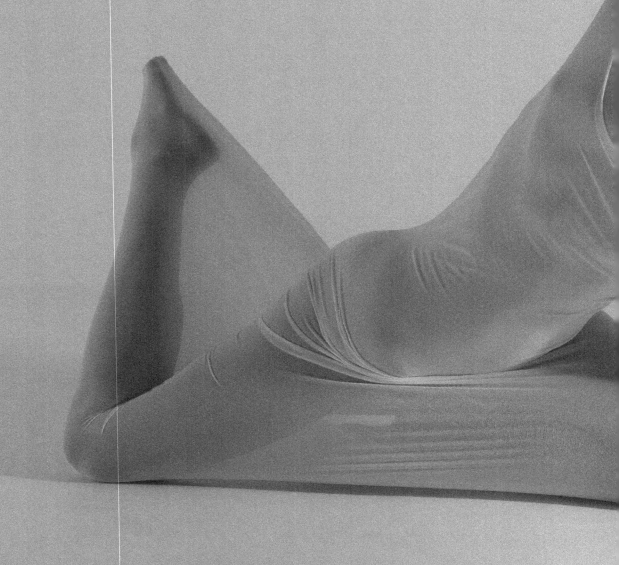

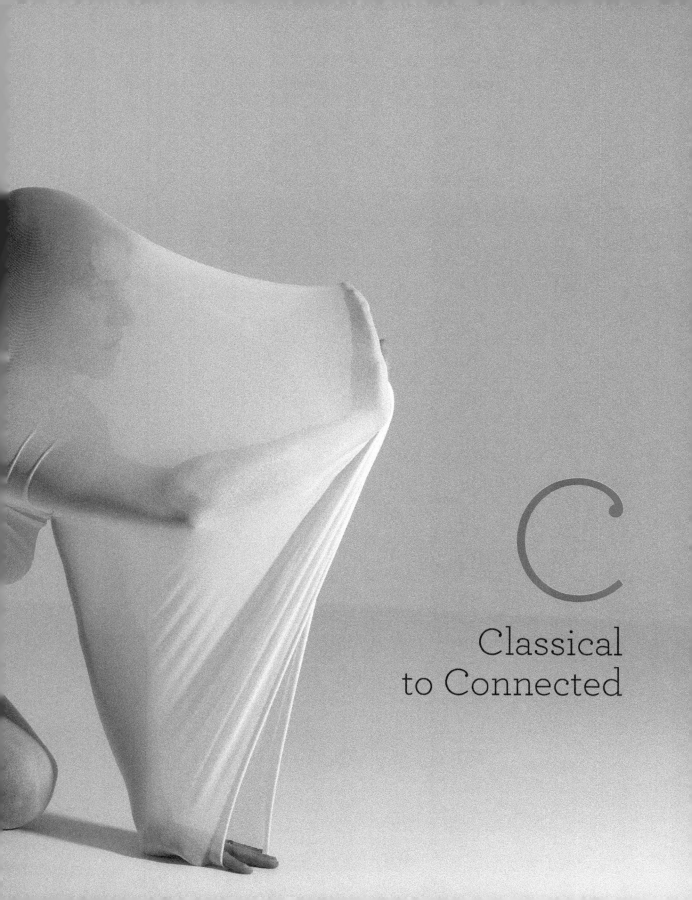

C

Classical
to Connected

Part C Introduction

The Compound Essence of Time[1]

"Put it where it belongs and call for movement".[2]

Dr Ida P. Rolf

The "compound essence of time" is a famous phrase used by Dr Ida P. Rolf, founding matriarch of Structural Integration (aka Rolfing). This refers to the nature of time as part of any process of learning movement, or healing, or treating clients practically as a movement or manual practitioner. Recognition of different time frames in the human body is a key to understanding how the magic of fascia works on every level. That is intellectual science, instinctive movement and intuitive self-aware, inner knowing (gnosis). John Sharkey refers to our understanding of fascia as "an appreciation of Temporal Medicine" and in this introduction we bring the notion of time into creating class plans and working in "real time" in the classroom. Essentially, in the physical realm, we are all working with the fascia, so it is worth considering what might appear metaphysical, but actually applies very literally in terms of learning and teaching. Class planning (Ch. 16) becomes a delightful creative exercise in this context. Have fun!

The fascia is omnipresent in the body. We have learned through the research into this "fascia-nating fabric"[3] that the design of our sensory selves is organised for listening more than doing (Ch. 5). We might say we are made of a listening tissue. At the level of social interaction, and certainly teaching, tuning in and listening can be richly rewarding.

The fascial system is, among other things, an intelligent means to sense where we are in space at that time. Speaking in a fascial dialect of body language, is it possible to expand our ability to listen kinaesthetically just by being still? Can we go beyond that too, to a place of intuitive sense? We might call it "pre-sensing" but it has little to do with "seeing into the future". Rather it seems to reside as a deepening of our ability to be aware and expand into the moment, rather than forward from it (see Fig. IntroC.1).

Three Aspects of the Breath

One of the fastest ways to bring ourselves into a state of presence and awareness is by giving our attention to the breath. Simply stop and notice your

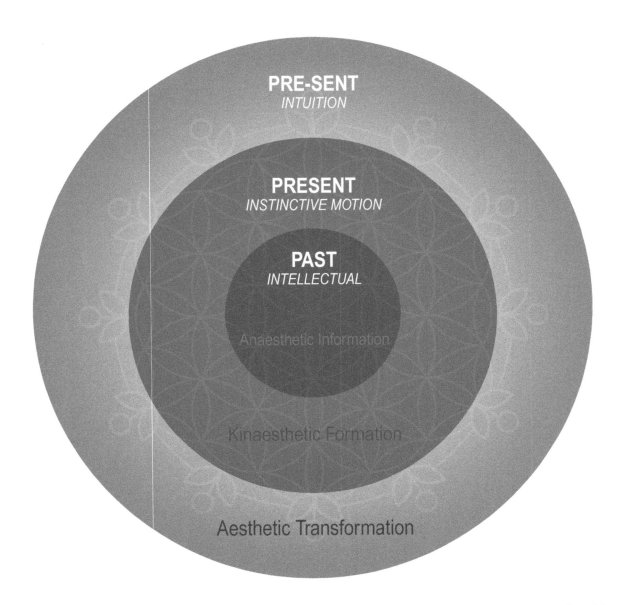

Figure IntroC.1

breathing, without imposing on it at all. It shifts moods and changes pace within a few moments.

In Chapter 11, we explored the elasticity of the breath as a simple way of nourishing the natural breathing rhythm. It provides a bridge to this next level of practice in more ways than one. We can approach working with the breath on three levels, just as we have approached the three parts of this book: intellectually, in physical practice and towards deepening awareness. We could say that the first is what we learn, the second is what we find out and the third is what we do not know. It is in the immeasurable domain of being (Fig. IntroC.1, outer ring). The ancient yogis had a profound understanding of these different levels and the subtle qualities they possess.

The Breath as Three Kinds of Knowledge

In the breath example, the first (inner) ring is the intellectual aspect of our understanding. It includes the chemistry, physics and biology of breathing. At this level we think it through. We activate the mind and learn about compliance, function and suitable ways to foster it in the fascial matrix. From a yogic point of view we can go further into the study of the subtle energies such as the pranas and vayus, gathering information to broaden our understanding of how fascial anatomy and yoga practice can benefit each other in practical and subtle ways (see Ch. 11). This relates to the past as we gather information and it becomes a part of our personal learning: our own historical database. We build upon it to become suitably qualified, expanding our learning as we go. We build the inner archives and their loading history by the physical process of learning. We think intently and attentively at this level.

In the second aspect (the middle ring), we put the books aside. We animate the information and data in present time. We do this by practising it and/ or teaching it. We can bring our attention to our own breath, to see how it moves us and how we can move it. However, even when we are not focusing on it directly, it works instinctively. Thus the information we acquired at the first level can be a means to explore at this second level. It accumulates into patterns. We can reflect upon and explore these patterns in ourselves and expand that enquiry with our students. At this second level, we work with integrating breath and movement so fluently (on the mat) that they become instinctively congruent. We do not have to think about it. In a movement field, drawing from that physical experience, we become our own resource through the experiential knowledge from which to teach. The inner ring is absorbed and we evolve to teach from both. Mind and body express their understanding in present time. (It is more than information at this level. It is incorporated into knowledge.)

In the third aspect (the outer ring), the practice can be taken to a deeper level. Here we can become quiet or still. It is less about either thinking or doing. At this level we focus inwardly, in periods of reflection or meditation, to feed the source of our ideas and inspiration, without necessarily knowing exactly what they will become. We pause. We can go within or beyond the techniques of Pranayama to being (and be-coming) the beneficiary. This is the benefit of expanding our awareness. This level – even harder to describe – is a deepening of the presence. It is hallmarked by the quietness of the conceptualising mind. It includes and transcends it. This is not a seeking of silence. It comes when the "seeking" stops. It is within the presence: a concentration of the source of being, when we have paused "doing" for a while. In this place of reflection the breath is exactly the way the breath is, at the time. This is the state of presence.

This state of presence (which could be described as joined-up pauses really) is the place from which the sense of "pre-sense" can be developed. It is the blank page upon which true creativity can occur: where inspiration comes in and can be recognised. We sense it.

The Blank Page

We first create the blank page (meditation) inside, in order to acquire the ability to find stillness. One purpose of the meditative part of yoga is to train ourselves, at least for brief periods, in stillness as actively as we do in motion. It might seem counterintuitive. When we are busy, the last thing we want to do is slow down. However, it seems to pay a different kind of dividend. It allows the inspiration to come to us or become visible, audible or tangible (however it comes to you). If we are preoccupied with thinking and achieving and worrying, it is difficult to see inspiration when it does come in: the "page" is too cluttered. Or if we are busy, we do not take time to be still. We can miss it.

The result of it is that creativity can seem to take less time to learn; in other words, it animates what we are doing. We find ourselves increasingly able to design, from within a class. Confidence and self-esteem can grow and we work with precision and, appropriately, from experience. Indeed, we can begin to trust something beyond our selves and our knowledge; something unmeasurable. We become able to witness our selves creating.

We "re-present" a class in present time for our students. We become the source that is their resource, while they learn. It is possible to work very intuitively (and rapidly) at this level. This practice naturally invites concentration (as in a more concentrated essence).

I have removed the meditation section from this book, in honour of the nature of meditative practice. There are links throughout the text referencing this vast field of wisdom and nurture, including resources for yoga Nidra and listening meditations[4] for you to choose from.

"while in samadhi, yogis and yoginis experience a powerful alteration in their sense of both time and space. I believe this is due to radical shifts in brain function (meditative states greatly increase alpha and/or theta activity). In these relaxed brain states, time seems more fluid and space often takes on strange attributes … What might last an hour in linear time may be experienced as lasting for eons or for just a moment."[5]

In essence, the power to generate presence is the ability to witness oneself witnessing. It is essentially uneventful and it takes honest and simple training to "be still", just as it takes honest and simple training to learn "to do" yoga. Sitting, standing or walking in meditation (or self-observation) is part of such a practice. It might just be a balance that brings a sense of quiet and ease to whatever you are doing at the time. It might be nothing more than a suppleness of spirit to match the same biomotional agility in the body.

Tissue Time Frames

Certain schools of ancient yogic philosophy believed that these three levels of awareness operate at three very different speeds. Thinking is the slowest, animated instinctive movement is considerably faster, and faster still is what we will refer to as intuitive awareness. This level has a sense of timelessness. It can bring us to a place of highly creative inspiration. One purpose of practising

Yoga refers to samadhi, the ultimate state of union that meditation is considered to assist us in reaching, if that is the goal. It is a state of being at one with the Divine force of life itself, no longer knowing our selves as separate from that original state of wholeness. It is considered to be the original state from which we emerged. Linda d'Antal[6] has an interesting way of interpreting this: Sama means same, Dhi comes from Dhiyana; meaning concentration and meditation. In this sense, concentration does not only refer to the focus of attention on an object. It also includes the concentration (as distinct from the dilution) of a substance into its purest essence. This is something about alchemy, in the symbolic sense of transformation. It refers to the pure essence of (the) being. In this way a broader or more subtle interpretation of samadhi is the one (same) concentrated essence. It symbolises the wholeness of the being and the collective union of the one and all at the same time, within us: animated by the essential living force. It is the elixir we call vitality. Perhaps meditation is no more than allowing ourselves to remember our essence, or replenish it, without thinking, by just being present. Could it be that the presence itself concentrates the essence? Or even that it allows the concentrated essence to diffuse out into our awareness?

all aspects of yoga is to bring all these different centres, or aspects of us, into congruent balance. We do not have to think about them; they become more of a facility that we can call upon, consciously.

We each have a tendency to favour one particular aspect, whether intellectual learning, kinaesthetic learning or the intuitive approach. No aspect is better than any other. The purpose of this work is to find balance and access between all of them, through learning, through practising and moving, and through pausing to acknowledge and assimilate the knowledge that is accumulating in the tissues of our body and being. This last part requires something beyond reasoning – which is where meditative or reflective practices facilitate our awareness. One cannot do it like mixing ingredients for a recipe, but by practising in the kitchen it becomes possible intuitively to create something delicious – eventually working without the recipe book.

Forward from the Future: Creating in Advance

Let us divide our experiences into three domains of time (see Fig. IntroC.1). Rather than past, present and future, we can put them into past, present and pre-sent – where what has not happened yet can occur as if given to us, or created in advance. It is something we consciously anticipate. We can design a class, then re-create it or "re-present" it, in the actual classroom. This could be referred to as "designing the future from the future", which, in a way, is what we do when we prepare a class beforehand. We are just adding the sense here that it has already happened and come from that, as we describe it to ourselves and choose what we will teach (or will have taught, if we imagine having done it, just for this exercise). Deepak Chopra refers to "waking up the wizard that is deep to all of us". He presents this way of working from the future symbolically and delightfully in his book, *The Return of Merlin*. The principle of designing the future by creating it from the power of your present imagination is a metaphor throughout the book:

"This is the wizard's secret: the spirit is never overshadowed by the form or the phenomenon. The wizard knows that to be truly alive, she must die to the past in every moment. To be alive now is to be dead to the past. To be alive now is to have life-centred, present-moment awareness. If you have your attention on what is, see its fullness in every moment, you will discover the dance of the divine in every leaf, in every petal, in every blade of grass, in every rainbow, in every rushing stream, in every breath of every living being."[7]

Anticipation

The past is a useful resource, an archive. Regular practice in meditation seems to enhance our natural ability to leave it there and draw on it when we need to. That enables us to be more present to what and where is right now. It can accumulate grace and responsiveness, while deepening our listening faculties in whichever situation we are in. Can it possibly enhance the vitality of the entire fascial matrix as if by listening to it? We actually do not think so much but act more congruently and intuitively, trusting the inner voice of intuition more. In yogic terms this would imply balance between the pranas. In experience of teaching, it can translate to a keener sense of what is happening in the classroom and an appropriate and swift ability to adjust and manage a group. We go beyond simply giving instruction and become free to participate and have access to this third domain of anticipation. The intuitive ability to "pre-sense" can be honed as a skill.

The vital experience of anticipation is one of pre-empting the potential future as a deepening of the presence, occurring from within it. It may be less of an esoteric notion and more what our fascial tissues are doing anyway. It is the basis of adjustments when we become instinctive in our practice: subtle interventions that can sometimes alleviate potential issues before they become a problem. We do not necessarily need to think about them, yet we are very attentive and conscious about making accurate, subtle suggestions. It is awareness, from presence, in action; a kinaesthetic conversation wherein the tissues speak directly and intuitively to each other in their astute sensory language.

"Intuition is neither the ability to engage prophecy, nor a means of avoiding financial loss or painful relationships. It is actually the ability to use energy data to make decisions in the immediate moment. I firmly believe that intuitive or symbolic sight is not a gift but a skill – a skill based in self-esteem."[8]

Intuition

"Intuition" is a subject that can often be associated with a sort of mystical ability to read into the future and see things for which there is little evidence in the physical world. However – and this is important in understanding fascia – it is a different rate of knowing rather than necessarily a special knowledge gifted only to the chosen few. The fascial matrix proprioceptively anticipates all the time. Far from needing special powers, these are specialisations of your body's powers of recognition and distinction. Your body builds up its movement repertoire in time. It constantly anticipates with such ease that you do not even think about it, unless the sense of anticipation "makes a mistake". In a yoga sequence, for example, the movements are completions (of the previous move) and preparations (of the next in the sequence), all at the same time. This proprioceptive ability occurs at a considerably faster rate than thinking. In a way, it recapitulates our original self-assembly. There was no manual!

Caroline Myss[9] (the source of the quotation above) refers to this domain of intuition as moving at a rate so fast it lives in our experience in "still-spin". Myss, a medical intuitive who has been tested under medical research parameters, claims we all have these powers. As we develop our instinctive skills of presence, something becomes available in the realm of teaching movement and practising manual therapy. This "something" is not entirely answered in books on anatomy or psychology. It lives in the stories of what happens in practice and how we (and our students, clients and colleagues) experience it.

Proprioception seems to embrace more subtle distinctions that we can incorporate through the sensitivity of our systems, crafting their art. Our art is yoga and it speaks to the value of practising whichever aspect of it that you wish to teach and develop in yourself and your students.

As yoga teachers, we live in the domain of the body moving (assuming you practise what you teach). We become profoundly familiar with the nuances of form and subtle gesture. So much so that after decades we develop a certain mastery that allows us to intuit more easily. Since the fascial system is a communicating and signalling network, perhaps we are highlighting the more subtle and articulate forms of that communication. Perhaps our tissues are "speaking directly" to someone else's, living matrix to living matrix, via our ability to sense and resonate beyond the purely physical and measurable.

This intuition seems to arrive in advance, a kind of "nous"; it is the intuitive recognition of a potential. It has a different quality to "knowing". It is merely a possibility, a "light bulb moment". When enough of these moments join up, there is a certain illumination that seems to come with confidence or enhance self-esteem. One can begin to trust oneself to know the accurate thing to do at the time. Its hallmark tends to be "volume", in that it can be experienced more like a quietly occurring awareness (a whispering expansion) than a loud moment of revelation. It is, however, invariably an individual experience.

Learning from Teaching

Teaching the postures includes far more than learning them. Part of the task is organising them, creating class plans, inviting students, being on time, making sure of the details and dramas that inevitably go along with the actual process of getting yourself in front of the room. To do that with participants to teach is (in a way) an act of creation, of going from nothing to something. As we become more agile and adept at creating the still, blank canvas, so it seems we can become more creative with the classes we have not taught yet and crafting the confidence to re-create them.

Being present, while it starts with being able to reflect and meditate, goes way beyond your own meditative practice. It includes the participants inside the circle you create called "the yoga class". You become a resource on many levels, so a practice for yourself that enhances your well-being and your calmness so that you enjoy it seems an invaluable tool. This is about feeding the source: the source of life force (Prana) and the source that **you** are in life.

Pranayama means expansion of life force, which might also be associated with expanding our sense of happiness, community and relatedness. Yoga practice at this level works quite simply: a few minutes every day simply being with (and awake to) that life force (consciously doing nothing, essentially). If the fascia is our tissue of relatedness, our inner matrix connecting our wholeness with the parts of us on every scale, then can loading stillness and quiet reflection into its history accumulate calm? Or even vitality? (As a counterbalance to movement, that is, not as a replacement!)

The fastest way to access presence as a sense is through the body. Asking a class participant to follow their breath, or making a subtle adjustment, brings the sensory awareness immediately into present time. Practising this entering into present time is like joining up numerous moments in repetition.

Joining up moments in repetition is essentially what we did in order to learn the yoga poses and sequences. It is much the same process for learning meditation and practising stillness. By connecting many moments of present awareness, we can join them up in meditation and become still, more readily.

Pre-sense within Presence   From this place, we can create class plans, by designing them in advance on the blank canvas of our listening, our presence. Recreation is the basis of having fun. This is where we create and recreate the potential for enjoyment: the active en-joy-ment (ananda) of working congruently, inviting our class participants to do the same. This is something more than writing a list of postures on the way to teaching a class. It is a conscious act of creating a field, one that can contain the ideas of "right doings and wrong doings"[10] and work beyond them. It can make for some fascinating classes and is an interesting domain to teach from.

In this section, we will consider some class plans from this creative place. We become the intuitive creative force, literally and symbolically drawing the circle for others to stand in. Enjoy creating your own Sacred Circles and may the force (and the Source) of your divine inspiration be with you.

Notes

1. A famous phrase used by Dr Ida P. Rolf, founding matriarch of Structural Integration (aka Rolfing), referring here to recognition of different time frames in the human body. John Sharkey refers to our understanding of fascia as "an appreciation of Temporal Medicine" and in this introduction, we bring the notion of time into creating class plans and working in real time in the classroom.
2. Another of Dr Ida P. Rolf's famous phrases, in teaching Structural Integration. It applies in the movement classroom too, since we are learning in Part C how to bring information in Parts A and B to life in practical application.
3. Robert Schleip signs his emails "fascianatedly yours"; Andry Vleeming refers to people in the field as "Affascianados", others prefer "Fascianistas".
4. https://www.joanneavison.com
5. *The Magdalen Manuscript*, by Tom Kenyon and Judi Sion: https://tomkenyon.com
6. Linda d'Antal, https://www.treehouseyoga.co.uk; Vinyasa Flow Yoga; Advanced Yoga Teacher Training, Head of Yoga Faculty at the Art of Contemporary Yoga Ltd 2008–2010.
7. Deepak Chopra, *The Return of Merlin*, Century London, London, 1995.
8. Caroline Myss, PhD, Medical Intuitive. Caroline Myss, *Why People Don't Heal And How They Can*, Bantam Books, London, 1998. For further information see https://www.myss.com or wikipedia.org/wiki/Caroline_Myss
9. Ibid.
10. See Chapter 1 for full [opening] quotation by Rumi (1207–1273): Jelaluddin Rumi, *The Essential Rumi*, translated by Coleman Barks with John Moyne, A.J. Arberry and Reynold Nicholson, HarperCollins, San Francisco, 1995.

13

Classroom Connections 1: The Basics: Sitting Up Curved

"the fascia may be viewed as a single organ, a unified whole, the environment in which all body systems function … The fascia is the one system that connects to every aspect of human physiology. Langevin (2006)[1] and Langevin & Yandow (2002)[2] suggest that the fascia is a metasystem, connecting and influencing all other systems, a concept with the potential to change our core understanding of human physiology."[3]

James L. Oschman

We arrive on the yoga mat much as we first arrive in the world, complete and pre-tensioned by our whole architecture-occupying space. We then explore moving, taking the ability to "feel our way into forms" through the postures and practices. They may be more sophisticated than our first attempts to move in the gravitational field soon after birth, but the movements themselves are nonetheless emergent responses in the moment. They accumulate as history of our form but they actually occur in present time.

To experience this physical event is quite different from activating the intellectual aspect of us, thinking about how we move. It occurs at a different speed, where the body behaves in its own field of animation. Even if several people are doing the same pose or sequence, they cannot experience it for each other. Nor will they experience it in identical ways. The physical intelligence of the moving body takes on a quality of awareness that can absorb our attention in a different way, unique to each of us but universal at the same time.

Intellectual Information

When we are writing or reading about our movements, we tend to sit relatively still, absorbed by acquiring the intellectual information. Once we are on the mat, however, we are invited to absorb the thinking process itself and expand to include it, while we pay attention to the animation of shaping the postures. Yoga was developed for Western culture in a particular way. The movements have a primary purpose of getting us out of our conceptualising thoughts and entering the moving "business". All the attributes of that world become available through being in it and participating.

There is an obvious parallel in the simple example of learning to drive a car. Think of a first driving lesson. Every stick, lever, wheel, mirror, pedal and direction seems

Instinctive Movement

to compete for your attention, with different instructions for each limb. Once you have *practised and repeated* a practice physically, however, something accumulates "in soft developmental strokes" (see Ch. 4) that has a resonance and a momentum of its own. Whether it is driving a car or doing yoga, or choreographing a dance sequence, over time, a process that is initially intellectual (which steps? which order?) becomes instinctive, so you can begin to do it without thinking about every little move. When that happens, you can begin to relax and your attention is not absorbed in remembering things about what you are doing. You can focus on the task in hand, the present situation (constantly changing),

Already Listening

and, with practice and experience, anticipate and respond rapidly and appropriately. You can recall and pre-empt with presence and prescience. This is the witness state in practice. This is yoga.

The Power of Listening

The question most often raised in teaching workshops is that of the optimal balance of theoretical to practical training. The practical sessions, even if they take up half the training period, are often experienced as *seeming* much shorter than the studying time. The instinctive movement centre learns at the speed of instinctive movement. It occurs much faster than thinking.

Movement is instinctive. However, human beings, unlike certain animals, can only learn to stand up and walk around independently over a period of time. Just like the developmental movement patterns, learning specialised movements, such as dance or yoga, can also become second nature. We can use the same method of imitation and repetition to establish new movement patterns throughout our lives.

There are a whole host of external variables you never imagined when you watch someone able to drive instinctively because they have done it for years. Experienced drivers appear to carry out the necessary actions seamlessly and without thought. What makes it even worse that first time is that you are also supposed to anticipate other drivers on the road. (Isn't there enough to do remembering the Highway Code and all these different mechanisms, without worrying about the future?) Until and unless the practice has been repeated enough times to become instinctive, the task can appear fragmented, complicated and full of conflict.

Yoga is an opportunity to practise animating our tissues intelligently, if we honour the innate wisdom of our physical body and act congruently with and from where the body is *at the time*. It does not discriminate with regard to size, age, ability, religion, health, or human performance. Yoga is much less of a noun in many ways than it is a verb. "To yoga" is to "practise at", and explore *unifying* in practice. It confounds the mind – and it is supposed to.

In the Landmark Worldwide education programme[4] (a public self-development forum) there are many distinctions, one of which takes us into the domain of practical yoga with grace. It is the concept of "already listening". When describing the mind, such a term refers to the past, like being "stuck" in a mindset. It points to a natural tendency of human beings to see the world through a prescribed filter made up of our expectations, interpretations and history (i.e. our previous experience). We do it all the time. We filter what we see through the mesh of what we are looking for. If you are looking to validate how muscles and bones move the musculoskeletal system and operate the machinery of the locomotor apparatus, guess what you will find?

In the domain of the fascial matrix, we can shift the context of "already listening" to a powerful recognition. The *fascial matrix is already listening proprioceptively*, in present time, all the time. (Recall the ratio of listening sensory nerve fibres to motor nerve fibres in Chapter 5.) It is a doorway to being present, a way of "changing the body about the mind".[5]

The essence of "already listening" for the body (as distinct from the mind) is that perhaps our form, with its preference for listening, is already aware of where and how we are, relative to ourselves and the world around us. It does not "talk" about it. It experiences it. The body is an intelligent, self-aware communication system, so we need to take care of it (and the art of moving it) with due respect, if that is a consequence of appreciating the fascial matrix as a primary organ of proprioception.

My favourite yoga class of all time was a workshop with Elizabeth Pauncz. We were learning her interpretation of the Egyptian Sun Salutation.[6] Once the postures had been explained and demonstrated and we had familiarised ourselves with the transitions, the choreography began to come together in the group. Elizabeth had stopped talking altogether. Despite the fact that there were over twenty participants at different levels of ability, we moved instinctively, as one group. The salutation to the sun was saluting itself. No words were necessary; by the end of the afternoon, it was more like a synchronised swimming display as everyone moved together, silently expressing movement in its own language.

Yoga is a rich and rewarding forum for exploring this respectfulness. However, it is a process of trial and error. Serge Gracovetsky suggests that we use a gauge of "how we feel the next morning" to guide our limits.[7] At one end of the extreme, if we sit on the sofa reading a book about yoga, nothing much will happen. At the other end, if we over-stretch or force movements, the body is likely to raise its proprioceptive voice the next day and point it out to us in no uncertain terms. Somewhere along this scale we have the opportunity to work out our own optimum. As teachers, we get to experience self-regulating our own balance points and then working with others to establish theirs. We gradually learn (one practice or class at a time) to recognise and communicate this ability to our class participants, if they choose to invite us. Teaching this is a process of imitation, repetition and mutual respectfulness that engenders more of the same (see Ch. 17).

Ground Control

What begins to happen as we surrender to and practise this instinctive aspect of our being is that we move towards less effort, more elastic (free) energy and more conscious awareness. This is vitality. It is essentially animated from the ground up, whichever way up we are.

"The pull of gravity under our feet makes it possible for us to extend the upper part of the spine, and this extension allows us also to release tension between the vertebrae. Gravity is like a magnet attracting us to the earth, but this attraction is not limited to pulling us down, it also allows us to stretch in the opposite direction toward the sky."[8]

When our movement practice spontaneously delivers this effortless quality of elastic recoil, it feels like a revelation. Scarvelli's reference is to a "revolution", which her original approach to yoga effectively provoked.

"We make use of the force of 'anti-force', which gives us a new flow of energy, – a sort of anti-gravity reflex, like the rebounding spring of a ball bouncing on the ground."[9]

This experience of expansion and elastic return is innate to our breath-in-motion. It points to the intimate relationship between movement and breathing that we explore in more depth in a chapter of its own (see Ch. 11). There is a natural and innate quality of elastic recoil available in every pose, as Scaravelli points out, "through the much more powerful wave … produced by gravity and breathing".

The reference also points to the rhythmical sense of the body moving. It reveals itself as a wave through the spine that is palpable from ground to crown in standing (Tadasana) or from sitting bones to crown in sitting. In a headstand the same sense can be found from crown to feet, since the body is inverted but the ground reaction force remains the same.

Our whole fascial form forms a responsive, closed kinematic chain, from moment to moment in every pose (Fig. 13.1). Between the two polarities (of the preparatory counter-movement and the release in the opposite direction) we find and contain our breathing space: neutral. Perhaps this is the joy of intelligent body-wise movement.

Living Tensegrity in Motion

Biotensegrity structures are economical space-containing mobile organisations. This is our breathing space, changing breath by breath from the inside out, the outside in, and through the middle of our structure. Its compliance and fluid transition hallmarks our yogic "performance". Locomotion and respiration are not separate in living organisms, and biotensegrity might provide a context that makes sense of both aspects of our physiology as it works in class. Yoga manifests this unifying context.

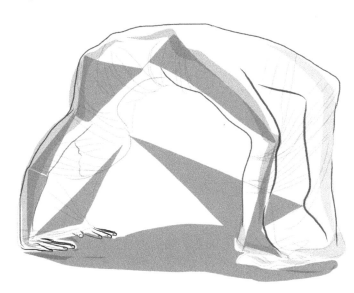

Figure 13.1

In this Wheel Pose (Chakrasana) the hands and feet press in a downwards direction to release the front body into an open upper curve, away from the ground. It is exactly the same the other way up in Dog Pose (Adho Mukha Svanasana), where the hands and feet go down to push the back body up.

Beyond Words

When you experience the quiet spring, or animated release into a headstand or a back bend, as if you are uncovering your own body's innate elastic integrity, its "already listening" motion-in-potential, it is a wonderful feeling and a striking experience of apparently effortless movement. One almost has to get out of the way to reveal it. It naturally springs. It is impossible to describe, even having experienced it, although you can recognise it immediately once you discover it for yourself.

Once on the mat we begin to feel and sense our way to the revolutionary thinking Scaravelli referred to thirty years ago. In essence, her teachings and work accounted for the natural elasticity of our (tensegrity) architecture. Our awareness of this architecture is partly in the living sense of a force and an anti-force united in neutral balance in any poised position. Those three aspects, unified, are the one and the whole together. It is so simple and yet can remain so very elusive to our academic way of thinking.

How do we see that in practice, and how do we foster it for our students' benefit?

Living Tensegrity
Architecture in Action

"All movement, of the body as a whole or of its smallest parts, is created by tensions carried through the living matrix."[10]

Whether or not we understand the tensegrity details of icosohedral or triangulated geometry in our human form, we can begin to explore the spring-loaded and adaptable nature of our tissues and awaken our spines in accordance with its natural laws.

There is an element of surrender in the practice, to an innate balance of forces. The tissues of our form are "already listening"; we cannot think that balance into place. It is a natural expression of our organisation. Having said that, "surrender" is sometimes taken to mean slumping, or be referring to a kind of soggy release. "Softening into a pose", as if one is giving up holding the body together by releasing tension, is a misinterpretation of surrender. It actually refers to a quietening of the mind and a permission to allow the natural forces of movement to do some of the work. It is the revealing of what is present; the revelation Scaravelli describes.

Somewhere between the extremes is a place Scaravelli refers to as "sending the spine away" in the opposite direction. It is achieved in sending the part on the ground down and releasing the part moving away from the ground, away. The space occurring between the two is effectively a sense of the spine releasing in two, opposite, directions simultaneously (down and up).

In order to experience this feeling of spaciousness and containment throughout the torso, we work with simple poses, such as sitting and standing. One place where we can "trip up" on semantics, however, is that we do not honour the spine by sitting or standing up "straight" (Fig. 13.2). We can honour the spine through a balance of curves, whether in the upright or supine position. We do not force the curves into flat planes or hold them in place

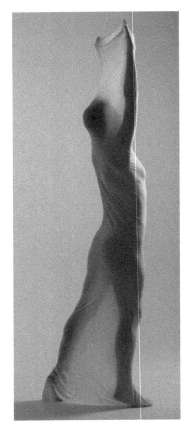

Figure 13.2

We stand in upright curves. The spine is not designed to be straight.

Model: Helen Eadie; Photographer: Amy Very. Reproduced with kind permission from Art of Contemporary Yoga Ltd.

The Sit 'n' Slouch Gym

rigidly. It is a more subtle distinction of *releasing compromise* rather than *controlling shape*.

We are poised in semi-tensioned potential at all times, **curved**. Our self-contained, breathing architecture is poised for motion and designed for mobility. We do not have to do it. Rather we can be with it how it is, and then explore, enhance and develop. If we can find it, it is available through experimenting with this sense of recoil, in person, on the mat. Ironically, it is not actually accessible from reading about it, despite the feeling of recognition if it "speaks" to you. You still have to work with it in participation.

Whatever style of yoga you favour, being able to stand or sit still in animated ease precedes being able to move into the postures comfortably. It allows us to restore ease in the natural, spring-loaded potential of our resting tension. Before we get to any extreme asanas, we can develop the practice itself to bring the simplest of movements to a place of ease. Yoga can deeply enhance the "middle way" of being relaxed in these apparently simple positions of standing and sitting. For although they may appear relatively effortless, they are not necessarily the easiest postures for everyone to be in.

Dynamic Stillness

There is a huge difference between conscious or dynamic stillness and a sedentary slump that might be described as "still", but only because it is not moving. Rather it expresses inertia. In yoga, we learn the value of stillness as an animated option, a personal choice, a vital aspect of any pose. In a way it is an expression of poised movement, repeated over and over. We practise the ability to restore this elusive, neutral condition of balance throughout the tissues, from speed to stillness and back again, developing the ability to adapt from one to the other in smooth transitions – and hold postures when we choose to.

Yoga has a significant contribution to make to our well-being if it only teaches us to sit in a way that does not build in sedentary slouch patterns. If they are not countered, these patterns, left in place as default positions, accumulate in the tissues and become our loading history. The cumulative effect over time can leave our ability to move around impaired by postural stress and compensation. Yoga can train us to sit and stand still in comfort, generating a state of quiet attentive awareness that is nonetheless restful. It is also promising a more optimal loading history to grow into and develop from, at any age.

If there is a twenty-first-century side-effect to the joys and benefits of driving, travelling and Internet communication (including but not limited to mobile phone use patterns), it is the consequences of sitting for long periods of time in *anything but* aware and attentive stillness (Fig. 13.3). The resulting "sedentary stoop" is a daily practice for a huge majority (and I include myself in this; it is hard to avoid). Consider the daily repetitions of this pose at the frequency many of us tend to do it. It is often the case that we are not sitting on our sitting bones as such but on the back of the pelvis and the sacrum. This inevitably changes the shape of the trunk (including the spine) and all things connected to and enclosed by it.

This is not rocket science. The body responds to loading patterns. If we load it in the fetal position for long enough it will adapt to it until that pattern becomes comfortable. This does not imply that it is optimal. It just means it becomes habitual and easier in the short term. It loads the position of the pelvis, the torso, the spaces between the spinal segments, the shape of the abdomen, thorax, neck and shoulder girdle, diaphragm, lungs and viscera; all change with the dominant slumping of the form. *They are designed to respond to and accommodate their loading history and adapt to it.* How can our organs function properly if the shape they reside in is distorted?

Are we structurally designed for quite so much stability or for the sedentary loading patterns of inertia, if they go on too long for our recoil ability to spring back? It is a time-dependent process. We have extraordinary range and potential, so an understanding of fascia's role in this invites us into a huge possibility for addressing health and performance. Practice (of useful loading patterns) gets us closer to optimising both these possibilities.

If we continuously fold the body in slump for long enough and carry on fostering it and expecting it to function by itself, it will not be long before it needs some help. At the very least, the tension–compression balance between front and back, spine and abdomen goes out. Of course, we adapt eventually but do we want to adapt function to optimise the slumping, or adapt the slump to optimise function? The choice is not complex if you have the health and mobility at your disposal.

Happily, it is not difficult to correct the default "sit 'n' slouch" training. The key is what you are sitting on. It does, however, take practice if you have become comfortable in a habitual slumped pattern. Just as a sub-optimal pattern is built in, so it takes repetition to build in a better one. There is a need to stay conscious of extended periods of sedentary slouching to avoid developing the disadvantages of the sit 'n' slouch training. (It gets reinforced over time by continuous micro-movements we do not even notice if our attention is fixed on screen, phone or managing an inbox. The body adapts if it can.)

Our optimal position allows the spine to move in all directions, safely. This is what we are designed for. The net results of this change are frequently described in the following terms: I feel so much less tired … I don't get headaches … I'm more attentive … I don't get indigestion … I can think more clearly … I breathe better … I'm more tuned in, it's as if my mind is clearer.

Part 1

Sit in a slouched position, on the back of the tailbone, with the spine curved as in Figure 13.3. (A commonly observed variation includes crossing the ankles and tucking them under the chair.) Keeping the slouch position in place, try to side bend, then to rotate. Note the range of motion, without going to extremes.

Next, change the shape of the seated posture with two movements: (1) place the feet under the knees and (2) sit "up" on the sitting bones, finding the front part of the pelvic base. Usually the lumbar and cervical curves "appear" naturally just by activating the sitting bones and placing the feet (Fig. 13.4). Pause a moment to feel the alignment of a balanced head, supported from below, relax the shoulders. Then repeat the side bending and the rotation. In most cases, these two small changes in reposition (of the feet and the sitting bones) give rise to a fuller range of motion through the spine in all directions.

Part 2

Next lean forward from the sitting bones. This activates a fold at the hip (instead of the mid-spine, as if we still had a dorsal fin or a dorsal hinge). If the desk is at the right height, and you sit on a cushion that slightly raises the hips above the level of the knee, this will allow an open angle at the elbow and a relatively relaxed head position.

In a therapeutic context, the benefits of training this in, as a preferable "default pattern", changing the "Sit 'n' Slouch" for the "Sit 'n' Smile" gym, are remarkable.

Figure 13.3

Many of us sit for long periods peering forwards to communicate or engage with the screen in front of us. There is a consequence to the posture. It is not complicated to rectify and it is important for optimal function.

Figure 13.4

In the upright position on the sitting bones (ischial tuberosities) the sacrum is free (rather than being sat on) and the torso can hinge at the hip, rather than the spine. The posture can honour the secondary curves (cervical and lumbar).

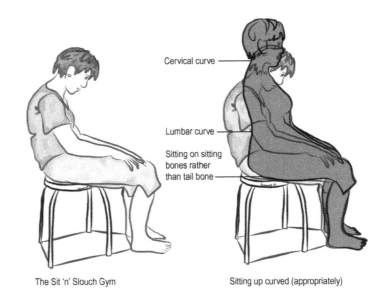

Cervical curve

Lumbar curve

Sitting on sitting bones rather than tail bone

The Sit 'n' Slouch Gym

Sitting up curved (appropriately)

Freeing the Tailbone

If we sit on our sitting bones, as they are designed, we honour both the fold at the hip and the lumbar curve (lordosis). The gluteal muscles are meant to feel "behind us". If we sit slumped onto the very back of the sitting bones, with the "tail tucked under", we are sitting on the sacral roof of the pelvis, instead of allowing the coccyx to float in its natural tensegrity architecture[11] and the tail bone (sacrum and coccyx) to be free. We are effectively following the primal instincts of an animal, wearing our "tail between our legs" in the same way as a dog that is unhappy or frightened.

By then throwing out the second secondary (lumbar) curve, since the spine is naturally an S-shape, we throw out the first secondary (cervical) curve and are obliged to recruit all kinds of neck and back myofasciae to pull the head up and peer forward. (The body will always seek relative balance, visually, to see the horizon line horizontally.)

The active need to lift the head up, out of a default slump, is effortful and, in its mission to save energy, the body will eventually accept and adapt to that loading pattern as a requirement, at least to save muscular effort of maintaining it. One day, after enough time has passed (and loading has accumulated), it will not elastically release and will become the norm. The tissues are then recruited for a less functional holding pattern. Therein lies the beginning of a negative feedback loop. Often pain (such as would be attributed to a chronic postural set) leads to less movement (note the way they can express an inverse relationship in Chapter 9), so we can get stuck in a cycle. If yoga can begin as a gentle restorative enquiry, to tease out (and ease out) habitual holding patterns, there is huge benefit to the smallest movements and sense of a more optimum position. (See Chapter 15 for a series designed specifically to train optimal sitting patterns for the spine.) We just have to repeat the optimal version little and often enough (once or twice a week might be enough, given the active attention on not building the less desirable pattern). As I have said, we are a continual work in progress, and we have power over which direction we progress towards (Fig. 13.4).

Finding your Feet

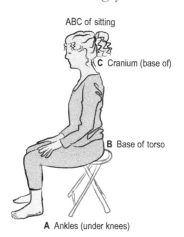

ABC of sitting

C Cranium (base of)

B Base of torso

A Ankles (under knees)

Figure 13.5

The **ABC of Ground Control:** This is a more formal format to the above exercises, as a basis for any preparatory work and a simple sequence to enhance sitting and standing postures. The exercises bring

The image shows the three sets of metaphorical "feet" we have to activate; the feet at the bottom of the legs, the "feet" at the base of the torso (sitting bones) and the "feet" at the base of the head (atlanto-occipital joint). The first two will give rise to the third.

Ankles

This refers to the space above the foot. It wants to rest over the foot in such a way that it is balanced and feels spacious and poised, directly under the knee. Thus the foot is able to feel the ground in its entirety, informing the upper leg.

Base

This refers to the sitting bones. They are designed to support the torso, biased towards the anterior aspect because that is how the pelvis is designed and organised to express our upright gait blueprint. This allows for a natural lumbar curve. If the hip joint is raised slightly above the level of the knee (with a cushion for example), it naturally encourages this posture. This frees the sacrum and coccyx to feel as if they "float" as they are designed to do.

Cranium

The "feet" of the cranium then align naturally with the sitting bones, and move in an appropriate way to balance the head, supported from underneath by the whole torso and neck. The structure is facilitated for the upper vertebral bones (atlas and axis) to work as they should, offering all kinds of subtle movements of the head. If the spine is drooped into one continuous primary curve, given about a naturally more comfortable place for the body, whatever poses are being taught. They are pre-poses in a way. Rather than simply focusing on the "right posture" for achieving specific asana shapes, we are bringing in awareness for the body in everyday life to enhance structure and function as a whole. Fascia responds all the time, so we can consider what we do in our default patterns as part of its training and loading history. Ignoring it all day and then remembering to "sit right" just for the yoga session, is asking a lot of that yoga practice.

Tom Myers nicknamed the levator scapulae muscles "capitis preventus going forwardus", and it is an apt description in the huge majority of cases I see in class or on the body work table. It is tiring to maintain a seated slouch position, with these key myofascial attachments around the neck and head straining to hold it up. Needless to say, there is always a reciprocal counter balance (compression) strain elsewhere in the body.

Relief can come from lengthening the front tissues and encouraging the client to sit up in this way, raising their position, to open the angle at the elbow. (It can also help to train ourselves to use the mouse on the other side and regularly alternate. Taking breaks helps too!) It frequently transforms the daily working demeanour and can make a huge difference to overall postural issues over time. If nothing else, it also allows for more optimal breathing patterns because the diaphragm is not squished. (This optimal posture can affect digestive function and visceral motility in a beneficial way, where the abdominal organs can move more appropriately.)

that the top of that curve is the head, then the relatively heavy cranial vault has to be actively lifted from behind to bring the eyes level with the horizon to see a screen. There is a natural tendency to shorten the back of the neck to compensate. When the torso is balanced, in natural support of the head, these extra "holding positions" are simply not recruited. The architecture leads naturally to a balanced head position, poised for its natural range of motion and attentive to all that surrounds it. Typically computer screens might need to be raised, just as rear-view mirrors in cars seem to be in the wrong place when people adopt this more optimal position.

This basic practice underpins all the seated yoga poses and helps all the standing ones, if we translate the "polarity" principle to all aspects of the asanas: down to go up, back to go forward, and so on.[12] We breathe more easily in the space between the two.

The levator scapulae myofascia and its surrounding tissues (Fig. 13.6) can get knotted and tensed as part of a story of sustained "dis"-integration and it leads to a classical condition I call "mouse shoulder". There are cases where the "lump" in the shoulder (initiated around the levator scapulae being trained for so long each day in the "hang-on-in-there" gym) is particularly clear and palpable on the side the client uses their computer mouse. (It can also be counterbalanced on the other side, so it is not always a simple compensatory pattern.)

People at desks with their elbow dropped below the height of the wrist often exacerbate "mouse shoulder". It is my repeated experience that by raising the height of the chair and the computer so that the hip and the elbow can work at a slightly open angle, while the eyes look straight forward, "mouse shoulder" and extraneous postural tension are relieved to the clearly related benefit of improved attention and biomotional integrity (Fig. 13.7). The feet become an active component of the seated posture. The body often seems to suffer less from being inert and enjoy these daily at-the-desk micro-movements that train the fascial loading history to accumulate a much more useful and varying pattern.

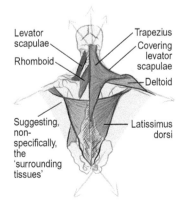

Figure 13.6

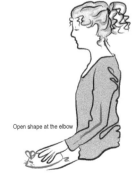

Figure 13.7

Back up

Sit (curved upright) slightly towards the front of the chair on the sitting bones (Fig. 13.8A), with feet placed comfortably apart (hip width) and flat to the floor, knees at right-angles.

Contain (or stiffen the body very slightly), rocking back on the sitting bones a little. This is a small movement: a slight rocking back before rocking forward as the feet are pushed down (to the ground), to *then* go up. It is one smooth transition, although repeating the rocking first can help. With practice the client may not need to use the hands at all.

The movement cue is "back to go forward and down to go up".

Feet off the ground as the body rocks BACK (holding the right-angle at the knee) (i to ii)

Rock FORWARD on the sitting bones, until the feet touch the floor (iii)

Press the feet DOWN as the tail lifts (iv)

Push into the feet to send the body/head UP in one fluid movement, to standing (v)

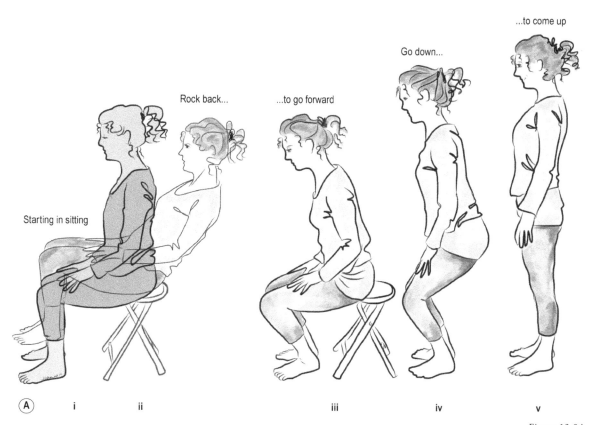

Figure 13.8A

Seated poses

Sitting postures on the mat can incorporate the use of blocks to begin with to open the angle at the hip slightly. This helps to learn to find graceful upright sitting, with comfort. (Please note, this is optimised if care is taken to avoid hyper-extending the knee; a half block is ideal, or a roll put in to the end of the mat, to slightly lift the sitting bones; see Fig. 13.10).

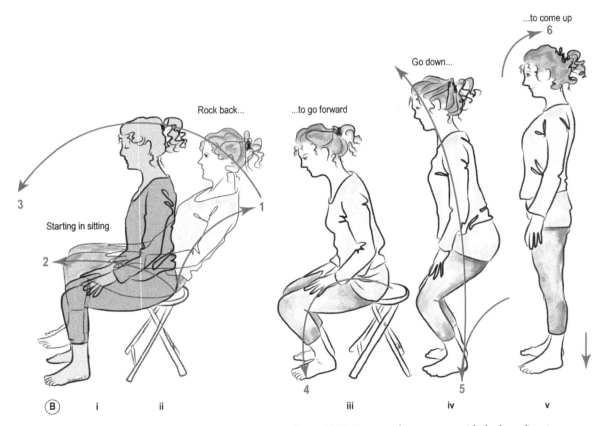

Figure 13.8B Sit to standing sequence with the force direction arrows

In terms of fascial elasticity, this principle, which Scaravelli refers to as a "rebounding" (ii–iii), is termed "preparatory counter movement". The basis is incorporated here: by rocking gently back to go forward; then pressing the feet down (iii–iv) to go up – there is a natural elastic recoil that is experienced as effortless movement. If anything, the participant has to "manage" the spring-loaded bounce to arrive steadily and sweetly into Standing Pose (Tadasana) (v). Sthiram, Sukham – the steady and the sweet – are ancient principles of the yogic postures.

In Between: The Sit-to-Standing Technique

As I work frequently with older people, I have observed that if the body is tired or aches, in order to stand up from sitting, a client will often fold forward, place their hands on their knees and press down hard on their (upper) legs to push themselves up from a chair. A lovely freedom arises from teaching this simple sit-to-standing exercise (Fig. 13.8A and B).

People are amazed how effortlessly they can move by containing the tissues, using this principle of polarity that animates living tensegrity principles, through the architecture as a whole. For the more agile, it can also be used to rise from a supine position to sitting up (Fig. 13.9). (For the very contained, it can be taken from supine to standing, via a squat position.)

Figure 13.9

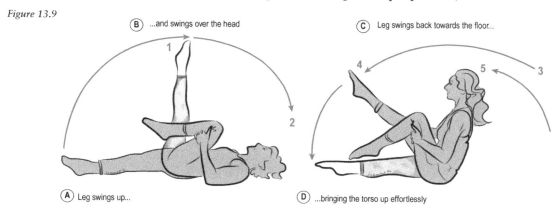

Ⓑ ...and swings over the head   Ⓒ Leg swings back towards the floor...

Ⓐ Leg swings up...   Ⓓ ...bringing the torso up effortlessly

When mature participants discover this, they become highly animated by their body's ability to move more easily than they imagined, just by using these innate elastic recoil principles to counterbalance from within. It invigorates and inspires them. It is great practice for many age groups (with the caveat that you are an experienced teacher, working with individuals you know and regularly teach and they have no spinal injuries; or you are working with a teacher who knows you).

Sensing the Curves of the Supine Spine

We have established the importance of the organisation of the spine in its primary and secondary curves (see Ch. 9). These play a key role in postural organisation, structural support and the optimal breathing patterns (see Ch. 8): all foundations of our fascial form in functional movement.

This simple preparation exercise can help participants to relax upon arrival in class and simply settle before the start. This preparation asana can be used to bring awareness and attention to the body and sense these curves in relation to the ground. It also helps in preparing the body with any supine breathing techniques as the ground provides sensory feedback. Our bodies change throughout the day, becoming gradually more compressed, and they usually decompress through resting overnight. Developing sensory refinement includes the time taken to be aware of how and when we practise. Forcing stretches rarely works but for different reasons at different times of the day.

Begin lying supine. One leg remains held as shown, both hands behind the knee with fingers interlocked. The leading leg swings up and over the head to gain the elastic momentum. As it swings back down towards the floor again, the head and torso lift from the ground into sitting. Interlock the hands behind one knee, take the legs back towards the body (and slightly up to lift the pelvis off the floor) and swing them back to go forward and down to go up (into sitting). At the same time relax the sitting bones down into the ground and it releases the torso up as the legs swing down, elastically. It feels completely effortless. (If it doesn't, it is recommended NOT to undertake without appropriate supervision.)

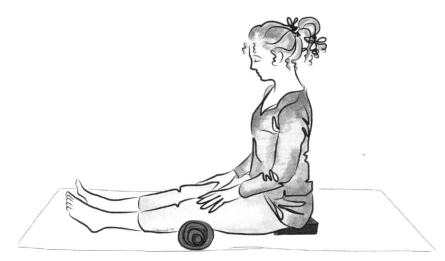

Figure 13.10

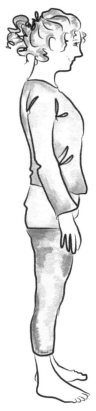

Figure 13.11

Encouraging gentle yawning stretches, after rest periods, primes the tissues and can serve us in accommodating these differences (see Ch. 10).

We find ourselves in a unique place that yoga can take us to. It is a place where there is nothing to do as such. It is a state of being, conscious of sitting and standing upright, curved. We can be in our form, responding movement by movement in subtle, pulsatory awareness of the ground, the shape we make from it and the heart-centred balance this awareness can bring us: simply sensing ourselves as a sensory, whole, animated architecture.

Supine Spine Curves (Fig. 13.12)

Lie on the back with knees bent, feet hip-width apart and toes turned inward slightly to allow the knees to drop softly together. This simply relaxes the legs and helps to release extraneous tension in the lumbar spine, pelvis and particularly the inner thigh myofascial organisation.

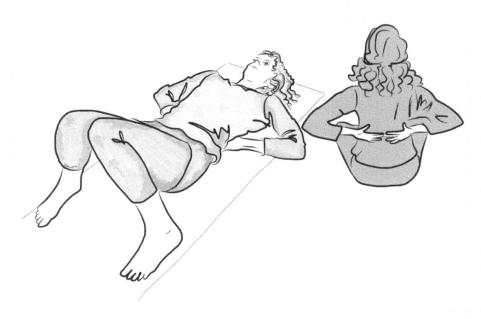

Figure 13.12

We start by feeling how the tissues meet and greet the ground to register them in our sensory field, thereby becoming more conscious of where we are in space.

Place the hands (palms down) under the back of the waist so that the middle fingertips touch. This allows the sense of a gentle lumbar curve, not so much that the back of the waist does not touch the back of the hands and not so little that they are pressed to the floor. (The hands can then be removed and placed comfortably on the floor or the abdomen, once this suitable soft lumbar-spinal curve shape has been found.)

This makes sensing of the primary curves very clear, from the toe tips to the crown, arching under the toes, the medial foot, from ankle to hip at the back of the leg, the lumbar spine and cervical spine.

Bringing gentle, subtle attention to how the curves change (if they do) as the breath moves through the body is a simple way to encourage sensory refinement, while the body remains relaxed and supported by the ground.

This also serves to bring an uncomplicated focus inward to begin a restorative style of class, if it is appropriate to your style of teaching.

PURPOSE: The purpose of this exercise is to sense and experience the arrangement of primary and secondary curves through the back of the body. This uses the ground as feedback.

SUPPORT: The body is fully supported by the ground, which can be further engaged as a sensory feedback mechanism for the breath. An appropriate support at the head can be used if a participant has a strong thoracic curve (kyphosis), such that they have to tip the head back in order for it to rest on the mat. A small block or cushion may be used so that they can clearly feel the back of the cranium as a primary curve. In general, however, I discourage use of a cushion or block under the head unless it is necessary. Neck discomfort is often alleviated by a rolled blanket or towel supporting the secondary curve at the neck. While the "automatic block support" might seem useful, it can also encourage the exact default habit we are seeking to transform. It really depends upon the individual and endorses the suggestion that this, or any postural guidance, is done with appropriate supervision of an appropriately skilled yoga teacher.

Notes

1. H.M. Langevin (2006) Connective tissue: a body-wide signalling network? *Medical Hypotheses* 66(6):1074–1077.
2. H.M. Langevin and J.A. Yandow (2002) Relationship of acupuncture points and meridians to connective tissue planes. *The Anatomical Record* 269:257–265.
3. James L. Oschman, "Fascia as a Body-wide Communication System", Ch. 2.5 in Robert Schleip, Thomas W. Findley, Leon Chaitow and Peter A. Huijing, *Fascia: The Tensional Network of the Human Body*, Churchill Livingstone/Elsevier, Edinburgh, 2012.
4. Landmark Worldwide education programme, http://www.landmarkworldwide.com/.
5. This was one of Tom Myers' strap-lines for the Kinesis Myofascial Integration (KMI) School) (visit www.anatomytrains.com for details of the training in Structural Integration). Now ATSI Anatomy Trains™ Structural Integration.
6. This is available through Helen Noakes, on video. It is a beautiful practice that can be downloaded via http://www.helennoakes.net/shop/.
7. Serge Gracovetsky, presentation at the Lighthouse Centre, Brighton, UK, September 2012.
8. Vanda Scaravelli, *Awakening the Spine*, 2nd edition, Pinter and Martin, London, 2012.
9. Ibid.
10. James L. Oschman, "Fascia as a Body-wide Communication System", Ch. 2.5 in Robert Schleip, Thomas W. Findley, Leon Chaitow and Peter A. Huijing, *Fascia: The Tensional Network of the Human Body*, Churchill Livingstone/Elsevier, Edinburgh, 2012.
11. See Stephen Levin, www.biotensegrity.com for an animation of the biotensegrity of the pelvic girdle.
12. In Fascial Fitness training principles this is referred to as preparatory counter-movement. R. Schleip, D.G. Müller (2013) Training principles for fascial connective tissues: scientific foundation and suggested practical applications. *Journal of Bodywork and Movement Therapies* 17:103–115.

14

"Prior to everything, asana is spoken of as the first part of hatha yoga. Having done asana, one attains steadiness of body and mind, freedom from disease and lightness of the limbs."

Hatha Yoga Pradipika (1:17)

Sthiram, Sukham, Asanam

Several years ago I read a *New York Times* article about investment in sports shoe technology. A doctor (and keen marathon runner) mapped the rise in shoe technology against injuries in elite athletes: injuries were not reduced. He proposed the foot mediates an intelligent listening to the ground, feeding-back to the body about the terrain. Wrapped in "smart" shoes, the feet and legs send/ receive inappropriate signals. The journalist, Chris McDougall, later wrote *Born to Run*. There is controversy about barefoot versus "shod" running. Research[1] suggests preference and training win over either: it depends what you are used to (congruent with the idea that fascia responds to our loading history). James Oschman[2] recommends walking on dew-soaked grass for a few minutes a day to animate the feet. Introducing people to their toes through yoga can improve balance and movement and all sorts of disabilities (see Fig. 14.19).

Sthiram means steady and *sukham* means sweet. *Asanam* refers to a position or posture that is both steady (firm, strong) and comfortable. In a way it echoes the simplicity Vitruvius bestowed upon architecture: *"firmitas, utilitas, venustas"*, making something strong, fit for purpose and beautiful (see Ch. 2). We are, of course, referring here to our natural physical architecture rather than to the built structures of Vitruvius. The postures presented in this chapter under the heading A Simple Practice are designed to naturally clear the energy channels and psychic centres. From the point of view of the fascia, they perfectly confirm the kind of practice that honours individual form and promotes elasticity and hydration. One purpose is to enhance proprioceptive and interoceptive awareness.

By focusing on the relationship of any posture to the ground, to start with, we naturally deploy our soft-tissue, tensegrity architecture to fulfil our multi-dimensional promise. This simple practice is an exploration of that. First and foremost is the technique of bringing ourselves "down to earth", and back to being in our bodies. Then we use our awareness and attention to develop our relationship to it in the simplest of ways.

The feet become our "ears to the ground" and since they have such a constant role in so many of the things we seek to do, there is a value in taking special care of them. These techniques are presented as a class. However, feel free to select what works. You will see exceptional results from 10–15 minutes at the beginning of any session spent on releasing and easing extraneous tension in the feet and "waking them up". They respond with enthusiasm by anticipating our responses to the ground and becoming more intelligent and aware. (See Exercise 8: Ears to the Ground (Fig. 14.19) for specific techniques.)

This sequence is designed as a useful simple and basic practice, though even very advanced yogis and yoginis have used it when they are travelling or working under pressure, with no time for a fuller practice. It is also extremely valuable after illness or injury, when the body is under stress. It allows for a deep strengthening and calming of the system. Counterintuitively perhaps, it can help to facilitate strength and speed on a demanding schedule and restores performance – deploying the elastic recoil principle of going in the opposite direction first!

A Simple Practice

DISCLAIMER: Participants have been able gradually to introduce the very subtle movements involved, even after surgeries or during pregnancy, under careful supervision. In this way, over a suitable period of time (which is unique to every case), they have been able to restore the valuable range of movement optimally available to them. It is advised that, in all such cases, an individual seek the guidance of a trained yoga teacher or yoga therapist, as a book cannot provide the watchful eye of an experienced witness. As a teacher, you are encouraged to practise and modify these foundational asanas to suit your own programme.

These asanas are used to prepare or relax the body and might be done just once per week to give the body permission to simply explore where it is and enjoy the kind of undivided attention that fosters self-regulation. I have used these asanas with people of various ages over long periods of time, at weekly intervals. The intention is to promote fascial glide and sensory refinement through the longitudinal aspects of myofascial continuities, with particular focus on the limbs. All the practices throughout this series are designed to animate the fascia matrix throughout the torso and axial body.

Fascia Muktasana for the Torso, Neck and Head

While freeing the fascia of the form, this Simple Practice also facilitates the breathing rhythm so the whole body is benefiting from gentle attention to the breath. The series presented later, in Chapter 15, invites more subtle movements for all the main joints to free the energy pathways or channels of the subtle body.

Table 14.1		
	Basic class with variations	**Notes**
1	Back to Earth (A and B)	Finding the ground
2	Filling the Space	Listening to the breath
3	Little Boat	Freeing the breath
4	Spinal Twist (A and B)	Two parts, including release
5	The Wave (A and B)	Two variations
6	Stretch-and-Squeeze	The elastic body
7	Fascia Muktasana (A and B)	Using myofascial meridians
8	Ears to the Ground	12 Toe and foot exercises
9	Honouring the Curves (A and B)	Three variations
10	Simple Standing Rotation	Gentle rotation and counter-rotation
11	Sun Salutation of your choice	See Chapter 16
12	Pranayama and Shivasana	See Chapter 15

1A Back to Earth

PURPOSE: The purpose of this is to kinaesthetically note the primary curves (touching the ground) and the secondary curves (not touching the ground) and bring the body into relaxed, but attentive stillness. It allows for life to be left outside the door and gentle attention to return inward for the period of the practice.

SUPPORT: There are schools of thought that place a support under the back of the head. This may be helpful in some cases; however, it is often even more valuable to support the back of the neck and allow the head to return to a more optimal position. A rolled blanket is ideal as it provides a minimal lift, but allows the neck to relax and begin to accommodate a more optimal posture. A small folded towel in the back of the waist can also assist in bringing a participant to a "felt" sense of their natural spinal curvatures.

TIMING: This position can be maintained for 2–12 minutes, with the caveat that at any time a participant can hug the knees to relieve any strain felt at the back of the waist. Its value is in slowing down the racing mind and bringing the attention back to the body.

- Lie on the back, feet hip-width apart, toes slightly turned in.
- Let the knees softly rest together allowing the body to rest down.
- Slide the shoulder blades downwards and slightly together.
- Allow the toe tips, ball of the foot and heel to soften down.
- Allow the pelvis, ribs, shoulders and head to feel the floor.
- Note that which is touching the floor and that which is not.
- Let the breath become relaxed and even.

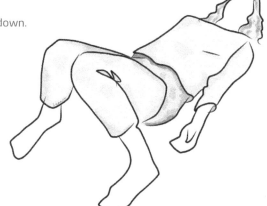

Figure 14.1

1B Back to Earth: Finding the Curves (as per Ch. 13)

PURPOSE: The purpose of this is to sense the primary and secondary curves of the back body from the crown of the head to the soles of the feet, including the heel, arch, ball of foot, spaces between the ball of the foot and the toe tips and the ends of the toes. We follow the "wave" of the curves using the ground as a reference for the whole length of the body – primary curves touch the floor, secondary do not. (The notion of pressing the back of the waist or the neck into the floor is actively avoided: a straight spine is not an integrated one.)

SUPPORT: This comes from the ground and is aided by the hands initially supporting the subtle and natural curve at the back of the waist.

TIMING: This can be at the discretion of a teacher, as a finishing pose, a starting pose, or a resting pose. If it is to specifically encourage primary and secondary curve recognition it can be used as a repeated reference.

- Place hands (palms down) under mid back, middle fingers touching (see Fig. 14.2B).
- Slide the shoulder blades together and down, resting into the floor.
- Feel the primary curves: head, shoulders, hips, heels, toes (Fig. 14.2A).

- The primary curves touch the floor.
- Now feel the secondary curves: neck, waist, back of legs and foot arch.
- Release the hands if preferred and sense the curves as a wave.
- Take attention to the sides and front of the body relative to the back.

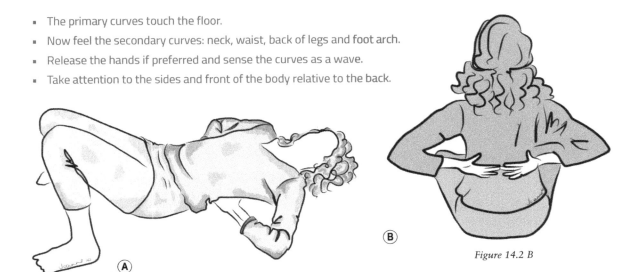

(A)

Figure 14.2 A

(B)

Figure 14.2 B

2 Filling the Space

PURPOSE: The purpose of this is to deepen the sense of elasticity that the breath can optimise. It is not to force the breath or induce fast or heavy breathing. Rather it is to familiarise the body with the sense of its biotensegrity architecture: inhaling fully to expand to the point of resistance, exhaling fully to squeeze to the tensional limit. In each case, the release returns the torso to its natural resting tensional integrity. This exercise can be repeated 2–12 times without force (and resting between cycles) (see Ch. 11). It is a preparation to invite tone to the torso as an overall value in any movement. It is enhanced by the specific breathing exercises in Pranayama practice; however, this is designed as an introduction.

SUPPORT: As for 1. Another benefit of this is to invite participants to feel the back and the front of the body, and fill into the sides so that they experience their three-dimensional "containment" of their own boundaries. The floor becomes an important resource and a feedback system as awareness is encouraged by "pushing the floor away" during the full inhale and surrendering to it during the exhale. It becomes an enquiry as to how that changes on the extra exhale and release during the three phases of the elastic breath cycle. Avoid forcing or inducing over-breathing.

TIMING: As below. At any time a participant can hug the knees to relieve any strain felt at the back of the body. This is usually done as part of the "back to earth" rest, once attention becomes inwardly focused.

- Allow the tongue to rest softly on the roof of the mouth.
- Breathe through the nose, inhaling and exhaling evenly.
- Gradually feel the inhale expand the torso, following it.
- At first let the exhale go and rest at the end of the exhale.
- Then explore the "extra exhale", squeezing the whole torso.
- Let that go and experience the inhale to release it.
- Explore this several times without force to become familiar.

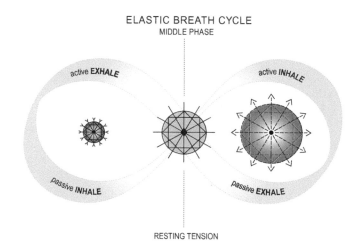

ELASTIC BREATH CYCLE
MIDDLE PHASE

active **EXHALE**

active **INHALE**

passive **INHALE**

passive **EXHALE**

RESTING TENSION

Figure 14.3

See Figure 11.3 for full size Elastic
Breath Cycle diagram.

3 Little Boat Variation (Pasva Pavana Muktasana)

PURPOSE: The purpose of this is to gently allow the spine to find its rotational ability, with the shoulder girdle and pelvic girdle rolling toward opposing directions. This should not be forced. It is a small movement allowing the spine to find its natural rotation, gently and cumulatively through the length of the spine. It is essential that this is done in a small and comfortable range, without force, as the breathing continues. Ideally the breath is inhaled at centre and exhaled toward the twist but this will become natural if the posture is not forced and allowed to find an instinctive rhythm. There is also a lovely bonus in "massaging" the long myofascial continuities of the erector spinae along their length on the floor. Fluidity of movement is more valuable than range in this asana.

SUPPORT: As for 1, although by this time participants often feel they need less support after the work of the first two parts of this preparatory sequence. The movement can be a micro-movement, so such a small range will not disturb the support under neck, head or lumbar spine.

TIMING: This postural twist can be explored for 1–3 minutes, as preparation for the fuller twist to follow. It is designed to relieve tension and improve range in a subtle way and at a natural speed.

- With an extra exhale to support the lumbar spine, squeeze and press into one foot to send the other knee to the chest.
- Wrap the hands around the folded knee and on the next exhale draw the other knee to the chest, releasing the lumbar spine.

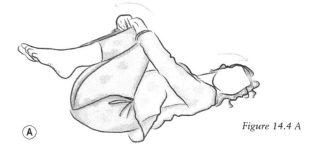

(A)

Figure 14.4 A

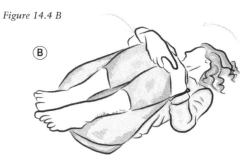

Figure 14.4 B

(B)

- Re-establish the soft curves of the back body, hugging the knees.
- Begin to rock the knees gently from side to side (a small range).
- Softly add the head to the movement in the opposite direction.

4A Lying Spinal Twist (Supta Matsyendrasana)

PURPOSE: The purpose of this is to gently deepen the spinal twist that number 3 prepared for. The invitation is to release into this posture as an opportunity to "unwind" the spine, using the breath to explore the spaces between the ribs, the "corners" of the lungs and sense the breathing in the neck, abdomen and diaphragm. A lovely cue is to imagine the right dome of the diaphragm as the wing of a dove (I do not know where this inspired idea first originated but it was not mine). The image of a dove opening one wing to let the sunlight (of the breath) through its feathers and allow that to release and open the breath is delightful. The weight of the pelvis and shoulder girdle will naturally facilitate the twist. DO NOT FORCE.

SUPPORT: Blocks can be placed on either side of the body to ensure the twist is within natural range. It is very common for the number of blocks to be reduced within a few weeks of practice if the participant honours their comfort zone and does not force the twist. Sometimes a block or towel between the knees is more comfortable. The angle of the knee can be adjusted for comfort too. Focus is "through" the spinal length of cumulative rotation evenly along the spine. There is no need for forced twist at the waist or neck. This can be detrimental and at the expense of subtle unwinding.

TIMING: This postural twist can be explored for a few breathing cycles. It is used to find the relaxed unwinding, not to be pushed into achieving a twist. The next pose is coming out of this posture safely, via the breath.

- Find the centre position (see 4B and Fig. 14.6) and take the right arm out to the side.
- Place the right palm on the ground, anchoring the pose.
- Inhale and do nothing, sensing the right arm moving downward.
- Exhale the knees towards the left, continuing the extra exhale.
- Rest both knees on blocks or the ground, as comfortable.
- When ready, gently turn the head to look along the right arm.
- Relax the body and explore the right side of the breath.

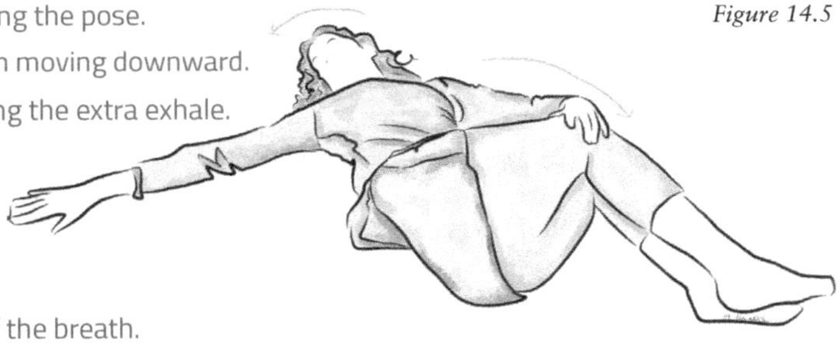

Figure 14.5

4B Releasing Lying Spinal Twist (Supta Matsyendrasana)

PURPOSE: The purpose of this is to gently return the body, without putting pressure on the lumbar spine. It also increases the proprioceptive sense of awareness regarding the distinct difference between left and right sides after doing the pose to one side. There is usually a sense of more openness, or that one side of the body is "lower" than the other. The pose also facilitates the subtle awareness of the breath and allows the tissues to be gently animated in a non-invasive but attentive way. The one rule of this posture is DO NOT FORCE. The range of motion will accumulate gradually over time and the benefits of increased breathing capacity will be naturally incorporated.

SUPPORT: As 4A.

TIMING: The rest between twisting from one side to the other is a matter of personal judgement. Usually a few breathing cycles while the participant appreciates the difference between left and right is sufficient to experience the value of this pose.

- Breathe in, do nothing. On the exhale return the head to centre.
- Breathe in, do nothing. On the extra exhale, squeeze and bring the upper knee back to the chest and allow the lower knee (closest to the floor) to follow.
- It is very common to experience a distinct difference between one side and the other.
- Having consciously noted that difference, repeat 4A to other side.
- Hug the knees and listen to the sense in the back of the body.

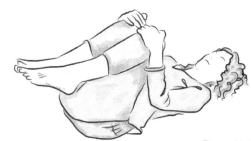

Figure 14.6

5A The Wave

PURPOSE: The purpose of this is to bring conscious kinaesthetic awareness to the spine in all its detail and synchronise breath and wave. To begin with there is often a feeling of sections of the spine moving together; however, this will foster micro-movements that eventually build a much more sensitive response, gently moving each vertebra and allowing the spaces between them to free up and bring more suppleness to the whole spine. The keynote of this posture is patience and allowing the spine to respond to the feet going down. One begins to surrender to the sense of a wave from coccyx to crown. It is a powerful preparation for shoulder stand but should not be forced at the neck. No tension is needed in the back of the body, as this is an exercise in less recruitment, not more. The buttocks do not need to tense to "push" the pelvis up. It is designed to encourage the wave of release through the spinal architecture, safely supported by the ground, as a response to the feet going down into it. One seeks fluid movement quality rather than height or force. A variation of this can be taken to the wall (5B).

SUPPORT: Ideally no support is required, as this posture need not be taken beyond a small sacral tilt if the participant cannot easily lift the weight of the pelvis. No force is needed. The purpose is to find or reveal a natural spinal wave, not perform a lift. Eventually it finds a breathing rhythm: breath and wave work together in synchronicity. This is the purpose of this practice.

TIMING: This wave can be done for several cycles up and down the spine.

- Return the feet to the floor so that they are parallel, knees bent.
- Find the ground and press the footprint down to move the sacrum.
- Explore and experience the subtle activation of this relationship.
- As the feet press the floor, the sacrum softly rolls back and forth.
- With legs and feet parallel, we explore this "down to roll up".
- One vertebra at a time, peeling the spine off the floor.
- Returning one vertebra at a time to the starting position.

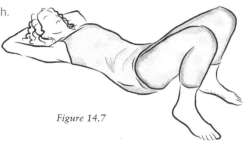

Figure 14.7

5B The Wave Inverted

PURPOSE: The purpose of this is to bring conscious kinaesthetic awareness to the spine in all its detail and to introduce inversion. For older participants inversion may not be suitable. However, using the wall allows any fear to diminish and increases confidence with a sense of the benefits of inverted poses. It also facilitates the lift of the pelvis. It can be easier to encourage an articulate spine from this starting position. Again, this will foster micro-movements that eventually build a much more sensitive response. Each vertebra is gently moved, allowing the spaces between them to free up and bring more suppleness to the whole spine. The keynote of this posture is patience and allowing the spine to respond to the feet pressing the wall. One begins to surrender to the sense of a wave from coccyx to crown. It is also a powerful preparation for shoulder stand but should not be forced at the neck. No tension is needed in the back of the body, as this is an exercise in less recruitment, not more. The buttocks do not need to tense to "push" the pelvis up. It is designed to encourage the wave of breath through the spinal architecture, safely supported by the feet against the wall. One seeks quality of wave rather than height.

SUPPORT: As for 5A.

TIMING: This wave can be done for several cycles up and down the spine.

- Press the feet to the wall so that they are parallel, knees bent.
- Find the wall and press the footprint into it to move the sacrum.
- Explore and experience the subtle activation of this relationship.
- As the feet press the wall, the sacrum softly rolls back and forth.
- With legs and feet parallel, we explore this "press away to roll up".
- One vertebra at a time, peeling the spine off the floor.
- Returning one vertebra at a time to the starting position.

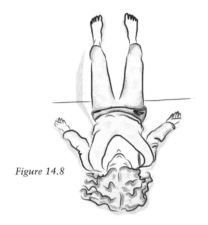

Figure 14.8

6 Natural Yawn

PURPOSE: The purpose of this is to bring the value of an actively loaded stretch to the whole body after having been on the floor for 12–20 minutes altogether. It primes the body and invites participants to remember how easy and how important it is to stretch-and-squeeze (i.e. yawn and stretch) after the tissues have been resting. Personally, I believe the minimum daily practice of spending a couple of minutes, even in bed, simply stretching and yawning and waking the body up (like most self-respecting animals) is a most valuable and forgotten resource. It serves the tissues but primarily it serves us to be conscious of them as we transition from sleep and rest to motion. Long periods of sitting in cars, not to mention at desks, are usefully countered with short yawning stretches.

SUPPORT: Rolling onto the right side of the body and using the hands to push up from the ground protects the spine as it rises to a sitting position. For some older participants, it is useful to go round onto all fours to bring themselves up without strain.

TIMING: Enjoying the experience of moving from supine to sitting in a different place mentally and physically, having paid attention to the body for a quarter to half an hour, encourages presence.

- Return to the mat and simply yawn and stretch.
- Yawning in class tends to be catching, so set up a wave!
- Encourage natural stretches one side then the other.

- Then opposite hands to feet, then same side.
- Gentle long arch and curls, feeling into the corners of the body.
- Reaching into the fingers and the toes, as they lengthen away.
- Roll onto the right side to push up into sitting.

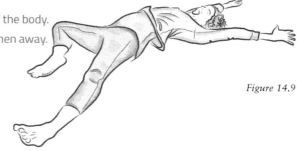

Figure 14.9

7A Fascia Muktasana (LEGS)

PURPOSE: The purpose is to bring more detailed awareness to the longitudinal meridians in the lower limbs and free the gliding capacity of the fascial tissues. It is important to practice this gently, with the sense of a yawning stretch, while remaining within personal elastic limits. Done with supervision, to avoid over-straining, this is the most valuable "flossing the tissues" experience. It frees the fascia at various depths, according to how it is in the individual. An excellent cue is to ensure the felt sense of pushing floor and ceiling apart (keeping the hip on the floor), so that the knee is not hyperextended and the spinal curves are not pulled. It is not about stretching the whole leg and folding it back to the head. For people who can do that easily, the task calls for more tensioning of the tissue, to experience the glide at varying depths. For those who feel shortness (which they may well describe as stiffness) or adhesion, it is important to do this slowly and inquisitively to find glide and length through the lower limbs, without forceful pulling on any meridian at the expense of any other.

It is also essential to pause, both knees bent, before doing the other side, to appreciate the difference resulting from freeing the fascia. Great benefits are reported from doing this for every age group, and it has been successfully used in rehab, as it can also be done sitting up. (See SUPPORT.)

SUPPORT: In standard practice, the ground and the other bent leg, with foot well placed on the floor, will provide the base of support. The fingers interlocked around the back of the leg prevent over-effort in the leg. It is an exploration of tissue glide rather than an exercise in strength or reach. Range expands as the layers free themselves. In seated versions, the leg must be fully supported, folding at the hip joint, and the back upright and supported if necessary (use a block to ensure comfort in sitting upright and have the back against a wall if that encourages an easy, seated pose).

TIMING: 1–3 minutes for each variation, taken relatively gently, will pay dividends, with pauses and releases as required throughout.

- Lie on your back (see 9A, Honouring the Curves).
- Press the left foot down into the ground to raise right knee to chest.
- Interlock the fingers behind the right knee and dorsiflex the foot.
- Relaxing back into the ground, press the foot towards the ceiling.
- Imagine pushing the ceiling away from the floor with the foot and ...
- Simultaneously press the floor away from the ceiling with the hip.
- This naturally opens the back of the knee, keeping foot flexed.
- Gradually reach the foot to the ceiling and towards the face.
- You will feel the Superficial Back Line (see Ch. 18) gliding (or not) through the back of the leg as you straighten it.

Figure 14.10

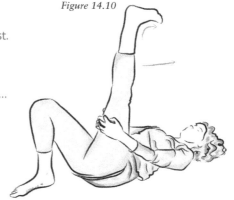

- Release the foot, with a soft bend at the knee, and repeat gently.
- Then point the foot (plantarflex) strongly towards the ceiling.
- Gradually reach the foot to the ceiling and towards the face.
- You will feel the Superficial Front Line (see Ch. 18) gliding (or not) through the front of the leg.
- Release the foot, with a soft bend at the knee, and repeat gently.
- Then flex the foot and invert it (face inward), reaching to ceiling.
- Take the foot across the midline of the body with a straight leg.
- You will feel the Lateral Front Line (see Ch. 18) gliding (or not) along the side of the leg.
- Release the foot, with a soft bend at the knee, and repeat gently.
- Then flex the foot and evert it (face outward), reaching to the ceiling.
- You will feel the Deep Front Line (see Ch. 18) gliding deep to the core leg as you reach up.
- Take the inner ankle bone (medial malleolus) across the midline.
- Keeping the leg as straight as possible and towards the face.
- You will feel the longitudinal "pull" of the deep leg compartment.
- Release foot, with a soft bend at the knee, and repeat gently.
- Hug the knee to the chest, stretch the other leg away and then ...
- Return both legs to the starting position observing the difference from one side to the other.
- Then repeat to other side.

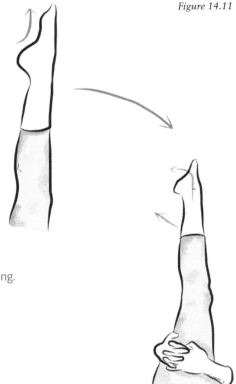

Figure 14.11

Figure 14.12

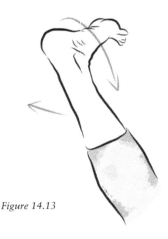

Figure 14.13

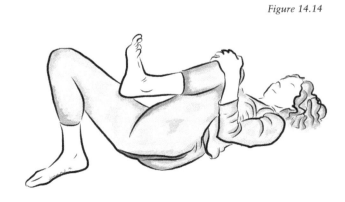

Figure 14.14

7B Fascia Muktasana (ARMS)

PURPOSE: To release and explore the limits of the arm tissues. This facilitates glide and mobility of the shoulder joint as well as releasing common holding patterns from seated postures and activities such as driving and working at a computer.

SUPPORT: In standing practice, Tadasana supports this pose. If done in sitting (on a stool with no back), be sure to be up on the sitting bones.

TIMING: 1–10 repetitions for each variation, taken relatively gently, will pay dividends, with pauses and releases as required throughout.

- Sit comfortably in an upright posture with space around you, or …
- Stand in Tadasana, with feet hip-width apart.
- Take the arms out to the sides at shoulder height, palms down (Fig. 14.15).
- Gradually rotate the hands behind (Fig. 14.16), leading with the thumbs.
- Keeping the length from hand to hand across the torso, as you rotate.
- Gently allow the thumbs to lead the breast bone up into an arch.
- Hold the elastic limit of the rotation and gradually reverse (Fig. 14.17).
- Leading with the little finger, reverse by turning the hands forward.
- Maintaining the length from hand to hand across the torso, rotate.
- Allow the back to round slightly.
- Feel the rotation of the hands curl the spine.
- Release the hands down by the sides and find centre in Tadasana.

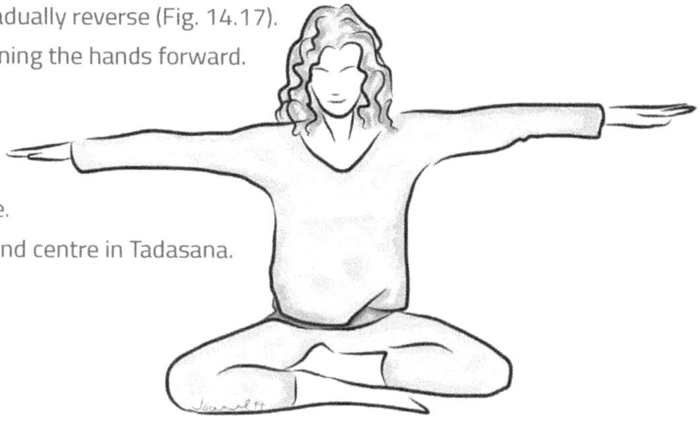

Figure 14.15

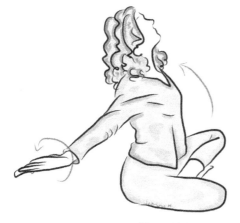

Figure 14.16

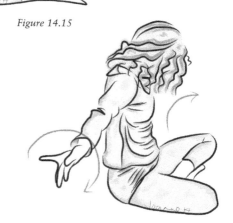

Figure 14.17

- Stand in Tadasana with feet hip-width apart (Fig. 14.18A).
- Clasp hands behind you at sacrum and interlock the fingers, forefingers together.
- Rest the hands on the sacrum, so that the elbows are bent.
- Inhale gently and do nothing, relaxing the arms and shoulders.
- With the exhale (Fig. 14.18B), begin to point downward over the sacrum and …
- Squeeze the wrists, elbows and shoulder blades together.
- Squeeze the breath, pressing the feet down and crown upwards.
- Release the breath with the arms and relax back to start position.
- Repeat as required (working up to 10).
- Variation on this includes folding at the hip in forward bend.
- Allowing the long arm position to continue to arc over the head.
- This is quite advanced so please move arms forward without force.
- Let the arms drop back before unrolling the body back to standing (Tadasana).

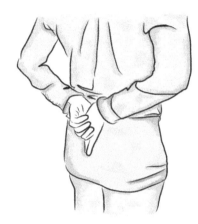

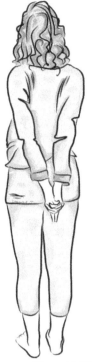

Figure 14.18A

Inhale

Figure 14.18B

Exhale

8 Ears to the Ground

PURPOSE: The purpose is to bring more detailed awareness to the feet and enhance proprioception and "ground control". The feet are our ears to the ground. The more detailed and "literate" they become, the more articulately they respond. We will go on to explore using the feet to guide us in activating the myofascial meridians. This preparation is valuable for gradually improving co-ordination of the toes and physical literacy in the feet. A 10-minute weekly practice of these exercises transforms the ability to do them over 3–12 months. They seem to provide a disproportionate confidence in the body, compared to the apparently small scale of the achievement. Since the feet have to "understand us" all day long, this offers an opportunity to encourage them to be more refined and detailed in their feedback signals to the rest of the body. I am convinced it prevents falling and, when a fall is inevitable, it seems to encourage bounce! Try balancing and rocking on the feet in standing before you do the other side. The difference is obvious and palpable between the two feet before/after.

SUPPORT: Ideally this is done barefoot.

TIMING: This can be done 5–10 times for each exercise.

- Use a block under the sitting bones to ensure comfort in sitting upright.
- Alternatively have the back against a wall to encourage an easy seated pose.

- Sit up on sitting bones, avoiding slump.
- Massage one foot in a seated position, including the whole foot and ankle.
- Place the fingers of the opposite hand between the toes and hold.
- Place one foot on the floor spreading the toes (A).
- You can hug the knee for comfort as you "talk to your toes".
- Lift and lower the big toe on its own, move side to side (B).
- Place the big and little toe down and lift/lower middle three (C).
- Raise all five toes up (D), lowering just the big and little toe alone.
- Attempt to move the second, third, fourth toes on their own (E).
- Drum the toes, seeking to lower them one at a time to the floor.
- Repeat on the other side.

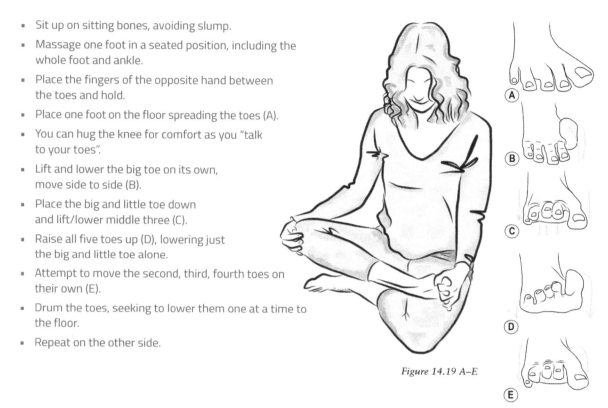

Figure 14.19 A–E

9A Honouring the Curves: Tadasana

PURPOSE: The purpose of this is to rediscover the sense of the primary and secondary curves in standing, to develop the self-sensing of a long torso, able to "create space" throughout its length. It also honours the subtle postural changes of the breath (see Ch. 17, Adjusting the Breath) and permits the confluence of breath and bones in their soft tissue architecture. It becomes relaxed and beautiful, without stiffness or discomfort. It takes practice but is worth exploring for the sensory refinement that naturally accumulates as the extra exhale is explored and released.

SUPPORT: This comes from the ground; the feet are consciously pressing into it but attentively, rather than forcefully. It is very rewarding, with practice, as the body quietly finds confidence and restfulness without strain, revealing its biomotional integrity in this natural and easy pose that actually is not so natural or easy at first.

TIMING: This can be at the discretion of a teacher but 1–2 minutes may feel a lot initially. Ensure participants are not over-breathing. This is a subtle animation of the previous asana and is, in some practices, considered to be an advanced pose. Stillness in standing takes practice. If it is to specifically encourage primary and secondary curve recognition it can be used as a repeated reference.

- Stand in Tadasana, with feet hip-width apart and activated.
- Spread into the toes and find the ground through the foot.
- Find the sense of going down (via feet) to go up (via crown).
- Imagine the pelvis as a tilted heart shape, slightly anterior (Fig. 14.20).

- Imagine the first ribs as a tilted heart shape (see image).
- Align the centres of the two heart shapes, over each other.
- Sense the curves as a wave from ground to crown and breathe.
- The inhale expands, the exhale waves and lengthens the torso.
- The "heart-shapes" stay over each other, their centres aligned.

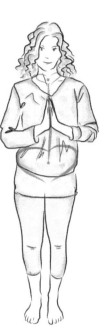

Figure 14.20

This is less fanciful than it might first appear. If you look at a classroom skeleton, the pelvic ring and the first ribs appear as tilted "Valentine heart" shapes if you stand in front of them. This cue is very easy for participants to follow and even inexperienced members of class can bring about a lovely and easy-to-remember poise in upright posture, standing or sitting.

9B Honouring the Curves: From the Diaphragm

PURPOSE: The purpose of this is to become conscious of the breathing, integrated psoas and diaphragm relationship. It also honours the lumbar curve and allows the somatic sense of the breathing movement to filter through the pelvis. This should not be forced. Again, these are micro-movements to encourage elasticity. The sensation is to allow natural elasticity at the hip to be revealed, gently observing the swing and breathing rhythmically.

SUPPORT: This comes from the ground under the standing foot (a block) and the hand on the wall or bar, resting gently so the body does not activate balancing as such. This is not a leg-raising or swinging exercise. It is a subtle observation of how we breathe down into the legs, via the lumbar spine, and experience the spine with their movements.

TIMING: This can be done for a minute or two and repeated, but is not advised for long periods on each side as it can, at first, feel unbalanced before both sides are animated.

CONTRAINDICATIONS: Participants should try this only after 9A, especially if they are sedentary or experiencing lumbar pain. It can help to relieve it; however, the return to standing must be cautious and attentive.

- Stand on a block, one foot centred, with a hand on the wall.
- Find an easy Tadasana, on the standing foot, knee "unlocked".
- Allow the other foot to hang off the block.
- The hanging foot often begins to swing very slightly.
- Feel the swing, the wave of the breath, and allow the foot to hang.
- Gradually find the sense that the foot hangs from the diaphragm.

- The swing is small, effortless, feeling the curves through the spine.
- Take attention to the length of the torso, subtle micro-movement.
- Release gently, standing down from the block to feel the two sides.
- Repeat to other side, preparing attentively and using the wall.

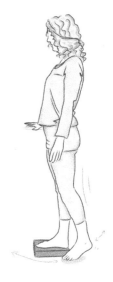

Figure 14.21

10 Simple Standing Rotation

PURPOSE: The purpose is to guide the body gradually into rotation to give the spine kinaesthetic information as to its rotational, elastic limits. Do not force any twist. Remain clear where the ground is and have the sense of rotating in a spiral to facilitate smooth gliding rotations throughout. Gradually, over time, this facility accumulates in the spine, without force and without compromising the natural lumbar and cervical curves. The effort is in fluid glide rather than range.

SUPPORT: This comes from the feet. The back of a chair can be used, releasing the leading hand (i.e. to the side or direction of the rotation) as the twist is completed and bringing it back to the chair by return and changing sides.

TIMING: Three repetitions or rounds, with a few seconds holding (as above), can be built to more with longer holds. However, the point is to free and release the spine.

- Stand in Tadasana, preparing to rotate up and down the joints as follows:
- Gently turn only the ankles over the foot, to the right …
- Then the knee over the ankles, the hip over the knee …
- Then the ribs over the hips, the shoulders over the ribs …
- Then the chin over the shoulders, cheek bones over chin, eyes over cheeks.

- Look around behind you, softening the stance, feet planted, and keep the breath even and soft.
- Hold for 30–90 seconds, relaxing.
- Return through the joints in reverse order; that is, eyes to centre ...
- Then cheeks, then chin, then shoulders, then ribs, then hips ...
- Then knees, then ankles over feet and back into Tadasana.
- Rest in Tadasana and repeat joint by joint to the other side.

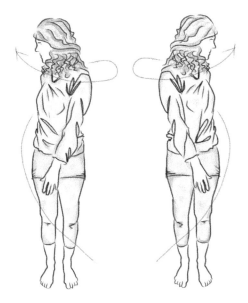

Figure 14.22   *Figure 14.23*

11 Sun Salutation (see Ch. 16)

PURPOSE: The purpose is to integrate all the different practices into a conscious sequence, with fluid transitions and integrated breathing movements. The body stays in communication with the ground and naturally responds to it. Speed accumulates; however, quality of movement through transition is paramount and will soon become more elegant as the body begins to move from contained relaxed structural integrity.

SUPPORT: This comes from the relationship that develops with the ground, through the hands and feet in all the postures of the sun salutation. It also becomes part of our torso strength and containment, as the breath is followed with fluid grace. Music can be very helpful to find the natural rhythm and help the body to drop into its instinctive movement.

TIMING: One or two rounds of Sun Salutation (Surya Namaskara) after a long practice can be very rewarding. Over time this can be built up; however, supervision is advised if any difficulty is experienced. Sun Salutation (Surya Namaskara) is a gift, rather than a challenge. It can bring energy to the awakened tissues and benefits from conscious preparation.

- Choose your own favourite Sun Salutation or use the one detailed in Chapter 16.
- Stand comfortably at the front of the mat.
- Carry out your favourite Sun Salutation (Surya Namaskara).
- Experience the congruent flow of the breathing and also ...
- The contained wave of the spine, from ground to crown.
- This is an opportunity to gently put all the above into practice.
- You can slowly increase the number of moves incorporated and the number of repetitions.
- Chapter 16 includes a Posture Mandala of this part of the practice.

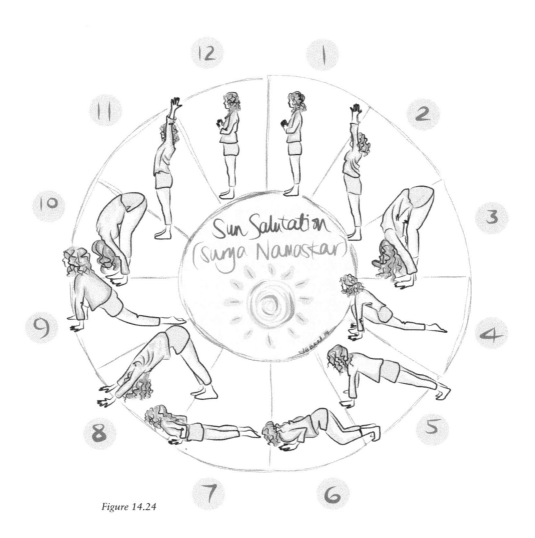

Figure 14.24

12 Pranayama and Shivasana

PURPOSE: The purpose is to begin the practice of stillness and contemplation as a preparation for meditation. It is partly to allow the body to simply "be": focusing the mind on moving the breath in subtle ways, while relaxing in a clear still position that eventually becomes effortless.

SUPPORT: This comes from the base position, the cross-legged pose or the block/cushion and/or the wall if it is used. Be sure to stay up on sitting bones, or even use a chair to start with, until the body is used to stillness. Meditation is not necessarily easy, however simple it may look. The body responds to loading patterns and it takes time to accumulate attentive stillness in a balanced body. That is the point.

TIMING: To begin with, this can be done for 3–5 minutes, building slowly. Supple joints and improved comfort in sitting are two of the many benefits of this deceptively simple series.

- Sit comfortably on your sitting bones, with legs crossed.
- Use a block for added comfort or lean against the wall, upright.
- Close the eyes and let the tongue rest on the roof of the mouth.
- Inhale and exhale through the nose, breathing gently, no force.
- Feel the coolness of the inhale at the tip of the nostrils.
- Invite the breath in, expanding upward to crown at the 12-finger point (Fig. 14.25).
- Hold the inhale for a moment, then allow the exhale to go, as if spiraling out.
- The sense is that the exhale spirals downward, squeezing the front of the spine to the ground, below the sitting bones, spiraling down/out, becoming roots, beyond you.
- Invite a quiet pause at the end of the exhale, squeeze the breath a little more.
- Release the breath (inhale) and continue smoothly through inhale cycle.
- Allow this to travel spiraling outward and upward, through the crown again to 12-finger point and repeat; sensing gently in the round, the spiraling nature.
- Pause for easy breathing at any point.
- Ensure that the eyes remain still, without following breath, quietly closed.

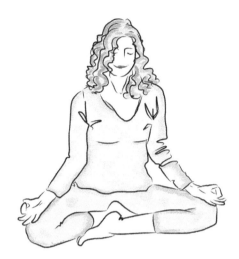

Figure 14.25

Shivasana

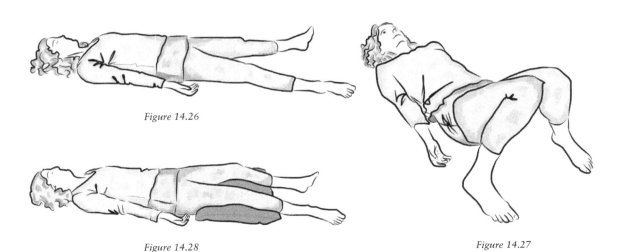

Figure 14.26

Figure 14.28

Figure 14.27

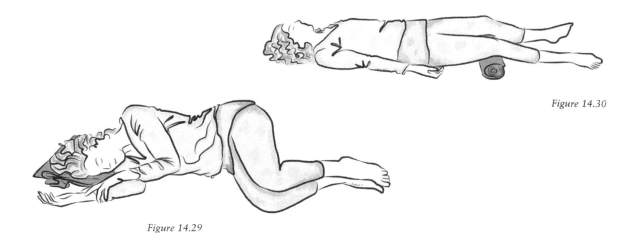

Figure 14.30

Figure 14.29

Ensuring the body will remain warm, lie down for Shivasana (Options: Figs 14.26–14.30).

If the back is at all uncomfortable after a class, a participant may prefer to return to the start position, with knees bent and softly resting on each other, or placing a cushion under the knees if they are lying supine. Otherwise side lying, with a small pillow at the head, may be preferable. If a participant has to leave a class early, it is recommended that they take a 3–5-minute rest such as this before going, rather than skipping this important stage of assimilation of the practice. A brief period of sitting up quietly to re-orientate after Shivasana is also recommended.

Please note, this sequence is part of a Restorative Yoga class and has been used thus for many years for people ranging in age from 8 to 89 years, including participants who are pregnant and others with a variety of conditions. However, there is a clear caveat that anyone suffering from disc herniation should not do the spinal twists. In all cases, any injury is specifically supervised and this sequence, like any other, does not replace the medical advice of a doctor or suitably qualified practitioner.

Notes

1. B.M. Nigg (2001) The role of impact forces and foot pronation: a new paradigm. *Clinical Journal of Sport Medicine* 11(1):2–9. Human Performance Laboratory, Faculty of Kinesiology, University of Calgary, Alberta, Canada
2. James Oschman, "Fascia as a Body-wide Communication System", Ch. 2.5 in Robert Schleip, Thomas W. Findley, Leon Chaitow and Peter A. Huijing, *Fascia: The Tensional Network of the Human Body*, Churchill Livingstone/Elsevier, Edinburgh, 2012.

15

Classroom Connections 3: A Subtle Practice

"*True yoga is not just doing a posture as dictated by outside robotic influences, but more an observation from within at what happens in the body along the journey ... No matter how still we think we are there is always a tiny movement somewhere inside, visible only to us, I think it is called life ... Just become quiet enough in the thinking brain to observe movement that is happening in the physical body. Relaxing – truly relaxing is becoming quiet, watching the pattern of the breathing and keeping your attention there until the pattern of the breathing takes over and governs the movement within. This is where the stillness in yoga comes from, not doing a movement but observing the movement that happens with the breath ... In the hustle and bustle of everyday life we don't have time to observe this deep movement, we're doing not being. It's like abseiling down the thread of breath.*"

Patricia Mary Sparrow (12 March 1935–13 April 2006)[1]

We can begin to "abseil down the thread of the breath" once we feel at ease enough to observe it and be present to it. This chapter is focused on the more subtle practices of yoga and seeks to provide a practice that can:

- free the internal channels of the subtle body, symbolised by the chakras (see Ch. 12)
- free the fascia of the joints to allow the subtle energies to flow more fluently and the tissue to glide and hydrate
- facilitate our sensory refinement through micro-movements and attention to the breath *at the same time* in rhythmic synchronicity.

The term Pawanmuktasana means "freeing the winds".[2] It refers to the vayus (winds) or pranas of the subtle body defined in Chapter 11. These form part of the practice of Pranayama and here they unite with the movements until the rhythm of the breath takes over. The actual techniques facilitate several things at once.

The gentle rotations, flexions and extensions through the joints free the fascia in every direction, without straining. When these movements are united with the breath, the respiratory rhythm can take over and we begin to

Foundation Practice	
1	Toes
2	Ankles A
3	Ankles B
4	Ankles C
5	Knees A
6	Knees B
7	Knees C
8	Knees D
9	Hips A
10	Hips B
11	Pelvis and Spine
12	Fingers
13	Wrist A
14	Wrist B
15	Elbow A
16	Elbow B
15	Shoulder A
18	Shoulder B
19	Arm Reach
20	Neck and Head A
21	Neck and Head B
22	Neck and Head C
23	Neck and Head D
24	Shivasana

There is no fanfare or celebration with this quiet approach. We are building a bridge between active postures and at the same time

The Practice

feeding the suppleness and self-containment needed to sit in meditative stillness. This happens as a result of the fascial matrix working in all its many aspects. It takes us towards attaining the natural ability to self-regulate and enjoy moving, breathing and stillness with quiet integrity, as appropriate. Perhaps there is a clear

be present to the motion. There is also a sense of stillness in those parts that are *not moving*. The exercise is to divide our attention equally between the moving and the still body, at the same time. Eventually the breath unites both aspects. Once that happens – when we arrive at this sense of "abseiling down the thread of the breath" – something else begins to occur. It is as if our vitality, the essence of the being, is nourished. It is a moment beyond words; perhaps the sense of an "eternal now".

By doing Pawanmuktasana regularly, the stillness of awareness and the dynamic balance of our attention are trained simultaneously. Each movement calls for attention divided between, on the one hand, the joint being gently and rhythmically released and simultaneously, on the other, the steadiness of the rest of the body to quietly support it. It is the physical practice in present time, bringing together all the polarities we have referred to throughout the book. We are becoming the witness; observing and facilitating *sthiram* and *sukham* together in present time: awareness and breath. Just breathe and be aware in rhythm with the ten movements in each set.

Resting tension, or elastic integrity, is naturally fostered by this first Pawanmuktasana series. Whatever one's age or level of skill, the result seems to be the same: a gradual improvement in seated and standing posture and in the ability to integrate the movements with the breath and develop a self-practice with ease. It is as if the fascia is freed from within, which is exactly the purpose of this subtle practice.

As participants become adept, the rhythmical breathing and movements begin to resonate in unison expressing exactly what yoga means. It is a deceptively simple and humble practice. It takes courage to bring the mind to calm and continue doing it on a regular basis. It is designed to draw the attention away from thinking and conceptualising and gradually invite the space (literally and symbolically) of our inner sense to develop in an ordinary and profound way.

We begin to find the spaces between our thoughts by transitioning along the breath and focusing gently on this, in rhythmical listening. If the mind wanders, as it is inclined sometimes to do, as soon as this is noticed, simply and gently return the attention to the breathing movements. Over time, the mental commentary switches off sooner and the body more readily stays in reflection. Then we have choice as to how we can be (still or in motion), at will.

This series has been devised partly as a result of working with the foundation postures described in the previous chapter and partly also using adaptations from the Bihar School of Yoga[3] series (see A Simple Practice, Ch. 14).[4] It has been taught to a variety of age groups and, once individuals can overcome the mind-chat and surrender to the rhythmical movements, natural comfort in sitting seems to be the most common experience.

This practice also demonstrates therapeutic value for a multitude of problems involving the shoulders, hips, neck and so on, by integrating parts of the body that have become isolated through pain or injury. Participants report an inner sense of calm and a greater ease or cumulative comfort with various correlation between the micro-movements of the body and the subtle awareness of the being? Yoga practice suggests this, and if the

Foundation Practice (Pawanmuktasana)

fascia is our largest sensory organ, it would naturally benefit from the soothing focus of these rhythmical movements. They begin to resonate in their own way, with the subtle rhythm of the compliant breath.

functions, from breathing and digestion to movement and sleeping. It is an excellent preparation for meditation, whatever your preferred meditative practice may be.

(Adapted from the teachings of Swami Satyananda Saraswati, Bihar School.)[5]

This foundation practice is recommended to begin with to bring any student into a place of self-awareness while reaping the benefits of strengthening the body. Regular resting periods between the postures are advised, sitting in the base position, observing the breath and pausing as necessary. It is also ideal as part of the preparation for (though not immediately before!) peak performance activities (such as sports or events like going on stage, for example) and after illness, particularly stress or tiredness. It is suitable for all age groups and all levels.

Physical sensations: At first there may be a slight "pins and needles" sensation from leaning back on the heels of the hands; if this happens, release the hands regularly and gently shake them out or rub them together, resting as frequently as needed. Also sit comfortably on a cushion, supporting the back of the knees if necessary with another, until the ability to sit becomes more established. It takes time but it is worth accumulating this quality of stillness in our loading history. The spine responds well and seems to be able gradually to enjoy sitting naturally and expressing its curved design in easy breathing. It is a subtle practice and, if the fascia responds to micro-movements in its loading history, this series optimises their beneficial resonance, gradually and efficiently from the inside out.

1 Toes

PURPOSE: The purpose is to bring more detailed awareness to the feet and free the joints of the lower limb. Have the arms straight but relaxed behind you and rest back supported by them. Remain long in the torso so the breath is clear and you can engage through the full elastic breath cycle (see Ch. 11) as you curl and flex the toes.

SUPPORT: This comes from the base position, particularly the hands. At first there can be mild pins and needles in the hands. If so, release them periodically and rest between the rounds. With regular practice, they will easily support you.

TIMING: To begin with this can be done 5 times with focus on the feet and 5 times more integrating the breath. As the choreography of this Foundation Practice becomes familiar, you can go straight to the integrated breathing and increase the number of rounds to 15.

The point is not to rush through and beat the clock. It is to experience the body freeing each joint and strengthening as it does so. Supple joints and improved comfort in sitting are two of the many benefits of this deceptively simple series.

- Sit comfortably on your sitting bones, hands behind you, as shown (Fig.15.1A).
- Have the heels resting a little more than hip-width apart.

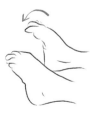

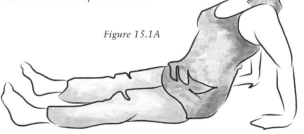

Figure 15.1A

Figure 15.1B

- Dorsiflex the feet so they are at right-angles to the ground.
- Focus on the toes and simply dorsiflex them together towards you.
- Then plantarflex them away from you, by curling them down.
- Isolate the movement to the toes only, if you can, for 5 rounds (Fig. 15.1B).
- Then add the breath, inhaling the toes up, exhaling toe curls.
- Do this in sequence with the breath for 5 rounds, working up to 10.

2 Ankles A

PURPOSE: The purpose is to bring more detailed awareness to the ankles and free the joints of the lower limb. Have the arms straight yet relaxed behind you. Rest back supported but long in the torso so the breath is clear and you can engage through the inhale and extra-exhale cycle as you move the ankle joint.

SUPPORT: This comes from the base position, particularly the hands. At first there can be mild pins and needles in the hands. If so, release them periodically and rest between the rounds. In time, with regular practice, they will easily support you.

TIMING: To begin with this can be done 5 times with focus on the feet and 5 times more integrating the breath.

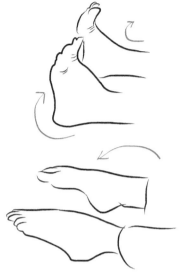

Figure 15.2

- Sit comfortably on your sitting bones, hands behind you.
- Have the heels resting a little more than hip-width apart.
- Dorsiflex the feet lengthening into the heel opening the back knee.
- Then point the toes in plantarflexion.
- Isolate the movement to the ankles only if you can, for 5 rounds.
- Then add the breath, inhaling in dorsiflexion, exhaling as you point.
- Do this in sequence with the breath for 5 rounds, working up to 10.

3 Ankles B

PURPOSE: The purpose is to bring more detailed awareness to the ankles and calves and free the joints of the lower limbs. Have the arms straight yet relaxed behind you. Rest back supported but long in the torso so the breath is clear and you can engage through the inhale and extra-exhale cycle as you circle the ankles and explore smooth movements. The key to this is finding smooth even movements throughout the range, rather than jerky, clicky motions. It takes practice.

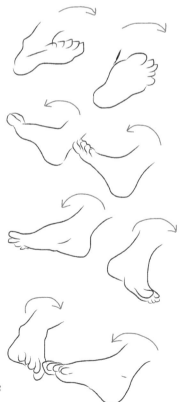

Figure 15.3

SUPPORT: This comes from the base position, particularly the hands.

TIMING: To begin with this can be done 5 times with focus on the ankles and 5 times more integrating the breath for each round. Eventually 10 times with the breath is sufficient. It is an excellent practice for strengthening ankles while maintaining suppleness.

- Sit comfortably on your sitting bones, hands behind you.
- Have the heels resting a little more than hip-width apart.
- Circle both ankles clockwise for a complete round.
- Circle both ankles anti-clockwise for a complete round.
- Circle both ankles away from centre for a complete round.
- Circle both ankles towards the centre for a complete round.
- Isolate the movement to the ankles only if you can, each 5 rounds.
- Then add the breath, inhaling the upper half, exhaling the lower.
- Do this in sequence with the breath for 5 rounds, working up to 10.

4 Ankles C

PURPOSE: The purpose is to passively encourage a meditative sitting position and free the joints of the lower limb. Have the right hand support the ankle and remain tall. Stay long in the torso so the breath is clear and you can engage through the inhale and extra-exhale cycle as you make the circling movements with the leg in this position.

SUPPORT: Support the ankle with the same hand and work gently but firmly with the opposite hand, encouraging range of motion without force. Support is in the torso now, so ensure you are sitting upright. (Use a block if it helps, preferably a low one to avoid hyper-extending the knee of the outstretched leg.)

TIMING: To begin with this can be done 5 times with focus on the circling motion and 5 times more integrating the breath. Later you can do 10 with the breath only.

- Sit comfortably on your sitting bones, or use a block to sit up.
- Take your right foot and cross it over your left thigh.
- Place your left fingers between your toes, or hold the foot.
- Gently circle the ankle, using the hands and relaxing the foot.
- Then circle the other way.
- Isolate the movement to the ankle only if you can, for 5 rounds.
- Then add the breath, inhaling the upper circle, exhaling lower.
- Do this in sequence with the breath for 5 rounds, working up to 10.
- Repeat to other side.

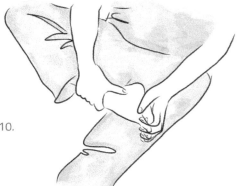

Figure 15.4

5 Knees A

PURPOSE: The purpose is to strengthen the upper leg and ensure support around the knee joint. Have the arms straight but relaxed behind you and rest back supported by them. Stay long in the torso so the breath is clear and you can engage through the inhale and extra-exhale cycle as you squeeze the knees.

SUPPORT: This comes from the base position, particularly the hands (see Fig. 15.1A).

TIMING: To begin with this can be done 5 times with focus on the feet and 5 times more integrating the breath. Eventually 10 with the breathing cycle is sufficient within the series.

- Sit comfortably on your sitting bones, hands behind in basic pose.
- Have the heels resting a little more than hip-width apart.
- Squeeze the knee caps up, so that the front of the leg engages (Fig. 15.5).
- Hold the squeeze for a count of 5.
- Then release.
- Isolate the movement to the knees only if you can, for 5 rounds.
- Then add the breath, inhaling and holding the breath on squeeze.
- Do this in sequence with the breath for 5 rounds, working to 10.

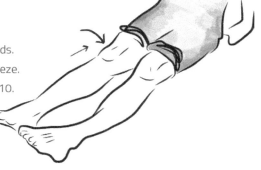

Figure 15.5

6 Knees B

PURPOSE: The purpose is to strengthen the legs and abdomen, integrating the breathing pattern. Eventually this pose can be done with both legs at the same time, finding "Boat Pose" (Navasana), but this should not be attempted until there is established strength and this version is easy. Please note the contraindication (below).

SUPPORT: This comes from the extended leg and the sitting bones and, eventually, from accumulated abdominal integrity. The arms are quite strong in this pose and should not be pulled into a slouched position.

TIMING: To begin with this can be done 5 times with focus on the straight leg and strong arms and 5 times more integrating the breath. The extra exhale is designed to help stabilise the lumbar spine and strengthens it by doing so.

CONTRAINDICATION: The advanced version of this practice with both legs is not recommended for people with weak abdominal muscles, lower back issues, high blood pressure or heart conditions. Over time, this sequence can strengthen the lumbar spine and abdominals but it is strongly advised that it is only attempted on one side at first and with few repetitions until strength is established.

- Sit comfortably on your sitting bones, hands round one thigh.
- Bend this knee, with foot flat to the floor, other leg flat and long.
- Straighten the leg out in front of you, holding it up with the hands.
- Focus on knee joint and hamstrings as you bend the leg to release.
- Isolate the movement to the knee and leg if you can, for 5 rounds.

- Add the breath, inhaling the foot down, exhaling it straight up.
- Do this in sequence with the breath for 5 rounds, working to 10.
- Change sides and do the other leg.

7 Knees C

PURPOSE: The purpose is to strengthen the tissues around the knee joint and assist its support structures, as it bears a great deal of weight and organisation. "These asanas rejuvenate the joint by activating the healing energies", according to the Bihar School.

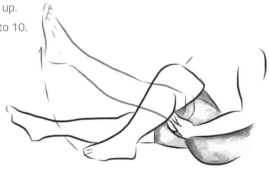

Figure 15.6

SUPPORT: This comes from the straight (other) leg and the hands. Use them around the leg you are working with, to "hold" the torso straight. You can interlock the fingers, or cross the arms, holding the elbows. The focus is on glide rather than range.

TIMING: To begin with this can be done 5 times clockwise focusing on the quality of the circular motion, and 5 times more integrating the breath. Then increase to 10 when you feel confident and the knee strengthens. Please avoid this practice unless specifically supervised if you have knee issues.

- Sit comfortably on your sitting bones, holding one leg up with the hands (Fig. 15.7).
- Describe a gentle circle with the foot without strain.
- Don't force the knee. This is designed to encourage movement.
- Focus on the circles, seeking to straighten the leg at the top.
- The upper leg and torso should remain still, the circles smooth.
- Isolate the movement, if you can, for 5 rounds each direction.
- Then add the breath, inhaling the upper half, exhaling lower.
- Do this in sequence with the breath for 5 rounds, working up to 10.

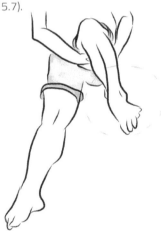

Figure 15.7

8 Knees D

PURPOSE: The purpose is to facilitate comfortable sitting positions, cross-legged for example, with freedom between the knee and the hip joint. After performing this exercise, take care to straighten the leg partially with the hands, bend it back to a folded position (heel at the groin if possible) and then straighten it out completely to ensure the knee joint is aligned correctly.

SUPPORT: This comes from the (other) straightened leg and sitting up on the sitting bones, without slumping in the spine.

TIMING: To begin with this can be done 5 times, with focus on the knee and hip relationship, while integrating the breath. Once strengthened and adaptable, this posture can be extended to add small pulses at the bent knee and an increased range at the "opened" hip joint. 10–20 pulses (not forced and not as strong as bounces) are sufficient to encourage the hip to release, if it can do so without strain.

- Sit comfortably on your sitting bones, one foot on the thigh, as shown (Fig. 15.8).
- Breathe in gently and lift this knee to the chest.
- Exhale and gently press it away from the body towards the floor.
- The torso remains still and no force should be used.
- The same-side hand does the work rather than the leg – it is passive.
- Do this in sequence with the breath for 5 rounds, working up to 10.
- Gently straighten the leg then place the heel against the inner thigh.
- Then lay the leg out straight and lengthen fully, to align the knee.

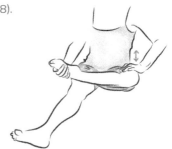

Figure 15.8

9 Hips A

PURPOSE: The purpose is to bring more detailed awareness to the leg joints and free the hip. As the knee and hip become supple, you can rest the ankle on the opposite leg and circle the knee with the hands. Stay long in the torso, so the breath is clear and you can engage through the inhale and extra-exhale cycle as you rotate at the hip.

SUPPORT: This comes from the base position and the hands/arms holding the rotating leg.

TIMING: To begin with, this can be done 5 times with focus on the hip circles then 5 times more integrating the breath, working up to 10.

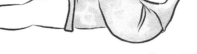

- Sit comfortably on your sitting bones, folding one leg.
- Hold the outside of that knee, cradled in the same side arm.
- Cradle the ankle joint in the other arm as above.
- Use the arms rather than the leg, which remains passive.
- Circle at the hip joint clockwise, then anticlockwise, 5 times.
- Isolate the movement at the hip if you can, for these 5 rounds.

Figure 15.9

- Then add the breath, inhaling the upper circle, exhaling lower.
- Do this in sequence with the breath for 5 rounds, working up to 10.
- Repeat on the other side.

10 Hips B

PURPOSE: The purpose is to prepare the body for seated postures and relieve tension in the groin from long hours of sitting, standing or walking. These postures can relieve tiredness after long hours on your feet at work.

SUPPORT: This comes from the base position, which gradually becomes optimal as the heels move closer to the pelvis. Be sure to sit up (using a block if necessary) and place the heels together in front of you where they are comfortable. As more range is introduced at the hip joint, they can come closer to the body.

TIMING: This must be done without force, always respecting the knees and hips and not pressing on them too hard. It is to invite and encourage a subtle impulse rather than a bouncing force. 30 times is a sufficient maximum.

CONTRAINDICATION: This posture is not recommended for anyone with sacral issues and/or sciatica.

- Sit comfortably on your sitting bones; place the feet together.
- Hold both feet in the hands, pressing the heels together.
- The heels should be as close to the perineum as possible.
- Relax the inner thigh muscles completely.
- Hook the fingers around the big toe to seal the posture.
- Gently raise and lower the knees 20–30 times, breathing normally.
- Gently press the knees down 20–30 times if you are comfortable.

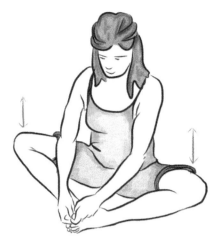

Figure 15.10

11 Pelvis and Spine

PURPOSE: The purpose is to feel the ground in the seated position and invite a rotation from it, without force. It can be nice to fold forward over the legs after this and rest for a minute or two, if that is comforting.

SUPPORT: This comes from the base cross-legged position. It is used to engage downwards and experience the upward sense of rotation. No force is required. It is an enquiry to ask how the spine is right now and encourage the optimal and natural lumbar curve in sitting.

TIMING: To begin with this can be done 5 times to each side, working up to 10.

- Sit comfortably with legs lightly crossed on the floor.
- Find the sitting bones and use the legs to sit up "tall".
- Inhale and do nothing. On the exhale, rotate the torso to the right.
- Gently continue until the head is looking over the right shoulder.
- Inhale as you come back to centre, then exhale the other way, till head is looking over left shoulder.
- Do not force this rotation. It is an enquiry not a challenge.
- Cross the legs the other way and repeat to each side.
- Do this in sequence with the breath for 5 rounds, working up to 10.

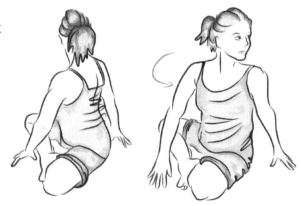

Figure 15.11 A   *Figure 15.11 B*

12 Hand A: Open and Close

PURPOSE: The hands are considered to be on the heart line, growing from the embryonic torso to wrap around it. This opens the energy meridians through the arm and thorax and it is surprisingly demanding. To add a variation to this asana, it can be done with the arms out to the side at shoulder level.

SUPPORT: This comes from the base position, particularly cross-legged. It is important to be comfortable sitting upright, so that the heart is open. If the arms tire quickly at first, rest them beside or behind you between practices.

TIMING: To begin with this can be done 5 times with focus on the hands and 5 times more integrating the breath. Work up to 10.

- Sit on your sitting bones, in base position or cross-legged.
- Use a block if preferred, to rest comfortably.
- Reach the hands out in front of you as shown (shoulder level).
- Stretch the hand and fingers apart, palms facing (Fig. 15.12).
- Then squeeze the hand into a fist, thumb inside the fingers.
- This is slow and deliberate but strong, for 5 rounds.
- Then add the breath, inhaling the hand open, exhaling closed.
- Do this in sequence with the breath for 5 rounds, working up to 10.

13 Wrist A

PURPOSE: The hands are considered to be on the heart line, growing from the embryonic torso to wrap around it. This opens the energy meridians through the arm and thorax and it is surprisingly demanding. To add a variation to this asana, it can be done with the arms out to the side at shoulder level. It is designed to facilitate glide at the wrists and strengthen the arms.

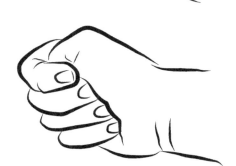

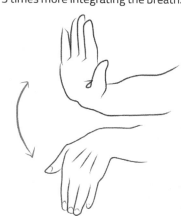

Figure 15.12

SUPPORT: This comes from the base position, particularly cross-legged. It is important to be comfortable sitting upright, so that the heart is open. If the arms tire quickly at first, rest them beside or behind you between practices.

TIMING: To begin with, this can be done 5 times with focus on the hands and 5 times more integrating the breath. Work up to 10.

- Sit on your sitting bones, in base position or cross-legged.
- Use a block if preferred, to rest comfortably.
- Reach the hands out in front of you as shown (shoulder level).
- Keep the palms open and fingers straight and touching each other throughout the practice.
- Press the hands up (as if against a wall) then point fingers down (Fig. 15.13).
- Elbows are straight and so are the hands. Do this for 5 rounds.
- Then add the breath, inhaling the hand up, exhaling down.
- Do this in sequence with the breath for 5 rounds, working up to 10.

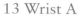

Figure 15.13

14 Wrist B

PURPOSE: The hands are considered to be on the heart line, growing from the embryonic torso to wrap around it. This opens the energy meridians through the arm and thorax and it is surprisingly demanding. It helps considerably if you have spent a long day at the keyboard, or working with the hands, as it relieves unnecessary tension and encourages gliding and hydration in the wrist joint.

SUPPORT: This comes from the base position, particularly cross-legged. It is important to be comfortable sitting upright, so that the heart is open. You can use the arm you are not practising with to support you from behind if it is easier. If the arm tires quickly at first, rest it beside or behind you between practices.

TIMING: To begin with, this can be done 5 times in each direction focusing on the hand and 5 times more integrating the breath. Work up to 10 for each hand.

- Sit on your sitting bones, in base position or cross-legged.
- Use a block if preferred to rest comfortably.
- Reach one hand out in front of you as shown (shoulder level).
- With a soft fist, thumb inside, rotate at the wrist clockwise.
- Reverse the rotation (anticlockwise) keeping wrist facing down.
- The arm should be still and the circles as large as possible.
- Then add the breath, inhaling the fist up, exhaling down.
- Do this in sequence with the breath for 5 rounds, working up to 10.
- Repeat with other hand. (Movement is isolated to the wrist joint if possible.)

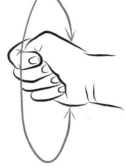

Figure 15.14

15 Elbow A: Flex and Extend

PURPOSE: The hands are considered to be on the heart line, growing from the embryonic torso to wrap the arms around it. This opens the energy meridians through the arm and thorax and it is surprisingly demanding.

SUPPORT: This comes from the base position, particularly cross-legged. It is important to be comfortable sitting upright, so that the heart is open. If the arms tire quickly at first, rest them beside or behind you between exercises.

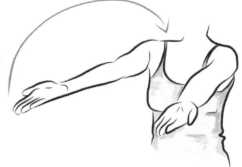

Figure 15.15 A

TIMING: To begin with, this can be done 5 times with the focus on the hands and 5 times more integrating the breath. Work up to 10.

- Sit on your sitting bones, in base position or cross-legged.
- Use a block, if preferred, to rest comfortably.
- Reach the hands out in front of you as shown (shoulder level).
- With palms facing up, bend the elbow to touch the shoulder.
- Then straighten the arms again, maintaining shoulder height.
- This is slow and deliberate but strong. Do this for 5 rounds.
- Then add the breath, inhaling the arms open, exhaling flexed.
- Do this in sequence with the breath for 5 rounds, working up to 10.
- Repeat the whole sequence, starting with arms to the side.

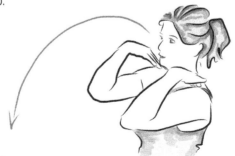

Figure 15.15 B

16 Elbow B: Rotation

PURPOSE: The hands are considered to be on the heart line, growing from the embryonic torso to wrap the arms around it. This opens the energy meridians through the arm and thorax and it is surprisingly demanding.

SUPPORT: With the other hand at the elbow joint, supporting the working arm to keep it steady throughout the practice, encouraging smooth circular movements.

TIMING: To begin with this can be done 5 times, with focus on the smooth movement of the elbow, and then 5 times more integrating the breath. Work up to 10.

- Sit on your sitting bones, in base position or cross-legged.
- Use a block, if preferred, to rest comfortably.
- Reach one arm out in front of you as shown (shoulder level).
- Support this arm, just above the elbow with the other hand.
- Bend the arm at the elbow, rotating the joint clockwise.
- The arm remains steady, hand brushing the shoulder.
- Do this for 5 rounds.
- Then add the breath, inhaling the arms up, exhaling down.
- Do this in sequence with the breath for 5 rounds, working up to 10.
- Repeat the smooth circling in an anticlockwise direction.
- Repeat the whole sequence with the other arm.

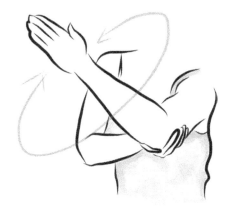

Figure 15.16

17 Shoulder A: Rotation

PURPOSE: The shoulder joints receive great benefit from this practice to relieve strain patterns from carrying bags, lifting, or sitting in relatively sedentary positions for work. This sequence can relieve the strain of driving and a variety of activities involving arm work.

SUPPORT: To begin with, the other arm can support the working arm. Once sitting up is comfortable and sustainable, both arms can practise together. The point is to encourage smooth circular movements through the full range so that the shoulder girdle can rest comfortably over the thorax and movement is isolated to the shoulder joint.

TIMING: To begin with, these can be done 5 times with focus on the smooth movement at the shoulder, then 5 times more integrating the breath. Work up to 10.

- Sit on your sitting bones, in base position or cross-legged.
- Use a block, if preferred, to rest comfortably.
- Reach one elbow out to the side, same hand on shoulder.
- Rotate this elbow in a large circle clockwise, smoothly, 5 rounds.
- Repeat in an anticlockwise direction, 5 rounds.
- Then add the breath, inhaling the arms up, exhaling down, in circles.
- This whole sequence can then be repeated with both arms.
- Left arm on left shoulder and right arm on right shoulder.

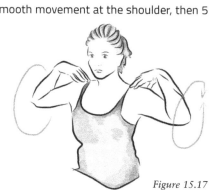

Figure 15.17

18 Shoulder B: Squeeze Forward and Back

PURPOSE: As in the Shoulder A exercise, the shoulder joints receive great benefit from this practice to relieve strain patterns from carrying bags, lifting, or sitting in relatively sedentary positions for work. It also helps to open the front of the body after long periods of sitting at a desk, at a computer or in a car, for example. This sequence can relieve the strain of driving and a variety of activities involving arm work and can be readily incorporated during work, as a brief interlude to prevent strain patterns.

SUPPORT: Both arms work together to sense balance of range between left and right. Ensure the spine does not fold forward when the elbows are drawn towards each other in front of the body.

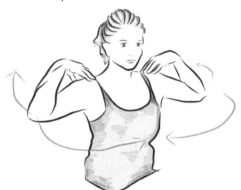

- Sit on your sitting bones, in base position or cross-legged.
- Use a block, if preferred, to rest comfortably.
- Reach each elbow out to the side, same hand on shoulder.
- Keep both elbows at shoulder height.
- Squeeze elbows together at the front, pause, then to the side.
- Take elbows in a smooth movement as if to meet at the back.
- Then add the breath, inhale elbows forward, exhaling back.
- Forward and back is one round; repeat 10 rounds.
- Maintain shoulder height for the elbows and pause as required.

Figure 15.18

19 Arm Reach

PURPOSE: The hands are considered to be on the heart line, growing from the embryonic torso to wrap the arms around it. This opens the energy meridians through the arm and thorax and it is surprisingly demanding. It ensures a full range of motion is encouraged at the shoulder.

SUPPORT: This comes from the base of the pose. It is recommended that if you are in a cross-legged position, you change the favoured side regularly throughout the practice.

TIMING: To begin with, this can be done 5 times with focus on the smooth movement of the hands up and down, then 5 times more integrating the breath. Work up to 10.

- Sit on your sitting bones, in base position or cross-legged.
- Use a block, if preferred, to rest comfortably.
- Place the hands together in prayer and reach them over the head.
- Bend the elbows softly until the heels of the hands touch the head.
- Lengthen the hands up, to position C, then return to A.
- The hands stay in line over the crown, 5 rounds.
- Then add the breath, exhaling the hands up, inhaling them down.
- Do this in sequence with the breath for 5 rounds, working up to 10.

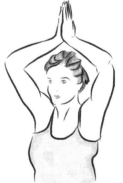

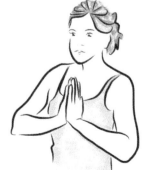

Figure 15.19 A   *Figure 15.19 B*

- There is a slight feeling of lift and extension through the spine.
- Hands remain palm to palm throughout. Rest in B as required.

20 Neck and Head A

PURPOSE: The purpose is to relieve tension and free the tissues of the neck. All nerves connecting the different organs and limbs pass through the neck and the myofascial layers and organisation can hold extra tension and be over-recruited by disorganised posture. These asanas are designed to free their mobility; however, they must not be forced. There are delicate structures in the neck and subtle mobility and sensory refinement is sought rather than length or range for the sake of it.

SUPPORT: This comes from the base position, particularly the hands. Be sure to use the hands for support if necessary. Otherwise sit up "tall" as the first secondary curve is essential to the natural efficacy of these movements.

TIMING: To begin with, this can be done 5 times with focus on integrating the breath and sensing balance. Work up to 10 rounds.

- Sit comfortably on your sitting bones, hands behind you.
- You can sit cross-legged if you prefer. Close the eyes.
- Exhale, taking the chin down to the chest, lengthening the neck.
- Inhale as you take the head up and backwards as far as is comfortable.
- Repeat 5 times and work up to 10; however, do not strain or force.
- Please note the contraindications for the neck/head practices (below).

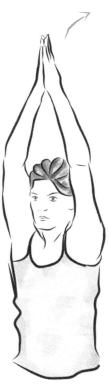

Figure 15.19 C

CONTRAINDICATIONS FOR ALL NECK AND HEAD MOVEMENTS:
These movements should not be performed by elderly people and those suffering from low or high blood pressure, vertigo or extreme cervical spine conditions, such as herniation or spondylosis. (NB: Cervical spondylosis patients must avoid forward bending of the neck.)

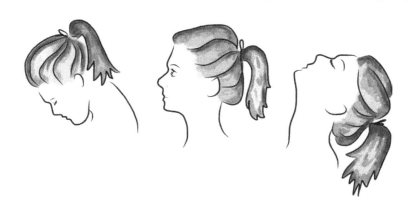

Figure 15.20

21 Neck and Head B

PURPOSE: The purpose is to relieve tension and free the tissues of the neck. All nerves connecting the different organs and limbs pass through the neck and the myofascial layers and organisation can hold extra tension and be over-recruited by disorganised posture. These asanas are designed to free their mobility; however, they must not be forced. There are delicate structures in the neck and subtle mobility and sensory refinement is sought rather than length or range for the sake of it.

SUPPORT: This comes from the base position, particularly the hands. Be sure to use the hands for support if necessary. Otherwise sit up "tall" as the natural spinal curves are essential to the efficacy of these movements.

TIMING: To begin with, this can be done 5 times with focus on integrating the breath and sensing balance and symmetry. Work up to 10 rounds.

- Sit comfortably on your sitting bones, hands behind you, as shown.
- You can sit cross-legged if you prefer. Close the eyes.
- Inhale in centre position, then exhale taking right ear to shoulder.
- Inhale back to centre, exhale left ear to left shoulder.
- Repeat 5 times; work up to 10. Do not strain or force.
- It is not necessary to get the ear to the shoulder.
- Please note the contraindications of the neck/head practices (Ex 20) and caution (below).

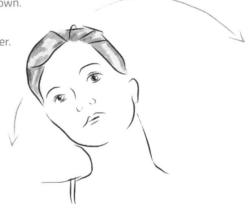

Figure 15.21

CAUTION:
If there are any neck injuries or disc herniation, then all neck movements should be done under supervision or with the advice of a doctor or physiotherapist. Where improved mobility is sought, these movements should be modified and minimised to micro-movements, gradually increased as range is improved.

22 Neck and Head C

PURPOSE: The purpose is to relieve tension and free the tissues of the neck. All nerves connecting the different organs and limbs pass through the neck and the myofascial layers and organisation can hold extra tension and be over-recruited by disorganised posture. These asanas are designed to free their mobility; however, they must not be forced. There are delicate structures in the neck and subtle mobility and sensory refinement is sought rather than length or range for the sake of it.

SUPPORT: This comes from the base position, particularly the hands. Be sure to use the hands for support if necessary. Otherwise sit up "tall" as the natural spinal curves are essential to the efficacy of these movements.

TIMING: To begin with, this can be done 5 times with focus on integrating the breath and sensing balance and symmetry. Work up to 10 rounds.

CONTRAINDICATIONS: See Ex 20 and 21.

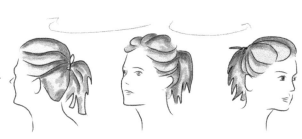

- Sit comfortably on your sitting bones, hands behind you, as shown.
- You can sit cross-legged if you prefer. Close the eyes.
- Inhale in centre, then exhale turning the head over the right shoulder.
- Inhale back to centre, exhale the head over the left shoulder.

Figure 15.22

- Repeat 5 times, work up to 10. Do not strain or force.
- It is not necessary to get the chin over the shoulder, keep head level.
- Please note the contraindications for the neck/head practices (see Ex 20 and 21).

23 Neck and Head D

PURPOSE: The purpose is to relieve tension and free the tissues of the neck. All nerves connecting the different organs and limbs pass through the neck and the myofascial layers and organisation can hold extra tension and be over-recruited by disorganised posture. These asanas are designed to free their mobility; however, they must not be forced. There are delicate structures in the neck and subtle mobility and sensory refinement is sought rather than length or range for the sake of it.

SUPPORT: This comes from the base position, particularly the hands. Be sure to use the hands for support if necessary. Otherwise sit up "tall" as the natural spinal curves are essential to the efficacy of these movements.

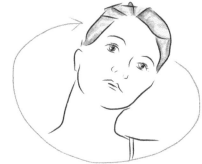

TIMING: To begin with, this can be done 5 times with focus on integrating the breath and sensing balance and symmetry. Experience the sensations of the head and neck and keep the eyes still, even though they are closed. (They do not need to move up and down with the head.) Work up to 10 rounds.

Figure 15.23

CONTRAINDICATIONS: See Ex 20 and 21.

- Sit comfortably on your sitting bones, hands behind you.
- You can sit cross-legged if you prefer. Close the eyes.
- Roll the head on the neck in a soft clockwise direction.
- Reverse the roll in the other direction, inhaling the head up.
- Exhale as the head rolls down, going back the way you came.
- Repeat 5 times; work up to 10. Do not strain or force.
- It is not necessary to pull on the neck. Keep it relaxed.
- Please note the contraindications of the neck/head practices.

24 Shivasana

PURPOSE: The purpose is to relax and let the tissues organise themselves, after having been invited to consciously move and hold a variety of positions. Pawanmuktasana allows the energy channels to open and flow. If this is done for the first time, there may be disturbance where tissue is being revitalised, the bodily fluids are reorganised and extraneous tension is released. Ensure that you drink plenty of water and take 2–5 minutes to rest the body in this pose.

SUPPORT: As above, ensure that you are comfortable. If there is any possibility of becoming cold after the practice, you are advised to ensure you have a light blanket over you during the rest period.

TIMING: This is arguably the most important part of the practice. If participants ever have to leave a class early, it is recommended that they stop 5 minutes before they leave to ensure some time in Shivasana before they return to the demands of everyday life. Opening the channels without giving the body time to assimilate and absorb can leave the body feeling unprepared and vulnerable, which depletes the rich benefits of this practice.

- Lie down comfortably on your mat.
- Ideally Shivasana includes the whole body resting supine.
- If it is more comfortable, either bend the knees (see Ch. 14, Ex 12) or place a cushion or rolled-up mat under the knees.
- Alternatively, lie on your side with a rolled towel, blanket or pillow.
- The posture is designed to allow the body to completely relax.
- Allow the breath to "breathe you" without force or effort.
- Rest while the postures integrate and the body assimilates.

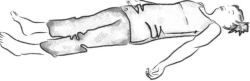

Figure 15.24

Postscript

This series is designed to bring the body into comfort in stillness. The mind eventually lets go and allows us to enter the "zone": a kind of timelessness, absorbed in the rhythm of uniting breath and motion. This practice may be used as preparation for meditation, gently bringing us to a place of awareness, where all the forms seem to be in a place where we can experience the formless. Whatever your chosen method of reflection, contemplation or meditation – enjoy. May the life-force be with you, Baruch Bashan (the blessings already are).

Notes

This beautiful practice was first shared with me by my dear friend and colleague Linda d'Antal.[6] Through her auspices the Bihar School of Yoga generously shared this work and I would like to acknowledge both Linda and the school (see Note 3 below) for their collegiate approach and generosity of spirit. Linda is a Senior Yoga Teacher and experienced Yoga Therapist and her work is beautiful. This can be found at her own Yoga Teacher Training school in Southfields, London, UK (see note 6).

1. From the personal diaries of Patricia Mary Sparrow (12 March 1935–13 April 2006), one of my most loved yoga teachers. Used with the kind permission of Stephanie Sparrow.
2. In Sanskrit, *pawan* means wind; *mukta* is to liberate, free, or release.
3. The Bihar School of Yoga was founded by Swami Satyananda Saraswati in 1964; https://www.biharyoga.net/.
4. Swami Satyanada Saraswati, *Asana Pranayama Mudra Bandha*, Yoga Publications Trust, Bihar, India.
5. See notes 3 and 4.
6. Linda d'Antal, https://www.treehouseyoga.co.uk; Vinyasa Flow Yoga; Advanced Yoga Teacher Training, Head of Yoga Faculty at the Art of Contemporary Yoga Ltd 2008–2010.

16

Classroom Connections 4: Class Mandalas

"I saw that everything, all paths I had been following, all steps I had taken, were leading back to a single point – namely, to the mid-point. It became increasingly plain to me that the mandala is the centre. It is the exponent of all paths. It is the path to the centre, to individuation. I knew that in finding the mandala as an expression of the self I had attained what was for me the ultimate."[1]

C. G. Jung

The idea behind the Posture Mandalas is primarily the preparation, in advance, of a Field of Grace in which to teach, the one Rumi refers to in Chapter 1: *"out beyond ideas of wrongdoings and rightdoings, there is a field – I'll meet you there"*.[2] It is also a field from which to teach and into which you can welcome your participants. It forms a kind of subtle, invisible "connective tissue" framework for the relationships you choose to present in real time, between postures. It is the field: your field to work from in your way. (I see it as creating a kind of Sacred Circle.)

The Circle

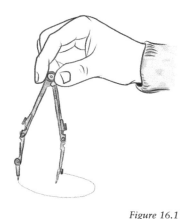

Figure 16.1

A circle to symbolise a Field of Grace within which to create a class.

This field is symbolised in the act of drawing the circle (Fig. 16.1).[3] This can become a ritual in itself. It is a quiet conversation between you and your own intuitive awareness, prepared in advance. The pair of compasses are used symbolically. One leg represents the positive, or active, force (Pingala) and the other leg represents the negative, or passive, force (Ida). The opening of the pair of compasses forms a ray of light, the Sun (Pingala) and the Moon (Ida). The point represents stillness while the pencil is the dynamic element, describing the "whole". When you remove the compass point, it leaves the mark in the centre – in yogic terms, the *bindu*. It is the dot, another tiny circle within the circle, representing the one and the all at the same time (Fig. 16.2).

The circle contains (encircles) the emptiness, the "no-thing" that zero represents. At the same time as containing the emptiness, with the boundary of the circumference the circle also represents "some-thing", emergent from the dot, becoming the line, to join and form into a circle. We saw (in Chapter 12)

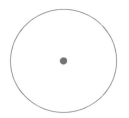

Figure 16.2

Drawing a circle is symbolic of an act of creation from (within) which the hidden geometries of life can all be found. The ancient yogis profoundly understood these forms in nature and included their resonance in many aspects of the deeper yogic teachings. In Chapter 12 we considered the chakras and the relationship of the geometries they represent to living tensegrity force transmission and our fascial architecture. They resonate literally and symbolically.

that the symbol of "one" is the Monad: a circle with a dot in it. Together the line enclosing the space it contains forms this symbol of the field that contains the opposites and presents them as united (the place beyond the polarities).

The mandala is then made by making another circle around the first one and dividing the circles into upper and lower halves horizontally. The outer circle is divided into 12 equal sections, six above and six below (Fig. 16.3).

The Class Plan

The simple premise behind these Posture Mandalas is pose and counter-pose, with two poses per direction of movement. It means that a series of postures in a class assure that the fascial matrix of the body enjoys different ranges of motion, in forward and back bending (flexion/extension), side bending (lateral flexion) and twists (rotation/counter-rotation). It is also versatile enough that these can be designed with postures of different levels.

In the centre you place the key or main pose you intend to teach, with its counter-pose underneath. We will use the example of Dog Pose (*Adho Mukha Svanasana*). In the top six segments we will choose two poses that emphasise each of the movement directions. Then a corresponding counter-pose will be placed in the opposite segment of the lower half of the circle (Fig. 16.4).

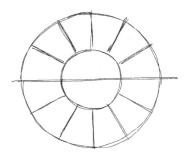

Figure 16.3

Above the line will be the poses and below the line the counter-poses.

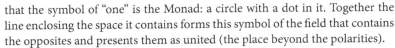

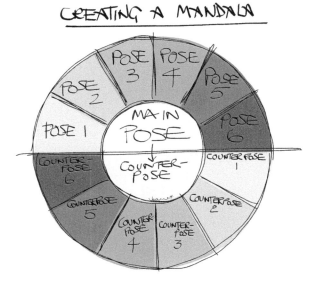

Figure 16.4

The Posture Mandala. This type of Posture Mandala has poses in the top half and counter-poses in the lower half. It is like a visual table of poses. This particular one is not presented as a sequence, but rather a visual teaching aid, to ensure that postures chosen for a suggested class plan are balanced overall. The elements include forward and back bend, side bend and twisting, each with pose and counter-pose.

Presenting a Balanced Class

This format invites a class design that honours overall equilibrium of the fascial body. It ensures that there is balance and variability of forces and directions of movement activated in a lesson, through the choice of postures. This is a common basis of any teacher training, although prior to a fuller understanding of myofascial anatomy in practice, priority is often given to the type of yoga rather than the type of individuals undertaking it.

Please note that a balanced practice includes all three "planes of movement" discussed in Chapter 9. Forward and back bending movements are just one direction, a counterbalance to each other.

Those forms of yoga that are biased to a particular repetitive sequence, emphasising one direction, can build strength and ability at first. However, from a myofascial point of view this can eventually become a repetitive strain pattern if it is repeated over a period of time without suitable counterbalance. By gradually introducing a counterbalancing sequence over a suitable period, the practice can be modified. If it is interspersed with all movement directions, in such a way that it is naturally balancing the tissue loading, such strain can be avoided. Balance and counterbalance, including the three directions, better ensure variety and elastic integrity within the level or ability of the participants or class being taught.

Posture Mandalas

Primarily these are a way of planning a class list in a visual format that can be read instantly, at the speed of a class. It offers a well-considered and recognisable template for you to develop.

What follows are three simple examples of this type of mandala, rather than prescriptions (Figs 16.5–16.7). The idea is to adapt them for your own style of yoga. This format encourages you to base the postures of a given class around an optimal design for tensional balance. As a teaching tool, they simply allow a creative class plan to be structured, saved and built into a portfolio as your experience and range of teaching develops or accumulates. It is really designed to encourage creativity and a balance of asana, adapted to work in a class, a workshop or over a term. They provide instant visual organisation, rather than a list in a notebook.

The idea of first drawing a circle is also a very practical way of working with the postures (in any order) to ensure a rounded, variable training programme per class, per term or per event. (It is scale free!). It echoes the theme of roundness, throughout this work!

The purpose of doing these is to create a clear and accessible way to:

- design a balanced class/lesson/personal practice to optimise fascial form overall
- ensure balance between the asanas chosen for either a general group or an individual
- contain a theme that can be carried through for an individual by session, or series of sessions (such as a term or course of work)
- retain a useful at-a-glance record of class plans and progress

- create a circle from your own intention, in advance, like the Field of Grace that Rumi speaks of (see the opening of Ch. 1).

These three basic class plans are themed around a main asana to base the class upon, such as Dog Pose (*Adho Mukha Svanasana*) (Fig. 16.5).

In this example (Fig. 16.5), Face Up Dog (*Urdhva Muhka Svanasana*) and Face Down Dog (*Adho Mukha Svanasana*) or Cobra Pose (*Bhujangasana*) could be used. They are placed at the centre of the mandala, one designating the main pose and the other the main counter-pose. The other poses chosen are put in for their value in contributing to the main pose and finding a suitable balance for the level of the class. The leading six postures are placed in the upper half, one in each of the six segments, and their respective counter-poses are placed in the lower half, in their opposite segment. Here the main poses are a Forward Bend and a Back Bend, so the other postures included are two twists, two more forward/back bends and one side-bending pose. The aim is to provide range of motion for the limbs (note the different arm positions and leg positions) as well as the spine.

Being creative does not necessarily require that your mandalas have to have perfectly drawn figures in them. Stick men (Fig. 16.6) and word cues will do. All the examples are designed to demonstrate this idea in different ways.

Mandalas do not have to have "goal oriented" postures in the centre. In this one (Fig. 16.7), the theme is one of resting the spine. The class plan animates

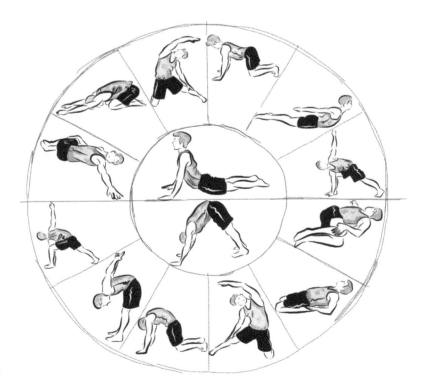

Figure 16.5

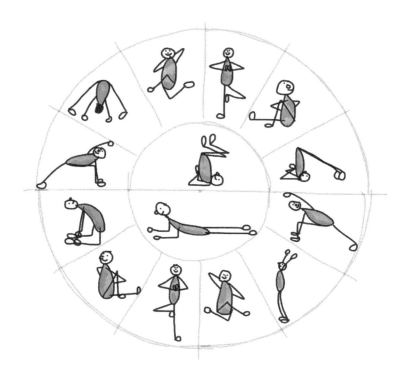

Figure 16.6

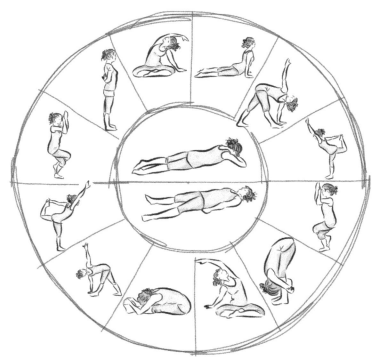

Figure 16.7

it in balance and on the ground, while the main feature of this class would be the comfort of rest and restoration. It could equally be done by swapping Lord of the Dance (*Natarajasana*) to either side, for example, with the prone and supine postures in the main centre.

Mandala Flows

In a Vinyasa Flow-based class, for example, or any sequencing programme, the postures can be presented as part of a flowing sequence. In this case, the same mandala can be used – but the postures work "around the clock" from one to the next (Fig. 16.8).

If you are teaching sequential classes, you may choose to design one biased to one movement plane, counterbalanced by another whole mandala biased to a different movement plane. This versatile format is based on common sense and the idea that the body responds well to range and variety as well as being trained by repetition. As ever, it is our task to find balance between these aspects of learning. It is for you to "pitch" the mandalas to the age, range, ability and scope of your particular practice and style of teaching. They can be used one-to-one to develop a particular participant, or for a class or group.

A well-known example of a flowing mandala sequence is the Sun Salutation (Surya Namaskar) (Fig. 16.9).

Posture Mandalas are an art form in their own right. They can be developed into class plans, workshop plans and term plans.[4] In the meantime, it is highly recommended that you take the time to draw the circles, make your

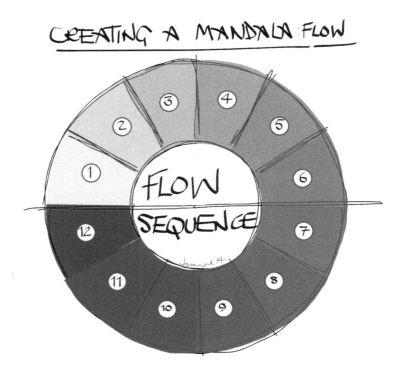

Figure 16.8

In a flow sequence, the numbers can start where you choose; it is a matter of personal preference. Some people prefer the numbering to follow a clock.

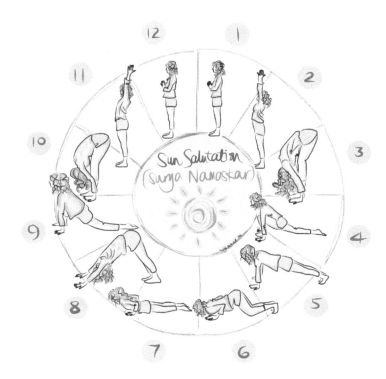

Figure 16.9

This sequence follows the numbering of a clock face. Sun Salutation (Surya Namaskar) Flow Mandala.

own templates and design your own class mandalas. Apart from being fun, they are a wonderful resource in their own right.

The mandalas are designed to bring you "present to" the class you intend to create, in advance of it being present-ed. It occurs in the domain of intuitive listening to the group, as an act of anticipational pre-sense. It can free you to be present to the participants as well as creative about what you will teach them. The mandalas can become a portfolio of your creative ideas. The circle symbolises that act of creation... Namaste.

Notes

1. C. G. Jung: *The Red Book of Carl Jung*: http://www.loc.gov/exhibits/red-book-of-carl-jung/the-red-book-and-beyond.html
2. Jelaluddin Rumi, *The Essential Rumi*, translated by Coleman Barks with John Moyne, A.J. Arberry and Reynold Nicholson, HarperCollins, San Francisco, 1995.
3. Image by Martin Gordon (www.mothmedia.co.uk).
4. www.joanneavison.com for details of courses teaching these elements of Classroom Connections.

17

Classroom Connections 5: Assessment and Adjustment Skills

"I have no special talent. I am only passionately curious"

Albert Einstein

In this chapter we consider some of the elements in assessment and adjustment skills, working in the round. It is designed to provide some distinctions, rather than formulae. These have emerged from experience that has grown and clarified in many and various classroom situations and one-to-one practice (in yoga teaching and yoga therapy).

These assessment tools are elements embedded in *manual* therapy. As *movement* teachers and therapists, however, if we have the licence to adjust, *with an understanding of the fascial matrix*, there are distinct overlaps between the two domains. Perhaps a broader and deeper understanding of fascia invites us into the world of Posture Profiling and *subtle* adjustment skills? Understanding fascia as a responsive, shape-shifting architecture also encourages us towards a certain mastery in self-regulation. If the invitation of professional adjustment is to foster such self-management, then it is hoped these ideas will inspire the curious and facilitate the journey along the path of safe and appropriate practice.

Posture Profiling

Posture Profiling is used to understand some of the general fundamental differences between different fascial "body architectural" types. The word "profile" is neutral; it implies neither right nor wrong, better nor worse. It exists relative only to itself. The value in Posture Profiling lies in finding suitable coordinates to guide appropriate change. This amounts to *accessing a starting point* and choosing a suitable direction *to move towards*. The caution is to beware of becoming too literal or using this to "brand" people, since that is precisely what Posture Profiling is designed to move away from. It suggests subtle direction, rather than bold or branded status.

The Ground Rules

We are not anatomists, carefully studying inert forms in miniscule anatomical detail. This profiling is for movement teachers, and more specifically yoga teachers, working *at movement speed*. Movement classrooms generally operate at a higher speed than manual therapy interventions. Although people might be standing still or resting during a movement class, we are often preparing for motion, if not actively participating in it. That occurs much faster than a manual therapy session where assessment occurs in a different time-frame for a client standing still or lying on a bodywork plinth.

Speed might be considered the other end of the spectrum to stillness – and in yoga classrooms we invite *both* dynamically. We are inviting individuals to discover more possibility, range and comfort for themselves, using these charts as a starting point to guide optimum direction *for them*. Part of our role is to provide useful feedback. However, we generally do so at a reasonable speed, just because we are working in a movement domain and Posture Profiling is designed to capture that, briefly and usefully. Clearly, in a Power Yoga or Vinyasa Flow class, it is towards the "speed end" of that spectrum and harder to interact in the moment. In any event, Posture Profiling is like fast sketching to an artist; you learn to see the essence of motion – rather than pin someone to a formula or static form. It is, of course, versatile enough to be applied in practices where postures are held for a while. Indeed, it is very valuable for that too.

Eventually posture profiling supports clients to become self-referencing in terms of their own balance and well-being and self-sensory refinement. It is, to some extent, an interpretive art that begins as a map, or a set of coordinates, based on fascia types. Using this map, our task is to recognise and place an individual on a useful, optimal, path of progress *for them*. It provides a sense of which direction to take them in, to foster *their* biomotional integrity, based upon *their* profile. It also expresses whole anatomy at the speed of movement, which is the realm we work in.

The information upon which this is based is founded on fascial and morphological body type, as a metaphorical sketch of a person in real life motion. It is not competing with scientific or academic charts. We are working in nature and non-linear biologic forms, animated by extraordinary, individual people being in an ordinary state of motion with comfort and ease. It is invaluable for ensuring different fascial body types can optimise and balance their training in a more personal or specific way.

These archetypal movement categories are considered to live within a range between the extremes of what Robert Schleip refers to as the "Asterix" cartoon character and the Indian Temple Dancer fascia types.[2] In this iteration we will call that range "Viking to Jungle" and make it the *x*-axis (see Fig. 17.1) for the horizontal co-ordinates.

Posture Profiling is not designed to be a substitute for such practices as Body Centred Psychotherapy, Hokomi or any of the many valuable protocols that speak in specific ways to the psychosomatic whole we live and dance in. It is an accessible, softly spoken framework, like a sketching template, for movement teachers. It captures a moment of the physical, connected, soft tissue, living architecture and places it in a temporal context with usable coordinates. It can facilitate adjustment through accurate reading of the individual form, from this basic logic. (It is also taught as a course, to hone and develop as a valuable teaching tool).[1]

The *x*-axis

Viking type: this is the build of the strong, resilient body that is capable of endurance, particularly at lower temperatures. The Viking body has mass and resilience and places a high priority on stamina, bulk and strength. The shoulders are broad, the fortitude is archetypally powerful. In terms of the elastic body, we would place the extreme Viking body towards the stiffness end of the scale.

This system has evolved out of a long training and teaching in archetypal patterning at the CMED[3] Institute and Body Reading at the KMI School.[4] It is not *based in* or endorsed by either. (Anatomy Trains™[5] body reading protocols are distinct and designed somewhat for static reading.) Please be sure to sense these types as *archetypal possibilities* to distinguish optimal practice. They are not designed to correct, criticise or reduce people's movement patterns, or suggest they would be "better if only ...". They could be described as an "optimisation guide" in recognition of fascial body types. They are not designed to restrict or diminish, merely to usefully identify, "tendencies towards."

The *y*-axis

These "somatotypes" were originally described in the 1940s by William H. Sheldon (1898–1977)[6] and were closely associated with different body types as regards their fat-storage tendencies and also psychological patterns. (This is reminiscent of Ayurvedic principles of how different types contain bodily fluids – see Hippocrates in Chapter 2.) They are used here in a very simple way and chosen for their association to shape (morphology), a keystone of fascial architecture. From a slightly different perspective we could also consider these morphologies from a sensory point of view. There are *all* highly responsive to the internal and external environment, whichever archetypal pattern it is filtered through. In this context, the distinctions are used to express movement *preferences*, in a neutral way, as much as they represent physiological tendencies or pre-dispositions.

Jungle type: this is a very different build to the Viking, representing the opposite end of that spectrum. Although it is no less powerful, it has a very different kind of agility. There is less bulk or brute force, rather a taught-limbed or sinewy kind of potential that might be associated with a warm or tropical climate and the symbolic ability to move silently through tangled undergrowth. In terms of the elastic body, this is the supple end of the spectrum.

There are many variations on these themes, of course. They live somewhere along this particular axis in terms of fascial types in a movement classroom. It is a soft motional interpretation and it is further defined by the vertical or *y*-axis.

At right angles to the horizontal axis is the *y*-axis that denotes shape. These somato-types are used as much for their general application in biology, referring to inner, middle and outer, as they are for any historical applications of particular personality or physiological traits.

On the *x*-axis, if Viking is West and Jungle is East, then Ectomorph and Endomorph take up North and South on this *y*-axis. Meso is in the middle and, just as in the embryo, it actually denotes the in-between (see Fig. 17.1).

We will use these categories and add some notes here for ease. Please expand them and add your own finer distinctions. It is as much to differentiate where someone *is not* as it is to assess where they are.

Ectomorph: the ectodermal layer comes from the Greek word meaning "outside" or the space beyond an external boundary – the outside of the shape. The ectomorphic type, in this context, denotes a sharpness of more active attention *outward*: an animal such as a bird, perhaps, or a squirrel, with a highly tuned sense of alertness to its surroundings. This type has a *tendency towards* a nervous disposition, staccato movements, high-speed bursts of energy and very finely tuned awareness and attention to detail. It might tend to focus on what is happening outside the body, while remaining sensitive to what occurs within.

Meso(morph): meso comes from the Greek for "middle" or intermediate. It suggests a halfway point but can also refer to something between the internal and external function and orientation – the middle of the other extremes. In some cases, this can refer to "moderate" and leads into the sense of mediator, as in finding the middle way. Here it suggests the place between the other main types but also one that can expand to include them. In tissue terms it is a balance of both outward and inward attention and awareness, possibly more inwardly focused than the extreme ectomorphic characteristics but less so than the more extreme endomorphic characteristics.

This type tends to prefer a balance of activity with thoughtful or reflective pursuits, needing to occupy their physical or instinctive body, with high regard for steady energy output. It sits in the middle, on the horizontal axis, because it can include both the strong, muscular body and the strong sinewy body of the Viking to Jungle extremes. At resting centre, it implies neutral balance.

Endomorph: this comes from "endo", meaning "within, internal", from a Greek origin. The endodermal layer of the embryonic structure refers to the internal gut tube, the forming of our digestively orientated systems and organs. This type can appear calmer or more reflective, certainly preferring a slower or more deliberating style of movement to the Ectomorph. It is not necessarily any less sensitive or fast, rather preferring a different rate of flow and a less staccato rhythm. If we were to use a sound scale, the Ectomorph would take the high notes, while the Endomorph would take the lower notes. Their focus might naturally be more on the inner world than what is happening outside the body.

We could say that we all have elements of all these morphologies; however, there is a tendency or preference towards one of them over others.

Centre: if someone appears to be perfectly balanced, both physically and in terms of their range of movement, then place them in the centre. For all people on the chart, the task is to consider training them from the opposite end of their spectrum, moving them *towards the central aspect* as it provides the optimum choice and range. If someone is already at the centre, then the game is to fill in the circle out beyond it and practice expanding in *all areas*.

Posture Profiling Chart: The Goal

Figure 17.1 depicts a Posture Profiling chart.

The goal is simply to move people from whatever point they begin at towards the centre. It is not to make everyone the same. Rather it is to invite a strong Viking type towards a greater range or balance, by increasing the suppleness-oriented movements of the Jungle body. The aim is not to turn the

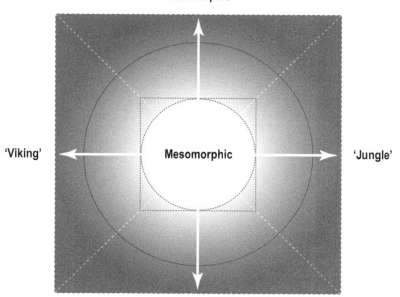

Figure 17.1

Using a broad brushstroke chart, we become artists more than scientists to "place" people on it and find appropriate coordinates.

person into a different type, but to recognise their default type and invite for them a greater range, a more optimal balance and elastic integrity.

A naturally very flexible Jungle body will be more likely to experience balance by considering more holding patterns, encouraging higher stiffness to ensure optimal containment and *biomotional integrity* in terms of tissue tone. That might include a more active or power-based yoga style. It might mean longer holding positions in suitable postures to tune the tissue for suitable stiffness, rather than suppleness.

A slower, more sedentary morphological type can "improve" by becoming more active and might find more vitality by attending a well-paced class on a regular basis. If they were placed towards the right side of the chart, then perhaps bringing in a holding focus would contain them and sustain their vitality. If they found themselves experiencing stiffness or having a naturally strong ("muscle-bound") build, then possibly encouraging suppleness would balance their particular profile, within its own parameters.

The ectomorphic type, which is associated with more staccato movements and a tendency to fidget, will want the opposite. For them, practising to enhance their ability to slow down a little and find the power of stillness might be of more value than focusing on speed and rapid change. They can benefit in finding the Middle Way, in their own particular way, through training a little more stillness or containment in the body. If they reside in the Viking side of the chart, it may be that longer, slower focus on becoming more supple, or more meditative, might be helpful.

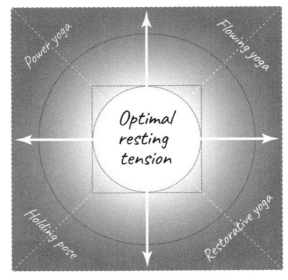

Figure 17.2

This is not a definitive chart of types of yoga, as many teachers interpret different combinations within a style. It is soft guide for interpretation, a framework to provide a context for recognising fascial body types.

Dose and degree of any (movement) "medicine" has to be grounded in common sense and softly implemented over time. The effect accumulates. Schleip recommends we have the approach of a "Bamboo Gardener" as the tissue changes over 6–24 months, while the fascial architecture responds fully to optimal loading patterns.[8] This tissue responds cumulatively over time. It resists fast and forceful sudden movement unless it is trained for it. It is *designed to* resist, in order to prevent injury. This is one reason why suitable preparation, or "priming the tissues", is so essential to prevent soft-tissue injury (see Appendix B).

Posture Profiling is swift and simple. It is designed to give a general cue to managing a class in which everyone is different. It allows us, as teachers, to optimise the fascial matrix of a given body type and assist that participant to find their balance in a way that is appropriate for them and the way their tensional matrix is generally organised. It is designed to improve elastic integrity over time, for the type they already, naturally animate. If the collagen matrix takes 12–24 months to change,[7] the purpose is to gradually accumulate a suitable loading pattern in a congruent direction for the person in question. It might mean choosing a different type of yoga entirely, based upon optimising a given pre-disposition.

This is not meant to be complicated. It is designed for ease of use and improved congruency, in terms of practice. Recognising fascial typing, as a component in choosing ideal types of practice or ways to encourage individuals of very different body shapes and tendencies, is valuable. Different types of yoga practice styles can also be usefully plotted on this soft graph. To start with they are simply placed in terms of the *x*- and *y*-axes. An individual is invited to try the style of yoga at the opposite end of their own place on the chart, to foster *their* elastic integrity, *gradually and occasionally* (Fig. 17.2).

Honouring the Individual

When I first came to yoga in my twenties, to manage post-childbirth and all kinds of aches and pains, I was at the base of the top right-hand corner of the graph, above the middle. Somewhat ectomorphic in terms of "highly tuned and sensitive", but very naturally bendy as my body tends towards hypermobility. Once I had learned to "hold back" from the extremes I could easily reach (not easy – thank you, John Stirk!), I discovered that stretching was detrimental and holding back before I reached extremes, was an asset to improve appropriate stiffness, to bring me to the "middle". I've always enjoyed a meditation practice since I was sixteen but sitting comfortably on the floor wasn't ever a naturally easy pose for me. Forty-plus years later, flexibility training is the last thing I would do; I can sense the energy leakage and it brings pain hot on the heels of a practice session. Using an awareness of living tensegrity forces and "squeezing in" or holding and compression biased motions maintain my vitality through meditative hours much more powerfully. Here is what my chart looks like (Fig. 17.3).

Having developed a sense for these general quadrants and positions, and where people "sit" at any given time in the squares, you can then hone the

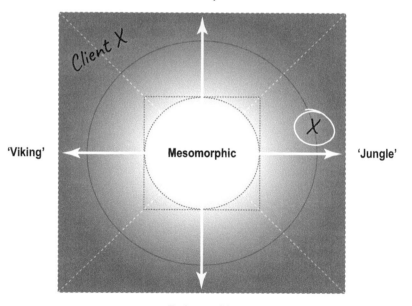

Figure 17.3

Example: Client X.

instinct for where they are relative to where they want to be. If we have the goal of optimal balance and variability, then we move in a general direction towards their opposite quadrant *via the middle*. This is done gradually over time. If someone is in an extreme combination, they will land in a square, outside the main (dotted) circle. The first task is to bring them inside the main circle at least. It takes time and practice to establish that first phase. The key thing is that it is unique to everyone and you are working with that individuality. Very small steps look like progress relative to the individual. For most people, progress in small degrees that improves their mobility and balance (relative to their ability at the time) is an achievement as well as an asset. That ability can change, so it is a valuable resource for gradual, safe progress in yoga.

Archetypal Movement Patterns – Nuanced Distinctions

There are nuanced distinctions within Posture Profiling. Taking yoga in general, from a movement programme point of view; it is generally a more flexibility-oriented practice than many other movement disciplines. Clearly, an Olympic shot-putter does not want to live at the centre; it is not optimal for them. They are in the Viking side of the *x*-axis and that is necessarily so; free to move with powerful force (and suitable bulk) as their main asset. However, they may gain *more power* (in terms of elastic recoil energy) in their overall fascial matrix from *occasionally* practising a more suppleness-oriented style (moving them towards the centre of the graph). This can optimise their flexibility and glide in the fascial architecture, *relative to their basic type*. Just a little. While strength-based training protocols might be their daily diet, yoga (albeit of a type focused on power and improving strength and speed to match their nature) might be ideal for them occasionally (if only to encourage a more supple overall approach to something more flexible than, say, weight-training, as an example). For people who have a morphology that lives firmly at one end of the spectrum (such as an Olympic shot-putter), however, even if they might secretly long to be an Olympic gymnast on the balance beam, it is archetypally beyond the scope of their fascia type. The mesomorph seems to naturally have the most choice, able to emphasise one style of practice over another, to affect changes either side of centre on the chart.

The value of this chart is that you look towards the centre. If you need to go up the *x*-axis, you are seeking more movement and possibly speed. If you need to go down it to get toward the centre you are seeking more relaxation and stillness and the value of slower, more deliberate and contained movements.

If, to get to the centre, you need to go right on the *y*-axis, you are seeking more flexibility and suppleness. If you need to go left, then it is more containment and compression-based holding positions, that are likely to optimise balanced tone in the tensegral architecture (or elastic integrity) of the overall form.

The point (and the value of this chart in terms of overall fascial awareness) is that giving someone who is hypermobile and tired a session of long, slow, flexibility-oriented movements might not optimise their tissue in the way that a faster and more powerful practice could. It may slow and tire them more. Although it may take time for them to be able to fully participate in a flowing, fast or strengthening class (e.g. Vinyasa Flow or Ashtanga or Power Yoga or one that holds the postures for longer periods), the value in starting slowly, to build up to it, might become clear in a few weeks to months of gradually strengthening their tissues by moving them *towards* (not to) a stronger and possibly faster-paced practice.

To add another, subtle dimension to Posture Profiling, this chart can deepen in relevance to contemporary yoga styles by incorporating the ancient

Table 17.1			
Yogic Trigunas			
Guna	*Related to*	*Tendencies or traits*	*Principle*
Rajasic	Ectomorphic	Active, animated, dynamic, seeking change, new light	Preservation
Satvic	Mesomorphic	Balance, order and clarity	Creation
Tamasic	Endomorphic	Inactive, dark, boundaried	Transformation

The principles of preservation, creation and transformation can be related to mesomorphic symbolism. Think of the hungry caterpillar – active, animated and driven to seek nourishment with urgency to preserve the species and progress towards freedom. It spins a thread towards the opposite state. At the opposite end of the scale, the next stage is one of darkness and inactivity, bound by a cocoon, a state of being retained and still. The result of these opposing forces combined is the emergence of the butterfly: able to walk on the ground, but also able to fly and express transformation. The butterfly lays the eggs that are the next generation, symbolic of the united forces of creation. It is important to recognise that all three forces (the one, the opposite and the combination) are present in all three gunas or tendencies. Like a tension–compression system, they all reinforce each other in honour of balance, order and clarity. A point in time marked by the cycle of creation: metamorphosis on every scale.

wisdom of the yogic *trigunas*. These are three tendencies that correlate to the ectomorphic, endomorphic and mesomorphic attributes on the vertical axis. The three gunas could be described as **rajasic, satvic** and **tamasic** *traits*. A guna literally refers to a "thread" in the metaphorical sense of a natural propensity or a tendency. They are used in Ayurvedic medicine and as such are not entirely unrelated to the "*humours*" of Hippocrates (see Ch. 2).

Translation from Sanskrit, which is a symbolic language, is much more subtle than the literal meanings we might try to ascribe. However, in this sense it is actually very useful here. We begin to find confluence between the manner of applying anatomy to understanding fascial form and yoga complementing each other rather than conflicting. They do not represent states and actions, but rather tendencies and innate preferences.

Innate to understanding the gunas is the respect for the theme throughout this work of balance between opposing forces, united to form a third state. Satvic means "being", the essence of the pure "is-ness", so it might be seen as the neutral centre. The gunas also encapsulate force and anti-force, both of which are needed to animate change or transformation as a balanced expression (Table 17.1). Thus, one is active and dynamic, one is more passive and still (associated with holding back) and balance is found by uniting them. It is precisely the same principles as living tensegrity is based upon.

Balance

When there is congruency in someone's movement loading, a balance of stiffness and suppleness or tension–compression resilience, their tissues have natural elasticity. It can be synonymous with vitality, which is why such emphasis is placed upon it. A participant can feel where it is missing and you can begin to see what style will be more or less optimal for their comfort and ability to do yoga to the extent they might like to. When the balance of practice is right for them you see it reflected in their architecture. It is different in everyone; expressed as the kind of poise and grace of movement that comes from being relaxed and at ease but free to run, if required, or ready to rest and be still in comfort. The principles of elasticity and biomotional integrity are reflected here. At its simplest, it is expressed as the ability to do a pose and a counter-pose with balanced ability to reach and return in both directions. This builds a congruent loading pattern and a certain embodied confidence.

What Next?

Once people are placed on the chart, ways of doing yoga get overlaid to direct the style of practice or the overall emphasis. They can choose which pathway to take, via strength and stiffening work or supple and softening work. What seems most suitable from your observation and their self-sensing awareness? It becomes clearer from recognising their movement archetypes. We can begin to put the two charts together. One distinguishes the participant (see Fig 17.3) and the other guides the practitioner (see Fig. 17.2).

This interpretive art also includes the teaching experience, the style of yoga and the length of time you have known the individual.

Developing your Skills

Once you learn to see many different bodies moving, observing as many classes as you can get yourself into, you will begin to build this intuitive sense. It is worth your time on every level because the reward is higher degrees of sensory refinement in your own Posture Profiling, assessment and adjustment skills. You will match a profile to a pose and a way of doing it that speaks almost instantly to the individual. It is transformative knowledge and it can literally alchemise the ability of the participant.

Once people are placed on the chart, you can use any other assessment tool that applies in manual practice. For a movement class, these are swiftly seen and sensed at speed when working to full advantage.

There are three major rules to follow to become adept at Posture Profiling. They are: *observation, observation and observation!*

You will learn to see subtlety and shadows, to interpret soft expressions of congruency and balance, reading movement signatures in individual "writing styles". You will even accumulate or refine the ability to anticipate imbalance. You can sense when you have taken someone beyond their comfort zone to their benefit, or if they need to hold back from their limits to become more contained, centered or stronger. These are the skills of top choreographers and teachers in elite dance, athletics and sports fields as well as in yoga. Experienced coaches recognize what is missing and call for something beyond what the individual *thinks* they can do, without compromising them. Not too much, in case they injure themselves, not so little that it makes no difference. Over time, optimal balance becomes available as a subtle asset.

Practising Posture Profiling

You can practice posture profiling anywhere that there are people. Ask yourself a series of questions and practice "pinning" randomly chosen people on the chart. Stay detached and work at speed. The essence of developing your intuitive impression is to work fast and observe yourself doing it. Suspend your judgement of yourself (the observer) and those you are observing. It is simply to practise placing many people on the chart for the fun of it.

A useful list of questions might be:

- What is your instant impression of where this person sits or lives on the chart?
- What made you choose that particular aspect?
- If they were in a line-up applying for an Olympic team, would it be weight-lifting (strength), gymnastics (flexibility), athletics (speed), a general sport (needing all the above, such as swimming, diving, field events), cycling (stillness and endurance) or would they prefer to watch it from the sofa and not participate? (This is designed to place them relative to the extremes on the chart.)
- Could they do all or any of the above?
- Make up your own questions.

This is for a soft impressionist sense of where that individual might be relative to the middle. Just playing this observational game will improve your skill in making more refined distinctions. It is as much about training you, the observer, as being accurate about those you observe. That will come with time, trial and error in accumulated strokes of experience.

Adjustment of the Postures and the Profiles

One of the useful applications of Posture Profiling for teaching yoga is in discerning when adjustment and modifications are optimal for a given student.

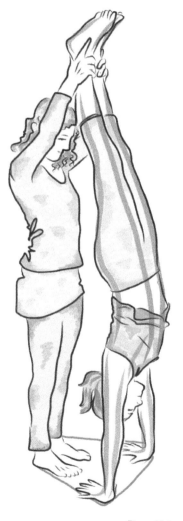

Figure 17.4

Facilitating balance between the front and back body.

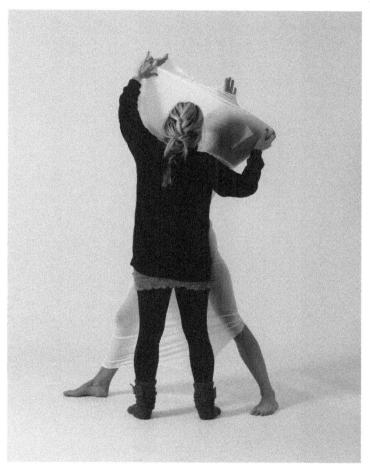

Figure 17.5

Even though this was for a photoshoot, the image makes the point about the imaginary kinesphere that helped the model to balance and self-regulate her architectural organisation. It helped her to stay very connected to the embodied sense of where she was in space. Adjustment was minimal.

(Model: Helen Eadie; Adjustor: Joanne Avison; Photographer: Amy Very. Reproduced with kind permission from Art of Contemporary Yoga Ltd.)

Figure 17.6

Working with the Fascia Sleeves gave the model a clear "felt sense" of feedback. Adjustment was a fascinating process of shifting the sleeve, or her weight, *so slightly* – that the whole feedback process was amplified throughout the fabric.

(Model: Helen Eadie; Adjustor: Joanne Avison; Photographer: Amy Very. Reproduced with kind permission from Art of Contemporary Yoga Ltd.)

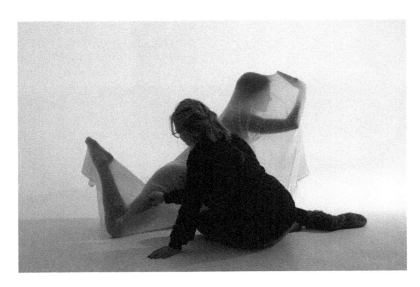

There is a "meet and greet" phrase in teaching manual therapy, when the trainee practitioner is taught to meet the tissues and match the energy of the client, as they "greet" them. Personally, I think this is amplified in the movement classroom, whatever the pose. My own experience of receiving adjustment at anything remotely forceful resulted in me sustaining permanent injury at the hands of my teacher. As a result, for a while, I erred on the side of non-intervention. However, I found in my classroom that participants could feel less "taken care of" when I used only verbal cues. Nevertheless, I find myself looking for the maximum difference for the minimum touch cue – and it is participant-centric and profile-specific. Posture-centric

Imaginary Shapes

adjustments make no sense to me, as so many people require a posture be modified to meet their particular profile, age, stage and agility. It is a skill and one worth practising. Given that the fascial body is already a sensitive, body-wide signalling system, we don't need to be heavy-handed to animate its appropriate response in finding forms, generated from within the participant, to assist self-regulation. In my experience the less force *added* from the teacher, the more the participant has to participate in finding their own

Once the type or style of yoga is confirmed for that individual, it can influence the way you assist them (if you do) and optimise the choices and options or requirements to modify a posture, to facilitate *their* optimal balance and natural range of motion.

Fascia research is shifting many of the parameters by which we measure and account for change in the body. Its impact on manual therapy has been considerable and subtle touch skills are a distinct asset in appropriate and well-placed adjustment. As we tune in to the sensory, body-wide matrix of the fascial network, it seems possible to appreciate how the most subtle, low-volume interventions can have profound impact to facilitate balance and poise.

Chapter 9 describes the standard classical biomechanical task of working from an imaginary axis, viewed as a straight pole or vertical line down the middle of the body. It acts as a reference point for the sagittal, coronal and transverse planes. What happens if instead of imagining a straight, linear pole we start imagining a volumetric tube enclosing the participant we view, literally and symbolically connecting them to the shape they are making? Let us call this imaginary "tube" the membrane between us and the "kinesphere" surrounding us. They are, perhaps, physical echoes of invisible energy fields around our soft-bodied volumes (in the round). It becomes a useful way to distinguish *the appropriate sense* of distance that we cross to adjust someone, if indeed they wish to be adjusted.[9] We shall refer to what is within the kinesphere as the "innersphere". This distinction facilitates a perspective of the postures from two dimensions into three dimensions; where they actually occur. It can provide access to a completely different understanding of adjustment.

equipoise. The kind they get to take away with them and use to sign their own movement signature, with a flourish, as a result (whatever the activity).

Proprioceptive Awareness

Sallie Brook is a graduate of anatomy science and the Laban school of dance. At the time of writing Sallie worked in the anatomy laboratory at King's College London. Her fascination with the fascial matrix led her to join my workshops and "kinesphere" was her word. It is a brilliant description of something that we can distinguish but not necessarily define in literal terms.

If we imagine a "kinesphere", it is a changing outline around a participant, in any pose (i.e. changing from moment to moment, just as we move). They are inside it, forming a tension–compression system that reflects the internal patterns, or geometries, that we cannot see.

Adjustment becomes more a story of proprioceptive invitation to self-regulation than an imposed position upon a body. Once body reading skills accumulate and become instinctive, the teacher can modify poses to enhance the sense of balance, according to the individual Posture Profile.

It is this field that each of us animates, that fosters self-containment and self-regulation, once we recognise its value and include it in our adjustment repertoire. Giving participants this kind of acuity is extremely valuable on a number of levels, not least of which is self-regulation and sensory respect for their own boundaries. If we imagine ourselves as having a kind of "energetic bank account", it is an advantage to us if we do not overspend or over-stretch our vitality and tempt injury while we are still expanding and deepening our investment. Self-containment is our balanced account and tiny adjustments, appropriate to the whole, keep that accountability as an asset.

"Nature always finds the most efficient way of doing things, and that includes geodesic geometry – the connection of points over the shortest distance, and the closest packing of objects together. Geodesic geometry provides the most economic utilization of space and materials and confers strength; it is at the heart of tensegrity with many easily recognized examples in biology. In two-dimensions a circle encloses the largest area within the minimum boundary which makes it a minimal-energy structure."[10]

Exploring this idea of an innersphere and kinesphere from which to see the postures gave rise to the images that were taken and developed inside tubes of fabric, as seen throughout this book. It is immediately obvious that these tensional surrounding "skins" provided sensory (kinespheric) feedback to the whole body; acting as a visual metaphor for what actually occurs from the fascial, sensory feedback system on the inside. The models reported a deep sense of confidence and responsive awareness from working within them (see cover image).

A New Perspective

The moment we touch someone, the two organisms combine to become one joined, closed kinematic chain. This is an important point. When you, the practitioner, adjust a participant you animate, at the next scale, the living tensegrity principle of three forces, re-iterated in yoga practice. That is, tension, compression and then tension–compression (as a whole trinity); or Ida, Pingala and Shushumna (arising from their combination); or negative, positive and neutral. There are two polarities and a third aspect of their

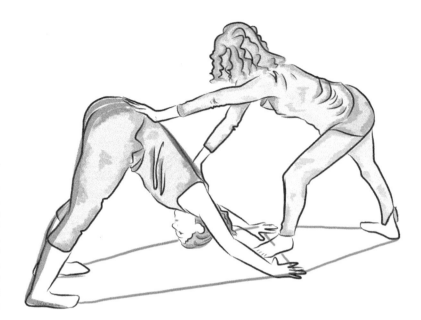

Figure 17.7

Example (1) of using a touch cue to adjust along the myofascial meridian or band being lengthened. In this instance, the facilitator is gently encouraging length in the back band (Myers' Superficial Back Line). As her body and the participant's form one whole shape, then the breath guides the response, via the ground, along that band (see Ch. 18).

combination, or *unity* – which is the meaning of the word "yoga". You join to become one enclosed kinesphere: one closed kinematic chain (see Ch. 9) with a larger ground print (Figs 17.9–17.10). The two distinct bodies become one architecture, with a different ground print and new emergent properties; the unity of the individual parts. That permits the smallest adjustments to foster equipoise and self-confidence.

A pose is not a suit of armour that a yoga participant is obliged to fit into. It is a reference for them to express and work towards, from within their body and their movement signature. By adding one or two informative links to improve their feedback system (their management of ground reaction force throughout their own matrix), you need very little action (i.e. adjustment). Two whole intelligent structures are now working together as one, both speaking the language of the body. One body does not become disabled while the ability of the other is relied upon 100%. Teacher and student are working at 100% capability plus 100% capability, as one whole information exchange. Just as our parts add up to something greater than the sum thereof, so too can the appropriate combination of two people, in mutual respect, bring about unpredictable possibilities and help to transform each other's practice. It is one way that we might go beyond our beliefs about our personal limitations, to the benefits of renewed confidence, in a momentary partnership, to facilitate balance and equipoise beyond our first attempt. Especially if the teacher can see a key point in the participant's balance that can be reinforced, or their weight transferred, or the angle of a foot slightly adjusted, or the curve of the spine, or a shift in attention, to make the difference. In this instance, the sum of the parts can bring about emergent properties, i.e. something unpredictable for each part, but available to their sum, with the least interference.

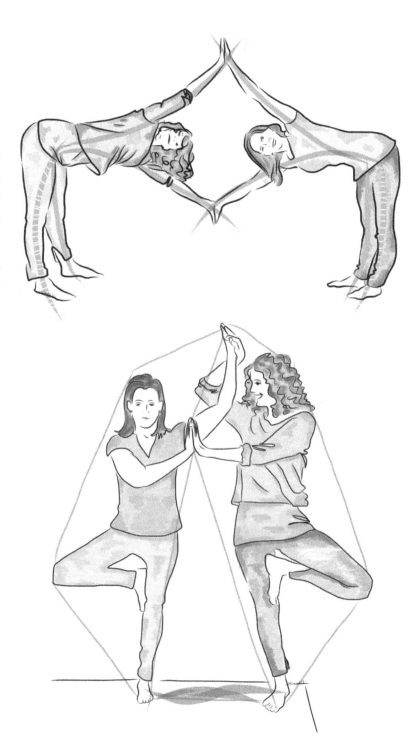

Figure 17.8

Example (2) of using a touch cue to adjust along the myofascial meridian or band being stiffened. In this instance, the facilitator is counterbalancing the stiffening required in the Front Functional Bands (Myers' Functional Lines). As her body and the participant's form one whole shape, then the breath guides the response, via the ground, along that band (see Ch. 18). The focus in a posture such as this is to "hold" the balance with sufficient structural integrity to do the opposite of stretching and releasing. Although the hands are stretched out, the structure is maintained through appropriate tensioning.

Figure 17.9

The facilitator or teacher (right) is mirroring the pose. The adjustment provides the counterbalancing force for the participant to counter-move.

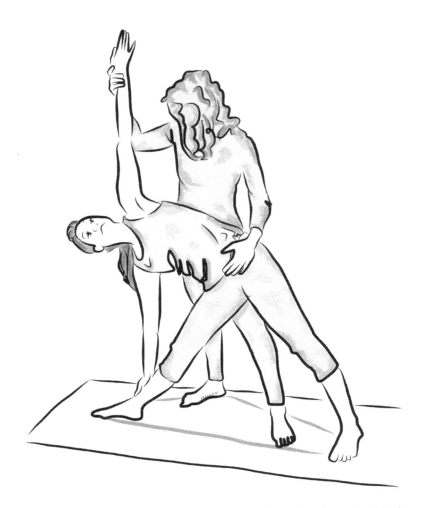

Figure 17.10

In this pose, the adjustment is expansive in the sense that it creates a broader ground print and supportive base – as if the participant has close access to four feet on the ground. The guiding hands are at the extremity of the upper hand and the apex of the shape made by the legs, as subtle support. The participant is not being pulled into shape, rather guided to find it.

Living Tensegral Adjustment becomes a relationship formed *with the ground* over a larger surface area (an extended ground print). There are more tension and compression struts (between the connected forms), joined at the point of engagement between teacher and student (practitioner and participant). In practice, this changes a few assumptions about adjustment.

The General Basis

Adjustment is a major topic in yoga teacher training programmes. Many books on the subject have three common denominators that our enquiry into fascia may shift or expand and possibly influence to some degree. The first of these is the emphasis on the posture, or asana, i.e. asana-centric; the second is assistance; and the third is placement.

1. **Posture being adjusted**. Authors readily acknowledge that the participants in a yoga class are all different. Nevertheless, the key or purpose of an adjustment is usually based on the ideal shape of the pose being

Table 17.2	
Classical Approach	*Contemporary Approach*
Teacher as guru	Teacher as guardian
Posture as perfect ideal or result	Postures as potential idea or reference
Separate definition of structure and function upon which form is imposed	Integrated distinctions of structure and function as united expressions of form
Pain as a signal of the nervous system	Refined sensory awareness as a pre-emptive guide to prevent pain signals
Adjustment seen as authoritative intervention	Adjustment seen as respectful invitation
Local directive of correct positioning	Subtle implication of congruent self-placement
Teacher as master of form	Teacher as midwife in formation
Leading hands	Listening hands
Performance induction	Pre-formance intention/preparation
Imposed correction	Exposed congruency
Body as linear, mechanical structure, governed by laws of linear relationships	Body as a self-assembled, self-organising non-linear biologic system of conscious awareness, attention and vitality
Competitive and striving attitude, toward goal-oriented perfection	Presence of inner stillness, enquiry and curiosity
Local view of joint angles in gravity	Global view of whole-body response as contained ground reaction force
Guidance to maximise stretch and reach goal of pose	Restoring sense of centre and self-containment to unfold into pose
Pose at all costs	Poise relative to postural limit
Controlled breathing to manage and present the posture	Freedom to breathe and express the posture appropriately
Maximised reach	Elastic integrity
Direct proximal adjustment	Subtle distal implication
Macro-movement	Micro-movement
External correction	Internal containment
Conversion from weak to strong forms	Conversation in balancing form
Assertive or zealous encouragement to achieve the pose	Gracious invitation to touch and move beyond limits towards the pose
Demand the best	Reveal the best
Achieve the asana	Accumulate the ability to explore asana

activated. Adjustment instructions are often based upon the ultimate aim of the particular asana and the correct form it predisposes (pun intended).

2. **Assisting the participant.** If someone in the class is aiming to complete a pose, to whatever level is appropriate for that class (beginners, intermediate, advanced, etc.), the idea is to provide aid so they can reach or achieve the posture by helping them to extend or (and this is the word most commonly used) "stretch" sufficiently.

3. **Correct placement for adjusting or assisting the pose.** Where do you place your hands or body in order to achieve the above, i.e. help the

participant organise or reach into the posture, the correct form, that they are seeking to emulate? Most books suggest the most appropriate positioning of the adjusting hands (or feet) in order to *achieve the pose*.

These may all be key components of adjusting. If someone is in a Warrior Pose, for example, and their knee is out of alignment, then a small adjustment of their knee can transform their ability to interact with the pose and find their optimum balance. However, in a different context, from a tensegrity-oriented point of view, the teaching hand upon their standing foot, or spine, might animate a *self-corrective alignment* response, so the participant naturally draws their own knee into a more appropriate place. This is the shift from adjusting the posture to adjusting the participant (see Table 17.2).

Robert Schleip's two-part series on "Fascial plasticity", published in the *Journal of Bodywork and Movement Therapies*,[4] considered some of the many questions manual therapists have about what exactly changes under their hands, when they effectively adjust their clients. From a viewpoint of living tensegrity, every connection forms a "chain reaction" in that the net, the internal net, the interstitial network within, is all continuous.

The recommendation here is towards an attitudinal shift that is clearly beneficial to both manual and movement practitioners. It errs towards fostering self-regulation as the purpose of any intervention, rather than creating dependency upon the teacher (Table 17.2).

The Adjustor

Touch skills are an essential part of teaching a physical movement form, if only because they occur in the same kinaesthetic language as the movements. Nevertheless, adjustment is a domain in which the power differential comes in to play and this is a hot topic for debate in manual therapy and more recently in yoga and other movement classrooms.

How can we serve our students, adjust appropriately, yet honour the self-regulatory advantages of a take-home wisdom for their personal practice? As practitioner, you can provide necessary feedback. How can that best serve the participant so they retain it and alchemise it for their own benefit?

Here, too, we need new distinctions and new definitions. Understanding fascia and tension–compression integrity, given its role in sensory refinement, calls for new views. The authentic exploration of structural balance can bring us an "upgrade" on the journey towards awareness and self-confident self-regulation. Is there an optimum way to consider this, between two intelligent systems?

Subtle Touch Skills

There are many working possibilities from the point of view of adjustment in different types of yoga. It is possible to use the Anatomy Trains™ examples to encourage balance between the bands or lines (as shown in detail in the next chapter). This ensures that a posture is not performed for one side at the expense of the other. As a useful overview we will highlight the main themes (see Table 17.3); however, this provides a summary of many hours of honing skills in training; it comes with practice!

Table 17.3	
Adjustment Theme	*Overview*
Ground control	Adjustment is based upon the ground print of the participant. What is the participant's relationship to the ground? By simply touching the part of their body engaging with the ground, you can facilitate a deepening sense of anchoring to the earth (Figs 17.11 & 17.12).
Spine design	Adjustment is focused on giving subtle feedback through the hands on the spine, to honour and support freedom of the primary and super curves, and the breath (Fig. 17.13).
Counterbalance	Adjustment is providing feedback to the opposite aspect of the movement. If the participant is working towards a back bend, then feedback from a counterbalancing hand implying a downward flexion can provide the most useful reference.
Expansive	Adjustment is based on a parallel movement that supports distal to the ground but expands the ground print (base of support) by replicating or increasing it.
Restorative	Adjustment is minimal but gives the limb "back to the spine" or supports the asana by resistance, the opposite of encouraging stretch. It restores the centre rather than encouraging movement away from it.
Anatomy Trains™ in yoga	This is developed based upon the Anatomy Trains™ principles by Tom Myers[11]: see Chapter 18 for how to work with them in motion to express volume. The adjustment is based on balancing of opposing bands (lines), encouraging the deep inner container to respond and hold its shape. See Chapter 18 for a variety of possibilities (and see also Figs 17.7 & 17.8).

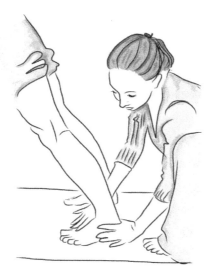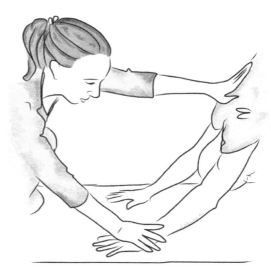

Figures 17.11 & 17.12

The feet and the hands are all engaged with the ground in this pose. By emphasising that engagement with subtle touch, the posture is anchored and the participant can self-sense to naturally contain their own fulfilment of the pose, down into and away from the ground, simultaneously, animating the Ground Reaction Force from it.

Adjustment invites the most subtle of touch skills. When we sense that we are touching an intelligent internal net (with an intelligent internal net), then any point will effectively communicate throughout and between the system(s). The most subtle resonance can be tuned into, like a radio frequency, to some extent. Adjustment can harm or heal, impose or invite; the hands are used

Figures 17.13

In this pose it would be easy to send the heels to the floor. However, balancing through the back bands (see Ch. 18, Superficial Back Line in Tom Myers' Anatomy Trains) allows a sense between stiffness and suppleness, a scale along which self-adjustment can honour the spinal curves. The adjusting hand enhances the sense of spinal freedom to *breathe and wave* through the natural spinal curves. The asana is dynamic, not static. The hand rests (on the spine at the back of the breath) to provide feedback. There is no pressure applied at all.

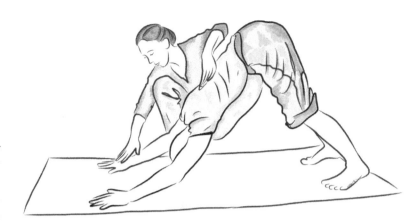

more as magnets than as hammers. Fingertips are eloquent tools and, depending to some extent upon the participant, suitable guidance might generally follow a "less is more" direction. Firm quiet hands give clear simple messages; kinaesthetic comments with signals designed to encourage self-organisation.

Inviting containment, steadiness and whole body participation from the ground to the extremes of the pose is a comment on integration rather than goal-seeking. The body usually loves finding balance within a smaller range, which can be gradually expanded (see Table 17.2).

We are fostering more refined understanding and transmission of movement forces, not forced movements. As such the language of adjustment is a softly spoken one and invites self-confidence to the practice.

Adjusting the Breath

There are many ways to "adjust" the breath. My preference is to use three key hand positions, illustrated here. The hands barely touch the body; they make just enough contact to feed back to the participant the sense of the movements/areas of breathing. The participant can focus inwardly, to feel the breath expand the torso, experienced as a volume in this exercise. The purpose is wide-reaching and beneficial. It allows the student to "fill" their structure and experience the omnidirectional possibilities of breathing a little more fully in three key "directions of breathing". The positions are shown below (Figs 17.14–17.16).

The three positions encourage fuller breath in the lower ribs, front-to-back body and upper chest. The student is guided to gently expand the breath, from the breathing innersphere – inside out. (As distinct from activating muscles to force breathing action from the outside in.)

Dose, Degree and Direction

The fascial matrix, and its highly tuned role in proprioception, shifts the foundations of traditional principles, so we need to change from a basis of biomechanical adjustment (based on correct form, angles of joints and so on) to something that can facilitate self-regulation. I like to call it "biomotional" interaction, which is based on respect for self-sensory "nous" (pronounced like "mouse" in English; it means "gnosis – a kind of knowing").

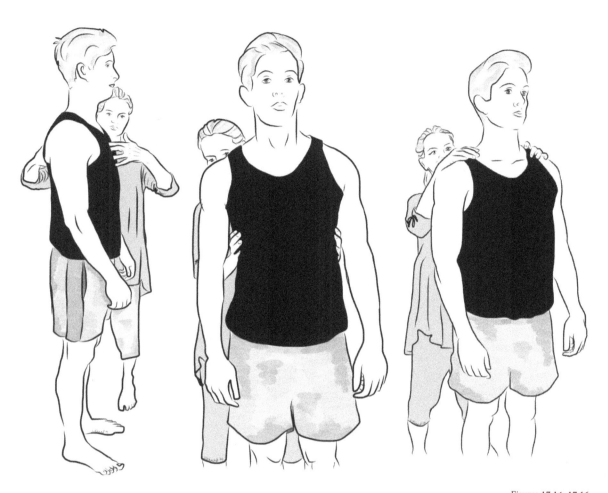

Figures 17.14–17.16

Breath adjustment hand positions for the practitioner. (See box below.)

Adjusting the breath

1. In Figure 17.14 the practitioner places fingertips on breastbone and spine to assist the sense of breathing them apart (inhale) and together (exhale) with the movement of the rib basket.

2. In Figure 17.15 the practitioner places palms on the lower back ribs to assist the sense of expansion in the back and sides of the body. There is also elasticity and glide between the fascial layers as the "bucket-handle action" of the ribs becomes compliant with the movement of the rib basket.

3. In Figure 17.16 the practitioner places palms on the shoulders to discourage over-recruitment of shoulders in the upper rib basket and encourage glide of the shoulder blades over it (i.e. with her thumbs lightly placed on the shoulder blades). Bringing the breath into the upper part of the rib basket is encouraged here (see Ch. 11 for detail).

Please note, these exercises are brief and gentle. Forcing the breath can cause distress and stimulate over-breathing. These exercises are kinaesthetic reminders to encourage fuller use of the breathing volume. They can be done in class in pairs with the caveat of wise direction regarding dose and degree.

If the fascia is the largest sensory organ of the body, the communication network from skin to brain and back, then adjustment raises some interesting questions.

How subtle a touch is needed?

We are not forcing movement so much as registering movement forces as an enhanced feedback system. The hands can be used as magnets, or subtle reminders of the ground, the centre, the spine or breath, etc. The least force can mean the most effective response in many cases.

Where should I touch, if the fascia is everywhere?

Using the categories of ground control, spine design, counterbalance, expansive and restorative, the purpose of a specific adjustment is toward optimum congruency for that participant in that pose and that point in time. As the fascia is everywhere, appropriate placement becomes specific to that occasion.

Are there key places that make a difference to every pose?

There are key meridians that are included in every pose, such as the Anatomy Trains™ lines,[12] which wrap the body (see Ch. 18), as one example. Acupuncture meridians would offer another guide, if you are familiar with them. The breath, the spine and the engagement with the ground arise as key places, common to all poses. However, as in the question above, this is occasion-centred, rather than posture-centred, since the state, day and anatomy can all be variable.

Are there fundamental principles that we should adhere to?

Integrity, subtlety and remembering one's own kinespheric balance, before combining it with the person being adjusted. It is a conversation between two intelligent systems that become one in that moment of adjustment. As Tom Myers points out: "The heart of healing lies in our ability to listen, to perceive, more than in our application of technique … interventions are a conversation between two intelligent systems".[13] While he is referring to the manual therapy of Structural Integration, it nevertheless applies to the subtle touch skills of yoga adjustment.

What is the point of adjustment; should we intervene at all?

It is to enhance practice for the person being taught and to develop their sense of their own containment and ability. If you cannot know you are doing that, then do not adjust.

If not posture-centric, then what guide or grid makes sense of poses?

See the details of kinesphere/innersphere and apply your heart-felt integrity, from your own sense of balance and experience of the posture being taught or recommended. Using or applying such systems as Anatomy Trains™ can be a useful guide, particularly at the beginning while you develop your own confidence. Simply bear in mind that the body doesn't work in a linear way!

Does fascia affect the biomechanics of adjustment as well as moving?

A Question of Ethics

Adjustment is necessarily part of an interpretive art. It is one of the many skills developed in yoga teaching. It is intimately related to the sensory faculties of the body, profoundly affecting them and affected by them. Effectiveness comes down to many aspects of integrity, whether in training, in teaching or transferring skills, on all levels. In Chapter 5, the sensory nature of all our organs is explored and yoga, given its approach, speaks eloquently in the language of our original heart-centred forming.

The most powerful question I have ever heard with regard to ethical

We might say it is the medium of translation, transmission and transformation.

The nature of the fascial matrix, given its living tensegrity architecture, means that every connection forms a "chain reaction" in the closed kinematic chain formation of the body. This means that (as we have said) the network of the connective tissue matrix – the internal net, the interstitial network, "the innerstitium" – is one continuous human fabric; formed and developed *under tension*. That makes the microcosm, the macrocosm and "us within the cosmos" based upon similar laws of nature and rules of self-assembly. It means we are a resonance field and when we touch another in adjustment, we "tune in" to become one resonance field. It invites an exquisite gift of nothingness: balance, or equilibrium.

Essentially that makes us instruments (see Ch. 7, excerpt by Mae-Wan Ho). We are literally and symbolically tuned *and in the process of attunement* in our practice. It is essentially personal and based in self-awareness, although the impersonal nature of our intention to teach allows us to work together. In the Hu-man Grace Field. If we assess and adjust from that place, we treat the mystery of the human body and the magic of fascia with the wonder and awe and curiosity with which it unfolds to us. May that subtle force be with you.

"Out beyond ideas of wrongdoing and rightdoing there is a field. I'll meet you there.

When the soul lies down in that grass the world is too full to talk about."

Rumi

practice around this point is "What is in your heart?". If you are intuitively intelligent enough to understand these movements and their integration, then you can use that same sense to know your own agenda. If it is not to adjust and assist your student to honestly optimise their own yoga practice, *with and for them*, then what are you doing there? Intentional integrity and tensional integrity are the same.

Notes

1. See https://www.joanneavison.com/ for further information on these courses.
2. Robert Schleip, various presentations on Fascial Fitness and Fascianating Fascia.
3. Caroline Myss Education (CMED) Institute Practitioner Training (Sacred Contracts) in archetypal patterns of the psyche and somatic resonance. 2002–2005 in Chicago, Illinois.
4. KMI (Kinesis Myofascial Integration) School: http://www.anatomytrains.com/at/kmi/.
5. Thomas W. Myers, *Anatomy Trains: Myofascial Meridians for Manual and Movement Therapists*, 2nd edition, Churchill Livingstone, Edinburgh, 2009.
6. https://www.britannica.com/biography/William-Sheldon
7. Robert Schleip (2003) Fascial plasticity: a new neurobiological explanation, parts 1 and 2. *Journal of Bodywork and Movement Therapies* 7(1):11–19; 7(2):104–116.
8. Ibid.
9. This article is very helpful regarding the use of and design of "consent cards" that give any participant in a class a means to inform their teacher of their personal preferences regarding adjustment. https://triyoga.co.uk/blog/yoga/triyoga-introduces-consent-cards/
10. Graham Scarr, www.tensegrityinbiology.co.uk, article: "Geodesic". See also: *Biotensegrity: The Structural Basis of Life*, Handspring Publishing Ltd., Pencaitland, 2017.
11. Thomas W. Myers, Anatomy Trains: Myofascial Meridians for Manual and Movement Therapists, 2nd edition, Churchill Livingstone, Edinburgh, 2009.
12. Ibid.
13. Ibid.

18

Classroom Connections 6: Maps: Anatomy Trains™

"All organs of an animal form a single system, the parts of which hang together, and act and re-act upon one another; and no modification can appear in one part without bringing about corresponding modifications in all the rest".[1]

Baron Georges Cuvie

Myers has challenged assumptions about the architectural organisation of the body. For a long time, his chapter "The World According to Fascia"[2] was the only available work on the fascial matrix that someone outside scientific research could use to begin considering the body as whole, including the context of connective tissue.

Before tensegrity was fully appreciated and tested to the extent it is now beginning to be understood, Tom Myers offered it as a possibility for considering how bodies occupy space and move in a way that makes sense of them, essentially as a whole. This is very different from reducing bodies to anatomical categories and theories of motion mechanics that feel reductionist in the context of a full-bodied yoga class, or an embodied participant. Myers is not, however, an anatomist so the poetic license of Anatomy Trains™ can be appreciated and forgiven, since it was designed pre-dissection. It is an upgrade from bits to bands, however it doesn't substitute the living wholeness of bodies-in-motion.

The concept of Anatomy Trains™, as laid out in the book of the same name by Thomas Myers, remains controversial. I have had the privilege of working closely with both the book and the author, first as a student and later as an assistant and teacher, so I remember the earliest challenges and efforts to translate anatomical continuity into some kind of manageable and meaningful portrayal for practical application.

Myers carved a path through a very dense forest and cleared the way for kinaesthetically biased people to travel more easily between the classical anatomy texts and the world of practice. It is one thing to do that for manual therapy and another to do it for movement professionals; used in a particular way, Myers' work is a resourceful contribution to both.

As we have seen, anatomy can become lost in translation somewhere between the page and the person it is being used to define (in real time and natural pattern). Myers has created a means to traverse that divide, articulately, in a kinaesthetically appropriate way, with some relevant and applicable guide-lines. The pathways of the Anatomy Trains™ are worth learning, if only to steer a coherent course between the cartoons of muscle units (as classically taught) and the schematic concept of continuity, even if lines (as linear by definition) do not *ever* explain 3D wholeness, or myofascial unity, as it is physically experienced. It has been a relatively uncharted route. Yoga postures occur as an expression of natural *continuity* (laterally and longitudinally, in the round), so this work is a valuable bridge from historical analysis to the contemporary classroom, as *guide-lines* towards a more continuous architecture. That is *if we remember* they are not functional, linear progressions in real life, ever.

As yoga practitioners, we seek lightness of foot and spirit, anchored in an articulate conversation with the forces of gravity, framed and explored in poses (asanas). Some of this resides in seeing the obvious: often things are not quite as cloaked in mystery as scientific reasoning might at first seem to imply. It is certain, for example, that movement does not happen in individual units of action (be that sectioned as muscles or myofascial meridians) that somehow organise themselves into the asanas done by the coherent beings that attend our classes. *People can already move.* Yoga is, among several other things, one of many ways to specialise, refine, practise and differentiate the details of our mobility or "motionality", if we can use such a word. Its very nature is joined up, as is ours: "these meridians [Anatomy Trains] girdle the body, defining geography and geometry within the myofascia, the geodesics of the body's mobile tensegrity."[3]

It is a very poetic notion, however Anatomy Trains™ do not, in *any way*, explain or represent the body's "Geodesics". Buckminster Fuller's geodesic domes explain the geometry of volumes and tetrahedral force transmission. Anatomy Trains™ is an essentially linear description of different longitudinal sections of a tube. (That's like taking a tape measure to work out how much water is in a pond; they don't relate well.)

Anatomy Trains™ is valuable and useful, however let us be clear what it is and what it is not, so that we don't forget we are round volumes, moving (ourselves) a-round as a whole; sur-rounded by gravity and sur-rounding our innate ground reaction forces. It is always useful to divide the body to study it (and read it) – and bands are an improvement on bits. However, we do not move around as different Anatomy Train lines.

We move around as close-packed, soft-matter systems, through whom the *forces of life* move in non-linear geodesic patterns. It is a huge and essential distinction in understanding Living Tensegrity architecture; it does not abide by Anatomy Trains™ rules and nor should the two distinctions be collapsed; they don't fit together. The Anatomy Trains™ were designed as a game, to help learn anatomy in "joined-up writing". As such, they are a valuable resource to get us from anatomical parts to anatomical continuities. However, they don't exist *as such* in the body – they are a **learning tool** and a **linear one**, that is carved in the cadaveric tissues, *not revealed*. It completely depends on how you cut it.

In our role as teachers, we are imparting ways of exploring what are strictly "girdles" or "slings" of tissue continuities. Our purpose is to make sense of optimal form, for the participant. Using Anatomy Trains™ to guide this, in terms of reading whole postural balance in asanas, is a useful tool to have if they are used in a particular way. It is a reference for finding the coordinates for an individual expressing a particular posture in their way. There are, however, a few points worth emphasising when applying it in movement.

The Anatomy of Continuity

Anatomy Trains™ provides a vantage point that yoga teachers can use to great benefit. It becomes particularly useful in adjustment (see Ch. 17).

A careful read of the many resources that Myers describes in his introduction to the second edition is highly recommended. In this section ("Laying the Railbed"[4]), there is a reference to the German anatomist Tittel,[5] who depicts

Anatomy Trains™ originated as a game, devised by the tutors at the Rolf Institute in the 90s, to help students of Structural Integration to see anatomical form in "joined-up writing", so to speak. The emphasis on continuity was a novel departure at the time from cut-up pieces of anatomical parts. It was designed to assist manual practitioners to assess the fascial body, with respect for the continuum in which the tissues grow and develop. Myers' work in presenting it is challenged by anatomical research, yet it was not intended to substitute fascial anatomy or define its continuity. Only to recognise and appreciate (particularly in comparison to classical anatomical reductionist views) how the human body balances as a whole, in a longitudinal pattern that matches, somewhat, the Meridians of Chinese Medicine. It does not pretend to represent functional organisation, if only on the basis that nothing in the human body is linear.

what he calls "muscle slings" in the active postures of athletic pursuits and dynamic movements. Myers refers to them as more "movement specific and momentary" as distinct from the Anatomy Trains™ fascial fabric connections, "which are more permanent and postural".[6]

The point is to recognise the echo of Blechschmidt,[7] perhaps, who suggests that even from our embryonic origins our muscles, tissues and bones were formed according to a plan that grew them as slings, in continuity (see Ch. 4). Given our basic human design blueprint, our expression of these "slings" in action is partially individual, as is our personal form. However, their continuity is, essentially, *global* and *universal*. As such, the Anatomy Trains™ suggest typical directions of force transmission, however *they are not the structural or the functional basis* of motion.

Both resources (Myers, Tittel and others) suggest the value of seeing in continuity and this is the basic premise of learning either view. Tittel did not name the functional bands he described, in the way Myers has; however, his depictions are visually very powerful in terms of making sense in the movement classroom.

We have to work in joined-up moments and once we develop appropriate ways to see in continuity of form, we can intervene wisely and sparingly to foster awareness and balance without imposition (Ch. 17). Other researchers[8] also refer to slings in specific therapeutic or pathological contexts, which are beyond the scope of this work. It is, however, a useful tool to analyse posture. It doesn't explain it, but it helps to map it, topographically, via the system of contours we could say it provides.

Using the Contour Map

It is a most valuable resource in any yoga training to see balance as a global possibility if we remember Anatomy Trains™ is a metaphor and hold the following four fundamental tenets in mind:

- Anatomy Trains™ is a particular kind of map that emphasises connectivity and connecting *longitudinal* pathways, at specific depths. It is nearer reality than many topographical maps but still not the territory.

- Myofascial Meridians are not synonymous with function. They are useful possibilities that suggest how refined balance might be explored in the whole structure. It depends how you apply them. They are an excellent platform upon which to stand while developing the art and the skills involved in seeing (reading) myofascial continuity.

- The rate of application is entirely different in a movement class to a manual therapy session, where the client spends much of the session (relatively) still and passive on the table, for assessment and receiving treatment. Herein lies the quantum leap we have to make as movement teachers: to harness the power of the tool and benefit from a particular aspect of its application, which we will explore (see below, for example).

- The body occurs in volumes (something Myers refers to in class) rather than in lines. If the metaphor of the anatomy train tracks is to be really useful in a movement class, **the tracks have to be considered (at least) in pairs, relative to each other**. Then they can be used for denoting form, rather than fixtures. Otherwise you need much more time to body read, thus leaving the realm of the active movement classroom and entering into the realm of therapeutic practice, and clients standing still for assessment. However valid that is in itself, it is not the remit of this book. In a movement class we are using this tool to read bodies in motion at speed and optimal alignment, in yogasana. Thus, we need pairs to acknowledge volume, as we will explore below.

Speed-Reading Prompts

I have personally dissected all the Anatomy Trains™ lines and while that does not make them "real" in the living form, it does make them valid for consideration as a way to represent continuity in our tensional body form. How they work for each individual is one thing. Whether they exist in the body as separate or distinct "entities" is another. They do occur in continuity, as continuous bands of composite tissues, just as individual muscles can be found in dissection. It is not their reality that is being discussed here, however, but *what we make them mean*. Essentially, we have to remember, **they are carved, not revealed** in the body forms that are cut up for demonstration. Continuity is relentless; we do not move the back body (or any other aspect) distinctly from the breathing volume of its depths.

Motional Modifications

An individual in motion cannot be globally defined at the speed of the class, whether using classical anatomy, biomechanics or Anatomy Trains™, since movement is not an intellectual process, particularly in real time. If we remember that Anatomy Trains™ is a guide (and an upgrade on single muscles-as-means-to-move), then we can now travel usefully into the territory called contemporary yoga using Anatomy Trains™ appropriately. It is an invitation to see in shapes and identify useful balance and less useful restriction, via a pose-in-progress.

Yoga does not really fit into (nor is it explained by) the Anatomy Trains™ lines (there are no lines, flat planes or perfect symmetries in the body; we do not all move the same, or slowly enough to read or be read as we move, nor are "lines of pull" the same in each person). Anatomy Trains™ can, however, be made to fit into yoga in an extremely intelligent and useful way. It helps join the dots; but it doesn't explain the non-linear territory.

You will need a broad brush, a relaxed "watercolour" style, and an eye for light and shadow and for "relative to". We will assume you have acquired the text of Anatomy Trains™ (or at least the posters for reference) as it is thorough and well-illustrated and an excellent resource for the anatomical definitions of each so-called "train" or "line", referencing the muscle units in their fascially continuous and bony integrations. (A summary of each is included here for ease of reference.)

Below you will find a few useful notes for working with Anatomy Trains™ in motion to optimise their application in a movement classroom:

- The "Deep Front Line" is a **container**, which at speed we read via the breath. It represents a volume and, since we cannot touch it directly, it may be that watching and cueing the breath can provide access. Breathing and movement integration (Ch. 11) are distinguished as a basis of optimal organisation and functional movement.

- The Functional Lines do not "function" as such in yoga, unless you include the feet and hands and continue the lines beyond Myers' defined limit of the elbows and knees. We do not move by hovering above the ground. *We integrate from it.* Whatever the argument for calling Functional Lines *functional* lines (like all the others, they are designated, topographical structural definitions), **they reach the ground in real life on the mat**. Hands and elbows (knees and feet) work in concert, so any line stopping at the elbow (or knee) does not get to be identified as "functional" in a movement context (unless it unfortunately *is* the distal end of that extremity, which would, at the very least, be considered pathological).

- Fascia *is not limited to* Longitudinal Bands such as defined by the Anatomy Trains. They are an extremely useful means to read overall body shape in such a way that gives us relatively fast access to seeing continuity of form and balance. To optimise assessment in motion, emphasis is on continuity and breathing rather than on any specific line *per se*.

There is indeed something like a Back Spiral Band! Many dancers (particularly ballet) and Yoga Flow practitioners animate the sense of the *exact opposite* of the so-called Spiral Lines (which are the most anatomically challenged in the research). There is a much more complex and integrated relationship between the front and back body in natural helical motion. The body

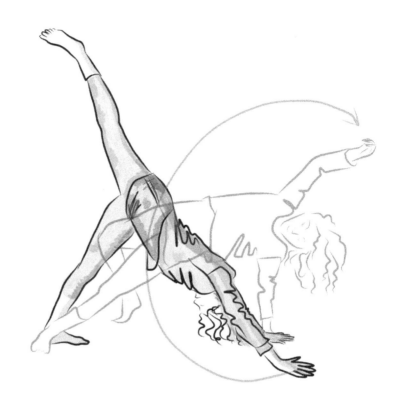

Figure 18.1

3-point Chakrasana.

Another useful work is *Dynamic Body, Exploring Form, Exploring Function*, by Erik Dalton.[9] Myers is one of the contributing authors to this book and his overview of Anatomy Trains™ is an excellent resource and introduction, without all the fine details of application to therapeutic intervention included in the full version of the original work.[10]

Movement comes through the body, rather than from it, at this level of performance. It also uses the ground and the gravitational field in a very instinctive way. A dancer leads with their head, moving forward from the back body, backward from the front, and so on. Dancers are trained in the polarities that become so refined they are only described by the body moving, in continuous transition in 360°. The analysis is only analysis. Freedom of expression using the kind of movement that a dancer can command can bring an audience to tears of emotion, a fact that is not easy to explain. It is something in and of itself that even

Starting Points for Anatomy Trains™ in Yoga

absorbs and transcends the dancer. *It can be as if dancing is dancing.* In Vinyasa Flow, which means "to place in a special way", it is expressed as continuous movement. The quality of "otherness" beyond analysis is harnessed and surrendered to, through practice. We do not move according to anatomy lines; as non-linear forms, we only move as volumes.

interprets sequential transitions in ways that are not always readily reduced to Anatomy Trains™ configurations. As Myers points out, Tittel offers bands that are related to "momentary movement" rather than postural set (Fig. 18.1). All motion takes place in time, so it works to climb the ladder the train tracks provide, without imposing the idea of them, as if they actually exist as forms.

These bands provide starting points, or references in the conversation between practitioner and participant. We will begin with showing the lines as sweeping impressions of continuities, or parts of continuous sheaths or bands, which is how they appear in the clothed participants that we see arriving in the classroom, presenting the impressions of each line in paired soft architectures to give an overall sense of fascial form, in motion at speed, relative to each other, emphasising that all the lines can be distinguished individually or collectively in any posture. They are very useful indicators in pairs, of restriction, balance or optimal shifts, working in wholeness. We will not go into the detail of all the depths, as found in Anatomy Trains™. Rather we will focus on relationships: seeing the front relative to the back, for example, such as we see in class.

Longitudinal Myofascial Meridians

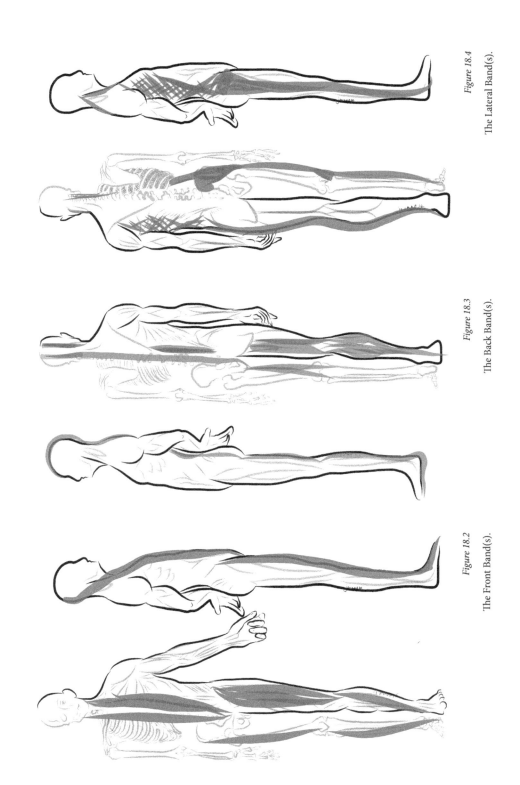

Figure 18.4
The Lateral Band(s).

Figure 18.3
The Back Band(s).

Figure 18.2
The Front Band(s).

Longitudinal Myofascial Meridians

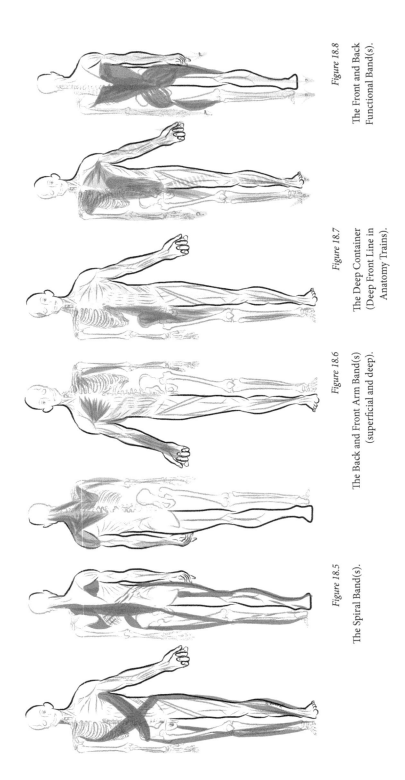

Figure 18.5
The Spiral Band(s).

Figure 18.6
The Back and Front Arm Band(s)
(superficial and deep).

Figure 18.7
The Deep Container
(Deep Front Line in
Anatomy Trains).

Figure 18.8
The Front and Back
Functional Band(s).

N.B. ALL the lines are relative to the Deep Container; it is seen via the breath, which gives us access to the structural balance between the lines (see Fig. 18.15).

Longitudinal Myofascial Meridians of Yoga Based on Anatomy Trains

Disclaimer: Please note these are broad brushstroke impressions of the bands that are detailed comprehensively in Anatomy Trains™ by Thomas W. Myers. These are in no way designed to replace or change the anatomy. They are provided here as a reference, without specific labels, as a guide to what is actually seen in the classroom and how we can work with them in natural motion. It is highly recommended that you obtain your own copy of Myers' book and/or posters.

Working in Related Pairs (Overview)

Using the Anatomy Trains™ definitions, arm bands are complicated by the fact that we can (as seen in Fig. 18.14) rotate our arms, such that the front and back can be twisted in yoga poses.

There is a great deal more going on in the fascial form at the different joints. However, this premise works extremely well at a "global glance" to facilitate balance in lying, seated, inverted, standing and bending poses, as well as twists (given our broad brushstroke, watercolour approach). If the spinal integrity of the primary and secondary curves is honoured, tension–compression balance

In the yoga classroom we are working with animated beings. These sketches are designed to give an overview of how to "see" the bands relative to each other balancing front-to-back, side-to-side, spiral-to-spiral and so on.

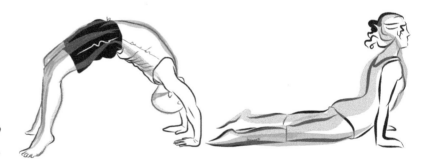

Figure 18.9

See the front relative to the back.

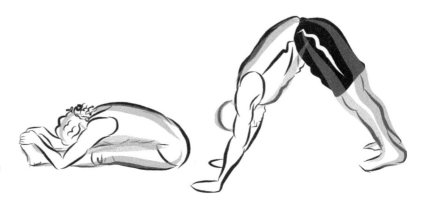

Figure 18.10

See the back relative to the front.

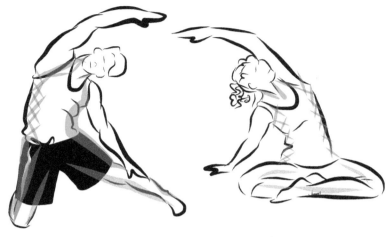

Figure 18.11

See the Lateral Lines relative to each other in the torso and to the Deep Front Line in the legs.

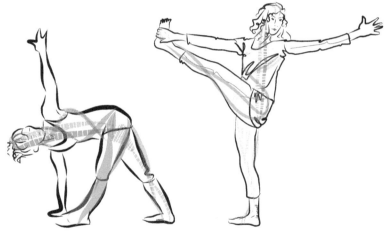

Figure 18.12

See the Spiral Lines relative to each other.

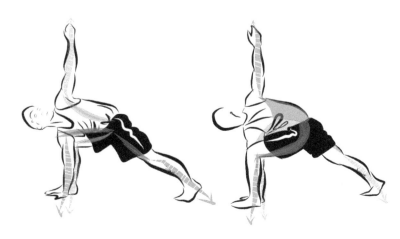

Figure 18.13

See the Back and Front Functional Lines (working from the ground to the other extremity).

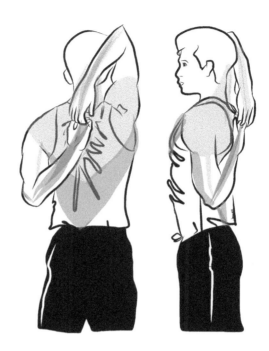

Figure 18.14

See the Back relative to the Front Arm Bands.

is fostered. The elastic integrity of the whole body can then be optimised as we work with the different practices (Classroom Connections in Part C, Classical to Connected, or those specific to your own style of yoga).

Worth practising

It may seem like a lot to learn for such a simple purpose; however, it is much more straightforward in practice and deceptively useful in assisting participants in your classes to:

- move honestly
- progress appropriately in relation to their own architecture
- explore postures from within their own limits
- sense their own balance; or develop at an appropriate rate for them
- gain confidence as the body feels safe in balanced polarities
- integrate sensory awareness and refine it
- animate focused attention in presence, whatever the pose
- accumulate elastic integrity as a resource, gradually over time.

As a teacher you can readily:

- deepen your ability to see and assess
- recognise movement forces expressed in each person
- confirm longitudinal balance relative to individuals

- ensure safe practice that is people-centred, not pose-centred
- manage progress at a suitable rate
- facilitate awareness and attention in neutral balance
- establish a basis for confident adjustments (see Ch. 17)
- become adept at optimising elastic integrity.

These features can expand your confidence as a teacher and the confidence a group has in you. Once this way of seeing becomes instinctive, you can (just as you did when you learned to drive, for example) relax about the applied anatomy and call forth the deepened breath, the moment of attention to a heel and the awareness of a part of the body in its context of the whole myofascial organised form. Just as with driving, eventually the knowledge becomes so instinctive it allows us to direct the class and anticipate at the same time, whatever your preferred style of yoga and your unique way of teaching it.

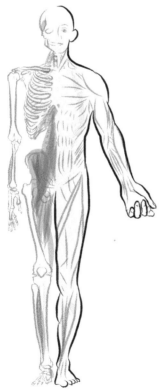

Figure 18.14B

DFL The Deep Container (Deep Front Line in Anatomy Trains).

The balance can be assessed between front and back, side and side, or rotation to counter-rotation. It is a fast way to identify someone forcing themselves into postures they are not ready for. Compromise shows up rapidly, as it shortens or squashes the cavities of the torso and the spine can then be forced to accommodate this. By recognising the longitudinal attributes, that balance can be quickly recognised and confirmed.

Going Behind the Lines

The essence of the Deep Front Line (Myers' term – I call it the Deep Container) and the foundation of the body as a volume in space are visible and outlined from every angle by watching the breath. We examined this further in Chapter 11, however it is fundamental to every aspect of the body in natural motion. Apart from anything else it may be that by breathing more consciously into a given aspect of the torso, we can bring it into conscious awareness and revitalise it through the breathing movements. When they are in congruence with our natural rhythm, shape is changed, posture and gait are enhanced and something light, an elusive spring, restores our step. I have seen it happen time and again. It arrives spontaneously when we stop striving and the posture becomes animated, from the inside expression – not the outside imposition. Trains or no, we use them as guides not formats.

Applying Anatomy Trains™ in Motion

The key to working with the Anatomy Trains™ idea, given that our form occupies three-dimensional geometry, is reading the balance between the "lines". They might appear as lines in that they are silhouettes in profile, but invariably around a volume. They behave as longitudinal coordinates of curved planes

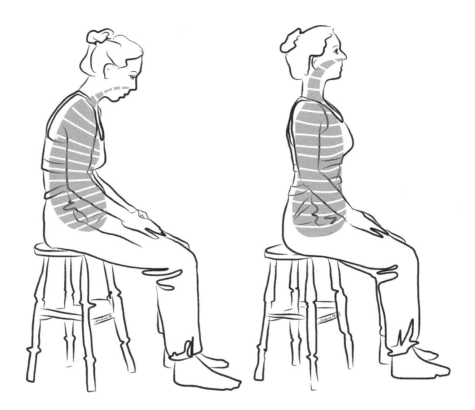

Figure 18.15

All the lines can be related to the idea of the breath "filling" the deep container.

and they are useful basic guides for movement and biomotional integrity, if we learn to read them in relation to (not in isolation from) each other.

The illustrations provided here simply denote where the lines would be on the body if it were static: captured in a moment in time. They can be used to guide both Posture Profiling and adjustment (see Ch. 17).

The Purpose

The purpose of putting the lines into pairs and reading the balance between the lines, or bands, is to ensure that movement of a given line, in a pose, is *not at the expense* of its opposite line. This will encourage the integrity of the volume that the lines outline, especially if you work with the breath as mediator. Essentially it is quite simple.

For example, in Cobra (*Bhujangasana*) it is one thing to simply lift the head, pushing the ground with the arms, tensioning the front of the body. If this lift over-compresses the back and is at the expense of freedom, volume and breathing through the back body, then it is less than optimal for that individual. The same can be said for forward bend – if it is achieved at the expense of a balanced back, or in counter to the natural curves, it is encouraging a less than optimal posture. This is clear in Figures 18.16 and 18.17.

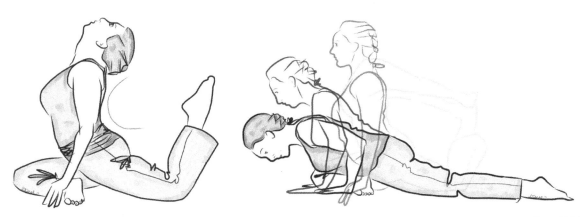

Figure 18.16

In the left-hand image, the posture is effectively over-compressing the back and tensioning the front (apparent "length" is achieved at the expense of the back body). In the right-hand image, the sense of elongation is achieved without over-compression or tension; the front and back bodies are in balance.

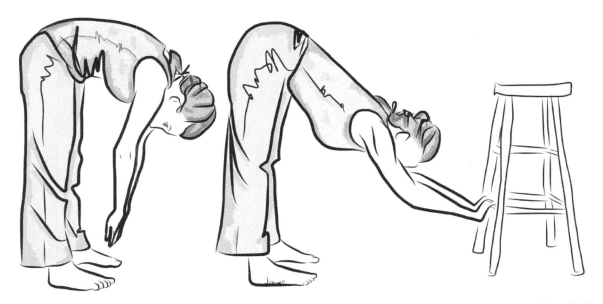

Figure 18.17

In the left-hand image, the posture is effectively over-compressing the front and tensioning the back (apparent "length" is achieved at the expense of the front body). In the right-hand image, the sense of elongation is achieved without over-compression or tension; the back and front bodies are in balance.

Notes

1. Baron Georges Cuvier, *Histoire des Progrès des Sciences naturelles depuis 1789*, vol. I, p. 310, quoted in E.S. Russell, Form and Function, 1916.

2. Ch. 1, "The World According to Fascia", in Thomas W. Myers, *Anatomy Trains: Myofascial Meridians for Manual and Movement Therapists*, 2nd edition, Churchill Livingstone, Edinburgh, 2009.

3. Introduction, "Laying the Railbed", in Thomas W. Myers, *Anatomy Trains: Myofascial Meridians for Manual and Movement Therapists*, 2nd edition, Churchill Livingstone, Edinburgh, 2009.

4. Ibid.

5. Thomas W. Myers, *Anatomy Trains: Myofascial Meridians for Manual and Movement Therapists*, 2nd edition, Churchill Livingstone, Edinburgh, 2009; Kurt Tittel, *Beschreibende und Funktionelle Anatomie des Menschen*, Urban and Fischer, Munich, 1956.

6. Introduction, "Laying the Railbed", in Thomas W. Myers, *Anatomy Trains: Myofascial Meridians for Manual and Movement Therapists*, 2nd edition, Churchill Livingstone, Edinburgh, 2009.

7. Erich Blechschmidt, *The Ontogenetic Basis of Human Anatomy: The Biodynamic Approach to Development from Conception to Adulthood*, edited and translated by Brian Freeman, North Atlantic Books, Berkeley, CA, 2004.

8. Introduction, "Laying the Railbed", in Thomas W. Myers, *Anatomy Trains: Myofascial Meridians for Manual and Movement Therapists*, 2nd edition, Churchill Livingstone, Edinburgh, 2009; D.G. Lee and A. Vleeming, "Impaired Load Transfer through the Pelvic Girdle – a New Model of Altered Neutral Zone Function", in *Proceedings from the 3rd Interdisciplinary World Congress on Low Back and Pelvic Pain, Vienna, Austria, 1998*.

9. Erik Dalton, *The Dynamic Body*, Freedom from Pain Institute, Oklahoma, 2011 (www.erikdalton.com).

10. Thomas W. Myers, *Anatomy Trains: Myofascial Meridians for Manual and Movement Therapists*, 2nd edition, Churchill Livingstone, Edinburgh, 2009 (see also 3rd edition, 2014).

Appendix A

Discovering the Interstitium

In answer to the author's question (June 2019–February 2020)

Please describe what inspired your work about Fascia and the Interstitium

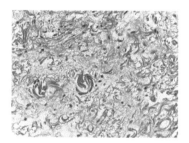

This is the tissue of the interstitium; the "in-between" that the research of Neil Theise and Rebecca Wells and their colleagues are able to demonstrate is part of the living fascial matrix.

(From Dr Neil Theise and Dr Rebecca Wells.)

Neil Theise is a physician and a scientist at the New York University-Grossman School of Medicine. While his clinical work arose through classical allopathic training in medical sciences, his scientific work has, for the most part, derived from his clinical observations to which he responded by applying scientific techniques. Thus, his science has derived first from observation and intuition which only then, later, begins to generate hypotheses that yield to experimentation. The result is an atypical career with diverse interests. His re-definition of normal micro-anatomy of the tiniest branches of the draining bile ducts of the liver confirmed that the human liver has stem cells and where the most important niche for these cells derives. That finding led to concepts of generalised stem cell plasticity throughout the body, *plasticity* meaning that cells are far more flexible than previously thought, being able to shift from one tissue- or organ-specific fate to another. This work was foundational for the transformation of regenerative medicine that began at the turn of the millennium.

Understanding the dynamism with which cells can move and change through the body led to further insights when stirred together with complexity theory. Complexity theory is the science of self-organizing systems. Stirring together dynamic cell motion and complexity theory inspired Neil to multiply the ways in which bodies can be conceived within the Western model. Western medicine and biology are "Western" as defined by *cell doctrine, that the smallest units of the body are cells and that cells always derive from prior cells*. However, while bodies may be considered self-organizing cells, as per cell doctrine, cells themselves may be considered self-organizing molecules in water. These in turn are self-organizing atoms which, in turn, are self-organizing subatomic particles, etc, down to the "quantum foam" that emanates from space–time. From such analyses, new models of the body can be derived, which are equally valid as cell doctrine, but perhaps have uses for explaining bodily phenomena that cell doctrine cannot explain, such as acupuncture or energy healing.

These musings unsurprisingly lead to ways of exploring the nature of consciousness: in collaboration with quantum physicist Menas Kafatos, Dr Theise has elaborated an *idealist* view of consciousness that sees Fundamental Awareness, or pure Awareness of Awareness, as the ground of being which emanates space, time, matter, and energy. This concept brings his work into direct dialogue with mainstream Western philosophy (e.g. Plato, Spinoza, Hegel, Whitehead) and illuminates scientific dialogue with metaphysical traditions, such as classical Buddhist and Hindu thought and Jewish mysticism. His delight is that such insights, in a logical, step-by-step fashion, derive from his first re-visioning of those tiny bile duct structures!

Most recently, using new techniques of *in vivo microscopy* – microscopic examination of living tissues – allowed visualisation of connective tissue depths of the body at the microscopic level. These observations showed that all connective tissue layers of the body are fluid-filled structures, long intuited and described by clinicians in diverse cultural traditions, but *excluded from allopathic concepts* since **the fluid evacuates through creating microscope slides**. The allopathic approach therefore ignored the dynamic, fluid aspects of connective tissue that other schools of thought embraced. This work on the "interstitium" of fibroconnective tissue confirmed the dynamism and fluidity of "fascia" in osteopathic and other fascia-based systems. It also suggests direct correlates with concepts from other cultures of healing such as those from China, Tibet, South Asia and shamanic healing.

The work, primarily in collaboration with Dr Rebecca Wells at the University of Pennsylvania, also extends concepts of fascia to include the connective tissue of the skin (dermis) and all the visceral organs (submucosal depths). While the interconnectivity of the connective tissue of the body has been recognized by researchers such as Franklin Mall and Andrew Still and is taught by all these diverse traditions, the continuity of the fluid-filled *spaces* within these structures has not yet been firmly established. Dr Theise's current work with Dr Wells focuses on confirming this continuity and exploring how fluidics of these spaces and electrical currents within the supporting collagen bundles are a dispersed, intra-body communication network.

Neil Theise

祖転 [SoTen]
הרשו רזעילא ןב דוד חנ לארשי

Fullest list of Neil Theise talking videos is at:

https://www.youtube.com/playlist?list=PLBYMng1cGWQ-Q-R7h8WAl-rUOttL7dY5WY

Current favourites of Neil Theise (consciousness, complexity, the nature of existence):

https://youtu.be/jaGuSZz-Fzw?list=PLBYMng1cGWQ-Q-R7h8WAlrUOt-tL7dY5WY

Appendix B

Stretching: The Faux Amis of Yoga – John Sharkey MSc, Clinical Anatomist, Exercise Physiologist

"Anyone who conducts an argument by appealing to authority is not using his intelligence; he is just using his memory"

Leonardo da Vinci (1452–1519)

Everything we do can be analysed and reduced to the smallest components. However, it is difficult to determine which level of analysis or which component one should focus on because every issue we are invested in can be represented as varying degrees of complication. To aid in discussions on complicated issues, most people nowadays seem to agree that words and language are important.

That being the case, let us analyse the ideological pre-supposition of what it means to "stretch" using inclusive language based on origin. Dynamic motion, dynamic stability, quiescence (or stillness) are valid, necessary utilities required for moving forward in life. My intention is to use science and reasoning to support my supposition that "stretching" (in the true sense of the word) of human tissues should, when possible, be avoided.

As a Clinical Anatomist I dissect everything. Having dyspraxia I have a deeply seeded cerebral need to dissect words to better formulate what it is I wish to articulate. Not happy with using a word without understanding its origins and true meaning has, for me, been a source of frustration and reward. For example, as an exercise physiologist I was, at first, intrigued when I discovered the meaning of the word "contract" means "to shrink". Contract is a word I use almost every day of my professional life and "to shrink" was thought-provoking, puzzling and a little baffling. More senior colleagues and tutors were of the opinion that the word itself (i.e. contract) was not so important and that I was making a mountain out of a molehill, hence the frustration. My early tutors expressed to me that the important issue was that everyone who used the word "contract" agreed a common meaning. This ensured continuity when sharing and discussing research in physiology and anatomy, hence the reward.

My goal from the earliest formative days of my life was to further my knowledge of the truth, based on evidence, science, reasoning and a sprinkle of imagination. "Shrinking", it seems to me, was imaginative if speaking about the concentric aspect of muscle activity. But then, what about the eccentric phase? It did little to ease my conflicts when I learned that "muscle" (from the Latin: muscularis) referred to "little mice". Little mice shrinking? Yes, it can be rewarding to have a common language and vocabulary for sharing and discussing research; however, frustrating problems arise when no-one has a uniform definition of the terms being expressed (a similar issue arises when discussing fascia).

A terse exploration of the internet reflects the very essence of the problem at hand, and the problem is complex. Attempts at defining stretch, or stretching, specifically in the context of exercise science, provides dictionary definitions such as:

1.　to stretch is to extend or lengthen something beyond the normal length (Vocabulary.com).
2.　to cause something to reach, often as far as possible, in a particular direction (Cambridge Dictionary)
3.　to pull something to make it longer or wider or to change the length of something (Macmillan Dictionary)
4.　(verb) be able to be made longer or wider without tearing or breaking (Oxford English Dictionary).

A more robust survey and research approach to the origins and etymology of the word "stretch" takes us back to the 1550s when the word expressed an intent "to enlarge beyond proper limits, exaggerate". Immediately, we can appreciate that the word stretch can conjure up images of taking tissue **beyond its normal length**.

Alternatively it could mean **lengthening while ensuring we avoid tearing or breaking the tissue**. This then raises the question "what is normal length?" and "at what point does human connective tissue tear or break?" I believe it is reasonable to state that most people stretch in an effort to make a tissue longer. Stretching is also commonly performed to *reduce stiffness and tension in a target muscle/s*.

Others believe that stretching will reduce risk of injury or improve performance.

This short annex cannot delve into the latter claims in detail. I can, however, inform you that peer-reviewed research suggests classical stretching has a trivial impact on performance and research informs us it does nothing to reduce risk of injury.[1]

We Homo Sapiens are material beings. That is, we are made up of atoms that combine to form molecules. Trillions of molecules made up from simple pairs of atoms, such as the oxygen molecule, which combine to form more complex organic structures such as proteins, nucleic acids, carbohydrates and lipids. Complex protein molecules make up filaments that are responsible for contractions in muscle fibres and fascia. Figure AppB.1 is a powerful educational image, with the skin and superficial fascia absent, revealing several examples of complex arrangements of human connective tissue. Now, take a moment to question what has passed as fact into popular culture concerning what it means to stretch. What exactly are we stretching? And what happens to living connective tissue when we truly lengthen (i.e. stretch) tissue beyond normal physiological length? It tears.

Recent research (in vivo and ex vivo experiments) has confirmed the highly anisotropic nature of tendons which exhibit a negative Poisson's ratio (see margin note) when "stretched" within their normal range of motion.[2]

It is easy to see why a reader would be confused when dictionaries inform us that "stretch" refers to "*lengthen something beyond the normal*

Poisson's ratio is a measure of the Poisson effect, where the expansion or contraction of a material is in directions perpendicular to the direction of loading. The value of Poisson's ratio is the negative of the ratio of transverse strain to axial strain or the **ratio** of the change in the width per unit width of material, to the change in its length per unit length, as a result of strain.

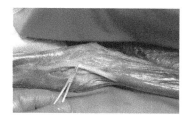

Figure AppB.1

Complex protein molecules make up filaments that are responsible for contractions in muscle fibres and fascia. In this image we are treated to a visual feast of speciality with tendinous tissue, perimysial tissue, muscle fibres, flat aponeurosis of the antebrachial fascia, intermuscular septa and associated neurovascular tissues.

(Image: J. Sharkey, Clinical Anatomist, 2019.)

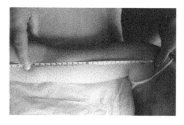

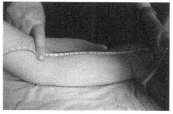

Figure AppB.2

These images demonstrate that the distance between the so-called origin and insertion of a muscle never changes. That is to say, the numerical representation of length remains constant (i.e. measuring tape length does not get shorter or longer) throughout the concentric (positive) and eccentric (negative) phase. One immediately notices a shape change in the gastor (i.e. muscle belly, as seen in B) of the musculotendinous complex.

length" yet research papers (e.g. Gatt et al 2015[2]) use the word "stretch" to describe moving within normal range of motion. So what is happening within the muscle belly (i.e. the gastor) during a so-called stretch? Are atoms, molecules, proteins or tissues actually shortening or lengthening at all? What happens to contractile tissue (i.e. myofascia) when we apply a lengthening force or what I refer to as *"a shape changing force in the direction of elongation"?* It increases its contractile state (i.e. "it contracts"). Muscles are never bi-phasic. That is, they are never "on" one moment and "off" another. Muscle actions are meticulously co-ordinated via integration by sensory neurons located in the dorsal root ganglia and motor exchanges within the central nervous system (CNS).

It is vital to appreciate that proprioceptively sensitive neurons (sensory Ia and II) instantly sense shape changes in resting muscle length and project this information, via axons, peripherally, to specialised muscle spindles and centrally to the intermediate neuron and ventral spinal cord. Here they form direct and indirect connections with motor neurons resulting in a proportional contraction of target fibers and inhibition to appropriate synergistic fibers as the terminal response.

Any attempt to lengthen a muscle, or a muscle fiber, will instantly result in a muscle contraction that is in direct proportion to the rate and speed of lengthening of a fiber or group of fibers.

This neurological phenomenon has been extensively studied as part of gold standard, peer-reviewed neural science research for many years.[3] It is commonly known as the monosynaptic reflex arc or the myotatic reflex. This, essentially, is the basis of all human movement. The monosynaptic reflex arc underlies how we digest food, how we breathe, urinate, defecate or move around in time and space. The last 100 years has seen many of the most respected physiologists, including Ruffini, Sherrington, Adrian, Katz, Kuffler and Hunt, dedicate their research to focus on the muscle spindle, also known as the stretch receptor.[4] Muscle spindles are located within, surrounding and between muscle fibers providing them ideal locations to detect the slightest change in resting length.

According to Valero-Cuevas et al,[5] shared information is occurring locally and systemically through fascial continuities. The Central Nervous System can be viewed as a slower parallel communication system. Primitive organisms without a Central Nervous System display a physical response to stimuli (i.e. sponges or Cnidaria. i.e. jellyfish). The Central Nervous System is more concerned with information gathering, cataloguing, and is therefore involved in longer-term decisions. Short, immediate-term decisions involve local biotensegrity mechanisms and communication informed by established small-world networks. For example, one bird in a flock or one fish in a shoal need only know what the birds or fish next to it are doing. There is no need to know what the bird leading the flock (if there is one) or the fish leading the shoal (if there is one) is doing. The biotensegrity model considers that all communal creatures work this way as do our cells and tissues.[5]

Stretching and Pandiculation

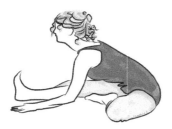

Figure AppB.3

The popular single leg hamstring stretch (variations on the theme of Janu Sirsasana) performed daily by millions of people across the world. In this position the hamstring muscles (and associated posterior muscles) are contracting eccentrically and isometrically.

Many authors assume that stretching and pandiculation are one and the same. Pandiculation is regularly performed by vertebrates, often after waking from sleep and usually accompanied by a controlled, decelerated yawn. Pandiculation involves elongating tissue (myofascia) while contracting stiffens and "wrings out" the tissues ensuring limbs stay within physiological and anatomical range of motion. Pandiculation utilises the monosynaptic reflex to full potential.

Analysing a popular exercise such as the statically held single leg hamstring stretch in Figure AppB.3 results in a neurologically informed truth that may surprise readers. Based on the model dependent reality of the monosynaptic reflex arc **any attempt to lengthen a muscle results in a contraction of that targeted muscle**. This undeniable fact means the muscle is in an eccentrically loaded, isometrically held contraction.

In Fig. AppB.3 the person is attempting to elongate the muscle while the nervous system is ensuring the muscle contracts to decelerate the moment. Few people would ever describe stretching in this way. If the reason for stretching a muscle is to reduce stiffness or tension in that muscle then the monosynaptic reflex arc confirms that stretching compounds shortness and increases stiffness. One could say we are "stretching the symptoms". Could it be that a muscle that feels stiff is simply the squeaky wheel and therefore the one that gets your attention?

To Conclude

"On the actions of muscles passing over more than one joint", a paper published by the *Journal of Anatomy and Physiology* in 1867 written by professor John Cleland, surgeon-anatomist and Chair of Anatomy at Queens College Galway, Ireland states:

"It is only by putting the limbs in positions uncomfortable, unusual and useless, that the shortness of the muscles is discovered. Thus, for example, the shortness of the hamstring muscles is illustrated by the difficulty of accomplishing one of the feats demanded of men on drill, namely, to touch their toes with their fingers, while the knees are kept straight; but this position is one which would never be assumed for any practical purpose, and although it may be ingeniously fitted for the torture of apoplectic soldiers, it is not likely to give freedom of movement in the proper use of the joints; being only calculated to stretch the hamstring muscles to a greater length than usual, which has not been shown to be any advantage".

The observation that the position utilised in such a stretch is one that *"would never be assumed for any practical purpose"* is an important principle in exercise science known as "specificity". If specificity is an accurate aspect of exercise science then any static stretch (if useful at all) is only useful performing that specific motion in that specific position. Simply put, there is no evidence to demonstrate a transference of any benefit from a static stretch to any other specific motion or activity. If you do manage to increase range of motion due to stretching, ask yourself the question "where did the extra range come from?" If you can answer that question with authority and confidence, and you are happy that the increase in range of motion has no detrimental effect on your joints, fine.

If not, perhaps it is advantageous to participate in movements from a deeper understanding of the human sensory organism and avoid "stretching the squeaky wheel". Food for thought.

Namaste, John Sharkey MSc.

References

1. E. Peck, G. Chomko, D. Gaz, A. Farrell (2014) The effects of stretching on performance. *Current Sports Medicine Reports* 13(3):179–185.
2. R. Gatt, M. Vella Wood, A. Gatt, et al (2015) Negative Poisson's ratios in tendons: An unexpected mechanical response. *Acta biomaterialia* 24:201–208.
3. A.D. Walkowski, S. Munakomi (2020) Monosynaptic reflex. [Updated 2019 May 3]. In: StatPearls [Internet]. Treasure Island (FL): StatPearls Publishing. Available from: https://www.ncbi.nlm.nih.gov/books/NBK541028/
4. O.P. Hamill (2010) A new stretch for muscle spindle research. *Journal of* Physiology 588(Pt 4):551–552.
5. F.J. Valero-Cuevas, J.-W. Yi, D. Brown, R.V. McNamara, C. Paul, H. Lipson (2007) The tendon network of the fingers performs anatomical computation at a macroscopic scale. *IEEE Trans Biomed Eng* 54(6 Pt 2):1161–1166.

Examples of scientific development and articles:

J. Sharkey (2021) Fascia and living tensegrity considerations in lower extremity and pelvic entrapment neuropathies. *International Journal of Anatomy* (in press).

J. Sharkey (2020) Site specific fascia tuning pegs and places of perilous passage. Myofascial consideration in upper extremity entrapment neuropathies: a clinical anatomist's view. *Int J Anat Res* 8(4.2):7823–28.

J. Sharkey (2021) Fascia the universal singularity- The dark matter of our inner cosmos. *International Journal of Anatomy and Applied Physiology (IJAAP)*.

J. Eyskens, J. Sharkey, J. Staring, L De Nil, J. August Appleton (2021) Quest for space: towards a novel approach in treating pain and fatigue on Earth. *International Journal of Biomechanics and Movement Science* (in press).

J. Sharkey (2021) Fascia and tensegrity. The quintessence of a unified systems conception. *International Journal of Anatomy & Applied Physiology (IJAAP)* 07(02):174–178.

J.B. Eyskens, J.J. Sharkey, J.A. Appleton, L.D. Nil, J. Staring (2020) Quest for space: towards a novel approach in treating pain and fatigue on Earth. *International Journal of Biomechanics and Movement Science* 2:002.

2019: 19th Congress of the International Federation of Associations of Anatomists (IFAA), London, England August 9th–11th 2019. John was the joint keynote speaker with Dr Carla Stecco, Professor of Anatomy in Padua University, Italy. Presentation is part of a Fascia Symposium regarding new research findings concerning fascia.

2018: Fascia Net Plastination Project in conjunction with the Fascia Research Society and the von Hagen's Plastinarium, Guben, Germany. Part 2, January 2020.

J. Sharkey (2019) Fascia Net Plastination Project. Journal of Bodywork & Movement Therapies 23(1):111–114.

Research Project by J. Sharkey. 2014–2019 Worlds First 3D Printed Model of the Fascia Profunda of Thigh. Supported by Fascia Research Society and 3D Life Prints, UK.

J. Sharkey (2019) Regarding: Update on fascial nomenclature-An additional proposal by John Sharkey MSc, Clinical Anatomist. Journal title: Journal of Bodywork & Movement Therapies 23(1):6–8.

J. Sharkey (2018) Anatomy matters. *Journal of Yoga and Physiotherapy*, 3(5).

J. Sharkey (2018) Biotensegrity – anatomy for the 21st century informing bodywork and movement therapy. *Journal of Massage and Myotherapy Australia*.

J. Sharkey (2016) Fascia and the fallacy of biomechanics. A three part research review and update. *Journal of Massage and Myotherapy*, Australia.

J. Sharkey, J. Avison (2015) Biotensegrity – powering the fabric of human anatomy. *Terra Rosa*, July, Issue 15.

Nan Zheng, Xiao-Ying Yuan, J. Sharkey et al (2014) Definition of the To Be Named Ligament and Vertebrodural Ligament and Their Possible Effects on the Circulation of CSF. August 2014. *PLoS ONE* 9(8):e103451

J. Sharkey (2010) Anatomy of Human Fasciae. A review of current literature. Presentation to academic board of studies, Dundee University.

J. Sharkey (2020) Tensegrity informed observations in human cadaveric studies: a clinical anatomist's perspective. Integrative Journal of Medical Sciences 7:260.

Please note that references to Figures are followed by the letter 'f', and Tables the letter 't'. References to Notes are followed by the letter 'n' and appropriate number.